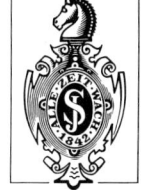

Urodynamics

Upper and Lower Urinary Tract

II

Edited by
W. Lutzeyer · J. Hannappel

With 243 Figures and 22 Tables

Springer-Verlag
Berlin Heidelberg New York Tokyo

Professor Dr. WOLFGANG LUTZEYER
Privatdozent Dr. JOSEF HANNAPPEL

Abteilung Urologie der Medizinischen Fakultät
der Rhein.-Westf. Techn. Hochschule Aachen
Pauwelsstraße, D-5100 Aachen

ISBN 3-540-15357-8 Springer-Verlag Berlin Heidelberg New York Tokyo
ISBN 0-387-15357-8 Springer-Verlag New York Heidelberg Berlin Tokyo

Library of Congress Cataloging in Publication Data. Urodynamics, upper and lower urinary tract II. Contributions resulting from a two-day workshop held in Aachen in 1983. Bibliography: p. Includes index. 1. Urodynamics–Congresses. I. Lutzeyer, W. (Wolfgang), 1923– . II. Hannappel, J. (Josef), 1942– . RC901.U747 1985   616.6   85-4765
ISBN 0-387-15357-8 (U.S.)

This work is subject to copyright. All rights are reserved, whether the whole or part of the material is concerned, specifically those of translation, reprinting, re-use of illustrations, broad-casting, reproduction by photocopying machine or similar means, and storage in data banks. Under § 54 of the German Copyright Law where copies are made for other than private use, a fee is payable to "Verwertungsgesellschaft Wort", Munich.

© Springer-Verlag Berlin Heidelberg 1985
Printed in Germany

The use of registered names, trademarks, etc. in this publication does not imply, even in the absence of a specific statement, that such names are exempt from the relevant protective laws and regulations and therefore free for general use.

Product Liability: The publisher can give no guarantee for information about drug dosage and application thereof contained in this book. In every individual case the respective user must check its accuracy by consulting other pharmaceutical literature.

Typesetting, printing and bookbinding: Konrad Triltsch, Graphischer Betrieb, Würzburg
2122/3130-543210

List of Contributors

You will find the addresses at the beginning of the respective contribution

Anger, K.   154
Bisballe, S.   95
Blok, C.   168
Bottaccini, M. R.   253
Boyarsky, S.   333
Coolsaet, B. L. R. A.   168
Djurhuus, J. C.   95
van Duyl, W. A.   20, 60
Gleason, D. M.   253
Gerlach, R.   102
Griffiths, D.   120
Hannappel, J.   13
Hertle, L.   30, 51
Hinman Jr., F.   241
Höck, F.   148
Laursen, H.   95
Laval, K. U.   148
Marberger, H.   246
van Mastrigt, R.   3, 126

Melchior, H.   317
Meyhoff, H. H.   253
Morita, T.   45
Mortensen, J.   95
Müller-Schauenburg, W.   154
Nawrath, H.   30, 51
Notley, R. G.   286
Ohlson, L.   69
Plevnik, S.   139
Rakovec, S.   139
Schmiedt, E.   203
Schulman, C. C.   292
Tanagho, E. A.   193
Turner-Warwick, R.   212
van Venrooij, G. E. P. M.   168
Vyska, K.   148
Vrtačnik, P.   139
Wieland, W.   203
Zinner, N. R.   263

Preface

The preface to *Urodynamics – Upper and Lower Urinary Tract* edited by LUTZEYER and MELCHIOR (Springer-Verlag 1973) mentions the self-evidence of using functional examinations in other medical departments: "It is self-evident that the cardiologist uses the ECG not just routinely, but continuously in an intensive-care unit, where it is computerized and always on call. It is self-evident, too, in gastroenterology and pulmology that a functional analysis is based on readings of different electronic probes. In urology, however, we tend to rely on optical control by cystoscopy, static data in order to reach a functional interpretation that is based on this information alone." Referring to the preface mentioned above, especially the upper urinary tract is said to be assessed mainly from an anatomic-morphologic point of view in the clinical routine, though in this case we are also mainly concerned with an active transport system.

Twelve years after the urodynamic meeting in 1971, which the above-mentioned volume was based on, a second urodynamic meeting took place in Aachen that was called and also dealt with "Reviewing the Aachen 1971 Meeting." Its purpose was to review which of the statements that had been made more than a decade before were still valuable, what had to be added or revised, and which experimental tests and results could be clinically applied. This was the reason that invitations to speakers were confined to those who had already displayed their results in 1971 and who in the past decade had had a significant influence on the development of urodynamics, based either on theoretical and experimental or on clinical and practical research.

Thus, TANAGHO reports that new findings concerning the morphology and function of the sphincter externus vesicae were achieved in the period between the two meetings in Aachen, and that in spite of the close evolutionary, anatomical, and functional interrelation between the floor of the pelvis and the external sphincter, both structures differ immensely in the properties of their smooth muscles. SCHMIEDT introduces an interesting new scrotal flap technique as an operative method for improving continence. An alternative is the new AMS-800 sphincter, whose implantation was demonstrated in a movie by GREGOIR. TURNER-WARWICK emphasizes the, meanwhile clinically accepted, necessity of differentiating between organic infravesical obstruction (like BPH) and functional obstruction caused by dyssynergic bladder neck obstruction. In this way uroflow measurement, a simple method of examination, has gained great importance. Recurrent infection of the uroepithelium is found in the borderland between urodynamics and immunology, whereby HINMAN differentiates between extrinsic and intrinsic defenses. MARBERGER and BOTTACCINI examine the loss of energy that occurs during bladder emptying in the region of the bladder neck and urethra from a clinical and engineering scientific point of view. ZINNER gives a summary of the development of our knowledge on the hydrodynamic bladder and urethral function. He states that „over the years the field has grown and now incorporates new components including neurophysiology, anatomy, pharmacology, and the like."

Essential items of the morphology described in 1971 have become approved during the past years (NOTLEY, SCHULMAN). Though the nexus have in the meantime changed their names and are now called "close approaches," the distribution of the ganglion cells and the existence of pacemaker cells are now no longer disputed. MELCHIOR describes the value of urorheomanometry introduced in 1971, comparing it with the recently developed noninvasive panurography. The last article of this collection, BOYARSKY's lecture "Ureteral Urodynamics, Past and Future," almost seems like an epicrisis, a review and a challenge for the future.

A two-day workshop on the upper urinary tract preceded the review meeting. On the first day the urodynamic laboratories of Aachen were open to the guests for in vivo and in vitro studies on experimental animals and of course for any kind of information. The second day offered a series of lectures concerning "Myogenic Control for the Upper Tract" and "Hydrodynamics and Mechanics of the Upper Tract." These lectures, which presented for many points new approaches, examination techniques, and results, precede the articles from the "Reviewing the Aachen 1971 Meeting." Thus, we hope to be able to offer the readers both a survey of 12 years of urodynamic research and clinical practice as well as new scientific findings on this research field which is expanding faster and faster.

Aachen   W. LUTZEYER

Contents

Workshop on Upper Urinary Tract Urodynamics

I. Myogenic Control for the Upper Tract

Passive Properties of the Smooth Muscle of the Pig Ureter
R. van Mastrigt. With 6 Figures and 9 Tables 3

Myogenic Function of Normal and Chronically Dilated
Pyeloureters
J. Hannappel. With 7 Figures 13

Modelling of the Propagation of an Action Potential
Along the Ureter
W. A. van Duyl. With 9 Figures 20

Voltage- and Agonist-Induced Activation of Smooth Muscle
of the Human Upper Urinary Tract: Different Mechanisms
L. Hertle and H. Nawrath. With 11 Figures and 1 Table . . 30

Effects of β-Adrenergic Agonists on the Action Potentials
of Canine Pyeloureter
T. Morita. With 4 Figures 45

Effects of Some Directly-Acting Smooth Muscle Relaxant
Drugs on Isolated Human Preparations of the Upper
Urinary Tract
L. Hertle and H. Nawrath. With 7 Figures and 1 Table . . 51

Search for Anisotropy in Specific Electrical Conductance
of Ureteral Tissue as a Measure of Muscle-Fiber Structure
W. A. van Duyl. With 5 Figures and 2 Tables 60

II. Hydrodynamics and Mechanics of the Upper Tract

Kinetic Urography
L. Ohlson. With 6 Figures 69

The Reproducibility of the Pressure-Flow Relationship
in the Normal Upper Urinary Tract of the Pig
J. Mortensen, J. C. Djurhuus, S. Bisballe, and H. Laursen
With 6 Figures 95

The Time-Distance Diagram of the Ureteral Transport
R. Gerlach. With 14 Figures and 1 Table 102

Mechanics of the Upper Tract
D. Griffiths. With 4 Figures 120

The Propagation Velocity of Contractions of the Pig Ureter
in Vitro
R. van Mastrigt. With 11 Figures and 2 Tables 126

Assessment of Ureteric Dynamics by Simultaneous Electric
Conductance Measurements at Two Sites
S. Plevnik, S. Rakovec, and P. Vrtačnik
With 10 Figures and 1 Table 139

Imaging of Peristaltic Urine Transport in the Ureter Using
^{123}Jodine Hippurate
K. U. Laval, K. Vyska, and F. Höck. With 4 Figures 148

The Nuclear Medical Space Time Matrix Approach
to Ureteral Motility
W. Müller-Schauenburg and K. Anger. With 5 Figures . . 154

Dynamics of the Ureterovesical Junction
C. Blok, G. E. P. M. van Venrooij, and B. L. R. A. Coolsaet
With 23 Figures 168

**Upper and Lower Urinary Tract Urodynamics –
Reviewing the Aachen 1971 Meeting**

I. Lower Tract Urodynamics

Innervation and Histologic Characteristics of the Urinary
External Sphincter
E. A. Tanagho. With 10 Figures 193

The Scrotal Flap Technique as an Operative Method for the
Treatment of Iatrogenic and Posttraumatic Male Incontinence
E. Schmiedt and W. Wieland. With 7 Figures and 2 Tables . 203

A Urodynamic Review of Bladder Outlet "Obstruction"
in the Male and Its Treatment
R. TURNER-WARWICK. With 9 Figures 212

Surface Factors in Recurrent Infection
F. HINMAN Jr. With 5 Figures 241

Causes and Consequences of Bladder Neck Obstruction
H. MARBERGER. With 9 Figures 246

Urinary Velocity: Twelve Years Later
M. R. BOTTACCINI, D. M. GLEASON, and H. H. MEYHOFF
With 4 Figures and 2 Tables 253

Review of Techniques to Evaluate Micturitional Performance.
Promises of 1971 Revisited
N. R. ZINNER. With 23 Figures and 1 Table 263

II. Upper Tract Urodynamics

Ureteric Ultrastructure – 12 Years on
R. G. NOTLEY. With 3 Figures 286

Innervation of the Ureter: A Histochemical and
Ultrastructural Study
C. C. SCHULMAN. With 26 Figures 292

Progress in Diagnosis of Ureteral Urodynamics
H. MELCHIOR. With 11 Figures 317

Ureteral Urodynamics: Past and Future
S. BOYARSKY. With 4 Figures 333

Subject Index 341

Workshop on Upper Urinary Tract Urodynamics

Passive Properties of the Smooth Muscle of the Pig Ureter*

R. van Mastrigt[1]

Introduction

It has been shown that there are large variations in the velocity of the front end of a urine bolus travelling down the ureter (Durben and Gerlach 1979). Since the velocity of this front end may be influenced by passive viscoelastic properties of the ureteral wall (Griffiths and Notschaele 1983), it should be possible to detect variations in these viscoelastic properties along the entire ureter. The purpose of this study was to investigate this hypothesis and also to obtain objective data on the viscoelasticity of the ureter. The variation in viscoelastic parameters along the entire ureter was measured. The isotropy of the ureter was investigated by comparing transverse and longitudinal sections, and the influence of metabolism on the viscoelasticity was evaluated.

Methods and Materials

Ureters were obtained from pigs which had been used for cardiac research. During the preparation of the ureters the in situ length was measured. The ureters were cut into eight segments of equal length. The segments were mounted in a specially made pneumatic straining device, see Fig. 1. This device contained sixteen clamps. The eight lower clamps could be moved simultaneously, using a pneumatic cylinder. The movement took place at a very high speed, about one meter per second, which is very fast in comparison to the time constants of the ureter segments (see Table 1). Therefore the straining of the eight ureter segments can be considered to be stepwise. The eight upper clamps were connected to eight isometric force transducers. Each segment was submerged in a modified Krebs solution (unless explicitly stated otherwise) (Coolsaet et al. 1975) in its own individual container. The solution in the individual containers was aerated, and was kept at 37 °C by submerging them in a larger container with heated water. The signals from the force transducers were amplified and fed into a minicomputer. One stepwise straining produced eight force responses. These were read into the computer for 1000 s. A viscoelastic relaxation

---

* Part of text and figures of this article were reproduced from Urol. Int. (1981) 36: 145–151 by kind permit of S. Karger AG
[1] Department of Urology, Erasmus University Rotterdam, P.O. Box 1738, NL-3000 DR Rotterdam

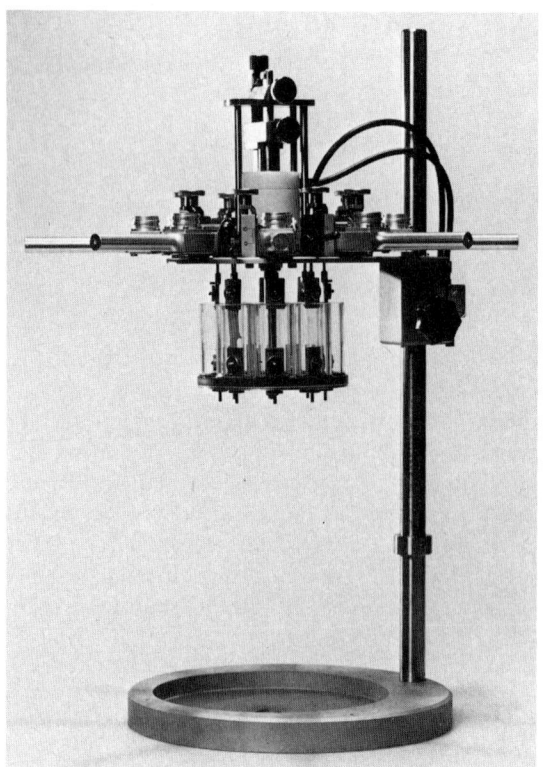

Fig. 1. Pneumatic device for the simultaneous stepwise straining of eight ureter segments in separate containers

curve, consisting of two exponentially decaying terms and a constant term (van Mastrigt et al. 1981), was fitted to the curves:

$$F = A_1 \exp(-\gamma_1 \times t) + A_2 \exp(-\gamma_2 \times t) + A_0, \qquad (1)$$

where F is the measured force as a function of time, A_0, A_1 and A_2 are coefficients, γ_1 and γ_2 are relaxation constants.

Three elastic moduli E_0, E_1 and E_2 were calculated from the three coefficients A_0, A_1 and A_2 and these were taken relative to their sum (van Mastrigt et al. 1978) to yield the relative elastic moduli e_0, e_1 and e_2. Since $e_0 + e_1 + e_2 = 1$ only two of these moduli are independent and carry information. However the sum $\bar{E} = E_1 + E_2 + E_3$ is now a new parameter. Altogether we obtained five parameters, i.e. the two relaxation constants γ_1 and γ_2, two of the three relative elastic moduli e_0, e_1, and e_2, and $\bar{E}$, from one stepwise measurement on one ureter segment. On average four measurements were performed on the eight segments of each ureter, yielding a total of 32 force curves for each ureter. In the first series of 20 measurements, variations in the measured parameters along the entire length of the ureter were investigated using eight successive sections from twenty ureters. In a second series of thirteen ureters, four transverse and four longitudinal sections of the same ureter were directly compared. In four ureters the segments were strained repeatedly to the same strain of 60%; in the other nine ureters the strain was increased.

Both sections were opened by a longitudinal incision. In a third series of eight ureters, the effects of EGTA, D 600 and a metabolic fluid in which all of the Na^+-ions were replaced by K^+ were investigated.

Results

Figure 2 shows an example of the force responses of six of the eight ureter segments to a stepwise straining. The other two responses were recorded on another strip-chart recorder. In a series of measurements on five ureters, the segments were repeatedly strained longitudinally to a constant strain level of 40%. The average values and relative standard deviations of these measurements are shown in Table 1. A variance analysis was applied in order to split the variance into two components, i.e. the variance within one segment and the variance between the segments of one ureter, and the F-test (5%) was used in order to test whether this second variance component was significant. Significance implies that there are real differences between the segments, and is indicated with a plus sign in Table 1. It can be seen that a significant difference was found in only one parameter for only one ureter. In Table 2 the results for another five ureters are shown. Here the segments were opened by a longitudinal incision and strained several times transversely up to a strain level of 80%. Significant differences between different segments can be seen in four parameters for three ureters. The higher strain level of 80% was chosen because it seemed that the segments were much more compliant in the transverse direction than in the longitudinal. In the next series of measurements, segments from five ureters were

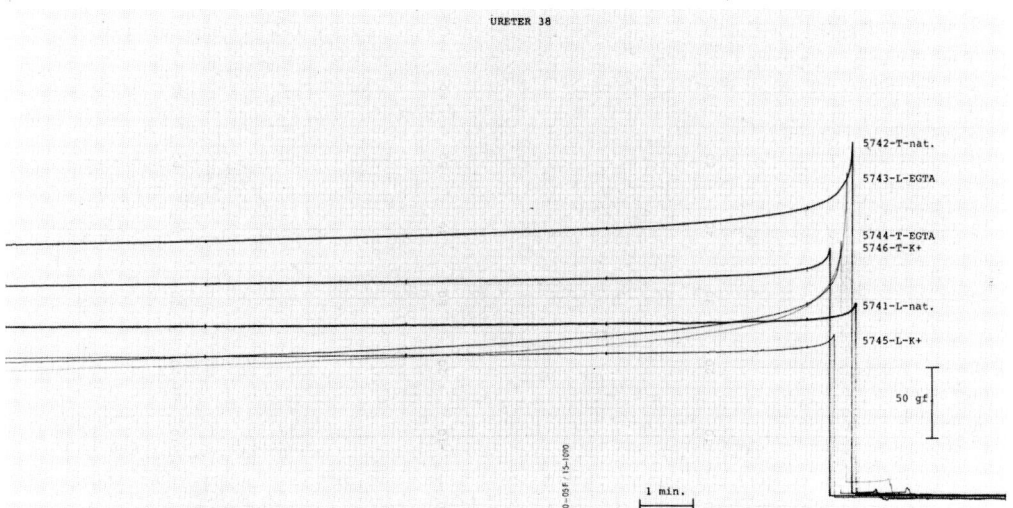

Fig. 2. Force responses of six ureter segments to a stepwise straining. Time runs from right to left. Each curve is identified with a unique number, T(ransverse) or L(ongitudinal) and a code for the metabolic fluid in which it was submerged (*nat.* normal Krebs solution)

Table 1. Averages, relative standard deviations (i.e. standard deviation/average × 100%) and results of F-test for the segments of five ureters, repeatedly strained lengthwise to a constant strain level of 40%

Number of measurements	$\gamma_1\,(\sigma)$ F (s^{-1})	$\gamma_2\,(\sigma)$ F (s^{-1})	$e_1\,(\sigma)$ F	$e_2\,(\sigma)$ F	$\bar{E}\,(\sigma)$ F $(N/m^2) \times 10^{-6}$
29	0.084 (64%) +	0.0025 (32%) −	0.15 (49%) −	0.18 (26%) −	0.26 (75%) −
27	0.12 (114%) −	0.0036 (161%) −	0.17 (91%) −	0.15 (37%) −	0.79 (93%) −
31	0.11 (103%) −	0.0025 (46%) −	0.15 (60%) −	0.15 (31%) −	1.18 (92%) −
27	0.095 (41%) −	0.0031 (34%) −	0.16 (58%) −	0.14 (39%) −	1.4 (95%) −
32	0.063 (28%) −	0.0027 (29%) −	0.14 (43%) −	0.13 (30%) −	1.3 (65%) −

Table 2. Averages, relative standard deviations (i.e. standard deviation/average × 100%) and results of F-test for the segments of five ureters which were opened by a longitudinal incision and repeatedly strained transversely up to a constant strain level of 80%

Number of measurements	$\gamma_1\,(\sigma)$ F (s^{-1})	$\gamma_2\,(\sigma)$ F (s^{-1})	$e_1\,(\sigma)$ F	$e_2\,(\sigma)$ F	$\bar{E}\,(\sigma)$ F $(N/m^2) \times 10^{-6}$
20	0.080 (38%) −	0.0032 (53%) −	0.18 (50%) −	0.14 (69%) −	0.14 (92%) +
16	0.061 (35%) −	0.0046 (71%) −	0.25 (22%) −	0.12 (45%) −	0.15 (110%) +
29	0.13 (133%) −	0.0048 (40%) −	0.15 (49%) +	0.11 (57%) −	0.095 (65%) +
27	0.074 (40%) −	0.0029 (59%) −	0.18 (40%) −	0.16 (55%) −	0.13 (108%) −
21	0.080 (33%) −	0.0030 (43%) −	0.15 (50%) −	0.11 (37%) −	0.11 (56%) −

Table 3. Averages, relative standard deviations (i.e. standard deviation/average × 100%) and results of F-test for the segments of five ureters which were strained longitudinally to strain levels increasing from 20% to 100%

Number of measurements	$\gamma_1\,(\sigma)$ F (s^{-1})	$\gamma_2\,(\sigma)$ F (s^{-1})	$e_1\,(\sigma)$ F	$e_2\,(\sigma)$ F	$\bar{E}\,(\sigma)$ F $(N/m^2) \times 10^{-6}$
25	0.11 (86%) −	0.0034 (39%) −	0.28 (21%) −	0.24 (11%) −	0.38 (78%) −
22	0.10 (29%) −	0.0033 (22%) −	0.27 (23%) −	0.23 (17%) −	0.12 (66%) +
26	0.10 (47%) −	0.0032 (37%) −	0.25 (31%) −	0.22 (31%) −	0.20 (80%) −
27	0.13 (51%) −	0.0039 (32%) −	0.29 (22%) −	0.22 (24%) +	0.25 (80%) +
32	0.073 (39%) −	0.0030 (35%) −	0.18 (22%) −	0.18 (22%) −	1.0 (46%) +

again strained longitudinally, but the measurements were taken at strain levels increasing from 20% to 100%. As can be seen in Table 3 there were significant differences between different segments in four parameters. Finally a series of measurements was made on transversely strained segments at strain levels increasing from 10% to 120%. As can be seen in Table 4, all ureters could then be differentiated by one or more of the parameters. Comparing the average $\bar{E}$'s calculated from Tables 3 and 4 (0.39 and 0.32 N/m²) only a very small and non-significant difference be-

Table 4. Averages, relative standard deviations (i.e. standard deviation/average × 100%) and results of F-test for the segments of five ureters, strained transversely to strain levels increasing from 10% to 100%

Number of measurements	$\gamma_1(\sigma)$ F (s^{-1})	$\gamma_2(\sigma)$ F (s^{-1})	$e_1(\sigma)$ F	$e_2(\sigma)$ F	$\bar{E}(\sigma)$ F $(N/m^2)\times 10^{-6}$
32	0.075 (21%) −	0.0033 (30%) −	0.15 (26%) −	0.12 (22%) −	0.40 (62%) −
29	0.085 (30%) −	0.0035 (31%) +	0.17 (41%) +	0.12 (21%) +	0.36 (47%) +
38	0.088 (42%) −	0.0034 (33%) −	0.22 (36%) +	0.16 (39%) +	0.17 (70%) +
32	0.078 (24%) −	0.0035 (22%) −	0.16 (23%) −	0.13 (12%) −	0.34 (68%) +
28	0.089 (24%) −	0.0035 (24%) +	0.12 (19%) +	0.11 (50%) −	0.32 (31%) +

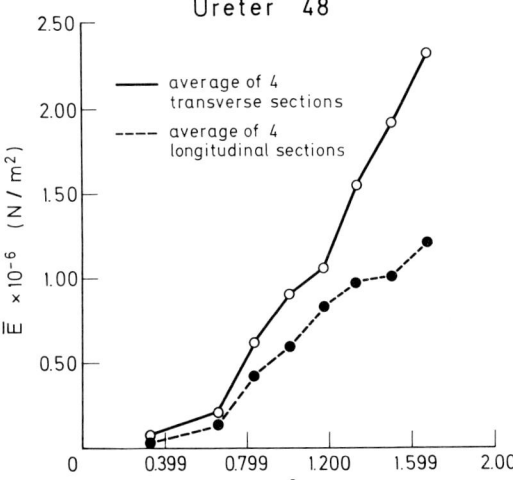

Fig. 3. Average total stiffness $\bar{E}$ as a function of strain for four longitudinal and four transverse sections of the same ureter

tween the two directions is found. Table 5 shows results from eight ureters for which four longitudinal and four transverse sections were directly compared. As can be seen, in all ureters except ureter 29 the transverse sections were stiffer, in five cases even very significantly. This effect was more pronounced in the sections investigated at increasing strain levels. As can be seen in Fig. 3, which is a typical example of similar results obtained from five ureters, the elastic characteristic of transverse and longitudinal sections differ, the former being steeper, i.e. the total elastic modulus $\bar{E}$ increasing more pronouncedly with strain. Table 6 shows a comparison between the e_0 parameters for longitudinal and transverse sections of the same ureter, bathed respectively in the normal Krebs solution and in a Ca-free solution with EGTA added. It can be seen that in the EGTA solution e_0 was always lower, in almost all of the cases even significantly lower. This means that *more* stress-relaxation was observed in these sections. Table 7 shows that in a number of these ureters the total stiffness $\bar{E}$ was greater in the EGTA solution. Therefore, for these ureters bathed in EGTA solution the stress-relaxation curves start at higher levels and relax to a similar or to lower levels than they do for ureters bathed in the normal solution (see Fig. 4). Table 8

Table 5. Averages, relative standard deviations (i.e. standard deviation/average × 100%) and results of F-test for the total stiffness $\bar{E}$, obtained from longitudinal and transverse sections of 8 ureters

	Ureter	Lengthwise section $\bar{E} \times 10^{-6}$ N/m²	Transverse section $\bar{E} \times 10^{-6}$ N/m²	Significance level t test
Constant strain $\varepsilon = 0.60$	27	n=16 0.33 (52%) F= 0.17	n=16 0.43 (57%) F= 2.6	90%
	28	n=16 0.24 (34%) F= 3.8	n=16 0.35 (50%) F=12.8	97.5%
	30	n=16 0.23 (43%) F=35	n=12 0.24 (21%) F= 0.9	–
	35	n=16 0.15 (49%) F=12.6	n=16 0.17 (40%) F=10.6	–
Increasing strain	29	n=16 1.8 (72%) F= 2.0	n=16 1.0 (53%) F= 0.6	97.5%
	31	n=20 0.7 (58%) F= 0.5	n=20 1.2 (54%) F= 0.4	99.5%
	32	n=18 0.50 (45%) F= 4.1	n=17 0.89 (67%) F= 2.8	99.5%
	36	n=20 0.49 (66%) F= 2.5	n=20 0.73 (109%) F=48	–

Table 6. Averages, standard deviations and significance of difference by Student's t-test for the parameter e_0, determined from sections bathed in normal Krebs solution and sections bathed in a Ca-free solution with the addition of EGTA, from 6 ureters

Ureter	Orientation of section	Natural solution e_0		EGTA e_0		Significance level t test
37	lengthwise	n=4	0.80±0.10	n=4	0.51±0.14	99%
	transverse	n=4	0.83±0.066	n=4	0.58±0.14	99%
38	lengthwise	n=3	0.82±0.10	n=4	0.60±0.15	95%
	transverse	n=4	0.77±0.064	n=4	0.59±0.10	97.5%
39	lengthwise	n=5	0.87±0.044	n=5	0.74±0.075	99%
	transverse	n=5	0.85±0.055	n=5	0.75±0.09	95%
40	lengthwise	n=4	0.86±0.075	n=3	0.71±0.048	95%
	transverse	n=3	0.80±0.12	n=1	0.52	–
42	transverse	n=4	0.85±0.073	n=4	0.69±0.14	95%
43	lengthwise	n=2	0.76±0.081	n=4	0.68±0.054	75%

Table 7. Averages, standard deviations and significance of difference by Student's t-test for the total stiffness $\bar{E}$, determined from sections bathed in normal Krebs solution and sections bathed in a Ca-free solution with EGTA added, from 6 ureters

Ureter	Orientation of section	Natural solution $\bar{E} \times 10^{-6}$ N/m²		EGTA $\bar{E} \times 10^{-6}$ N/m²	
37	lengthwise	n=4	0.13±0.029	n=4	0.60±0.40
	transverse	n=4	0.08±0.013	n=4	0.21±0.14
38	lengthwise	n=3	0.12±0.049	n=4	0.28±0.17
	transverse	n=4	0.33±0.21	n=4	0.25±0.13
39	lengthwise	n=5	0.11±0.013	n=5	0.05±0.016
	transverse	n=5	0.26±0.013	n=5	0.24±0.051
40	lengthwise	n=4	0.16±0.035	n=3	0.07±0.017
	transverse	n=3	0.18±0.047	n=1	0.19
42	transverse	n=4	0.27±0.043	n=4	0.08±0.037
43	lengthwise	n=2	0.06±0.002	n=4	0.10±0.026

Table 8. Averages, standard deviations and significance of difference by Student's t-test for the total stiffness $\bar{E}$, determined from sections bathed in normal Krebs solution and sections bathed in a Ca-free solution with the addition of D 600, from 3 ureters

Ureter	Orientation of section	Natural solution $\bar{E} \times 10^{-6}$ N/m²		D 600 $\bar{E} \times 10^{-6}$ N/m²		Significance level t test
40	transverse	n = 3	0.18 ± 0.047	n = 4	0.11 ± 0.025	97.5%
41	lengthwise	n = 1	0.09	n = 3	0.10 ± 0.023	–
	transverse	n = 4	0.17 ± 0.033	n = 3	0.09 ± 0.008	99.5%
42	transverse	n = 4	0.27 ± 0.043	n = 4	0.15 ± 0.022	99.5%

Table 9. Averages and standard deviations from the total stiffness $\bar{E}$, determined from sections bathed in normal Krebs solution, a solution in which all Na⁺ was replaced by K⁺, and a solution with extra K⁺/Na⁺

Ureter	Orientation of section	Natural solution $\bar{E} \times 10^{-6}$ N/m²		Extra K⁺ $\bar{E} \times 10^{-6}$ N/m²	
37	lengthwise	n = 4	0.13 ± 0.029	n = 3	0.17 ± 0.054
	transverse	n = 4	0.08 ± 0.013	n = 4	0.43 ± 0.046
38	lengthwise	n = 3	0.12 ± 0.049	n = 3	0.21 ± 0.056
	transverse	n = 4	0.33 ± 0.21	n = 4	0.13 ± 0.024
39	lengthwise	n = 5	0.11 ± 0.013	n = 5	0.31 ± 0.023
	transverse	n = 5	0.26 ± 0.013	n = 5	0.12 ± 0.013
40	transverse	n = 3	0.18 ± 0.047	n = 1	0.17
42	transverse	n = 4	0.27 ± 0.043	n = 4	0.20 ± 0.031
43	lengthwise	n = 2	0.06 ± 0.002	n = 4	0.19 ± 0.025
				Extra K⁺/Na⁺ $\bar{E} \times 10^{-6}$ N/m²	
41	lengthwise	n = 1	0.09	n = 2	0.07 ± 0.005
	transverse	n = 4	0.17 ± 0.033	n = 2	0.17 ± 0.040
44	lengthwise	n = 3	0.14 ± 0.017	n = 4	0.25 ± 0.041
	transverse	n = 4	0.13 ± 0.028	n = 4	0.14 ± 0.033

shows that in a Ca-free solution to which we had added D 600 the stiffness was usually significantly less, while Table 9 shows that in a solution in which Na⁺ was replaced by K⁺ the total stiffness of longitudinal sections was nearly always greater, but that of transverse sections was usually smaller than normal.

Discussion

The first series of measurements performed on 20 ureters, the results of which are displayed in Tables 1–4, show that, by performing several measurements at increas-

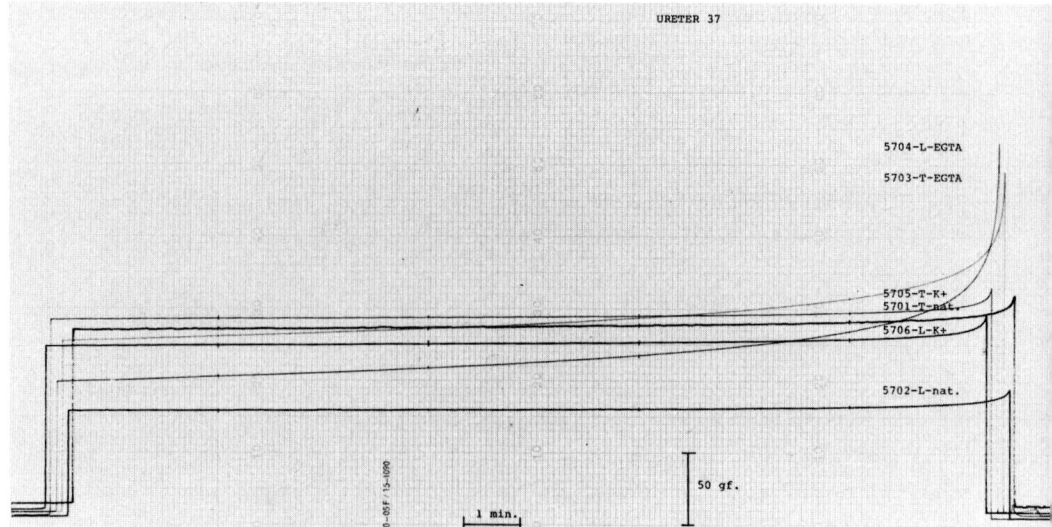

Fig. 4. Force responses of three longitudinal and three transverse sections of the same ureter, bathed in normal Krebs solution (*nat.*), a Ca-free solution with EGTA added, and a solution in which all the Na$^+$ was replaced by K$^+$

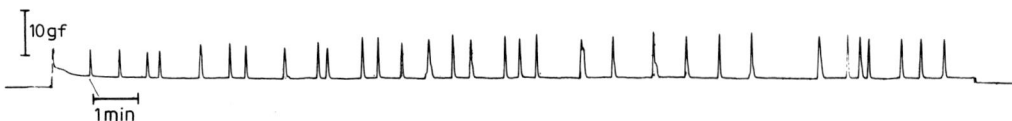

Fig. 5. Measured stress relaxation curve with superimposed spontaneous contractions. Time runs from left to right

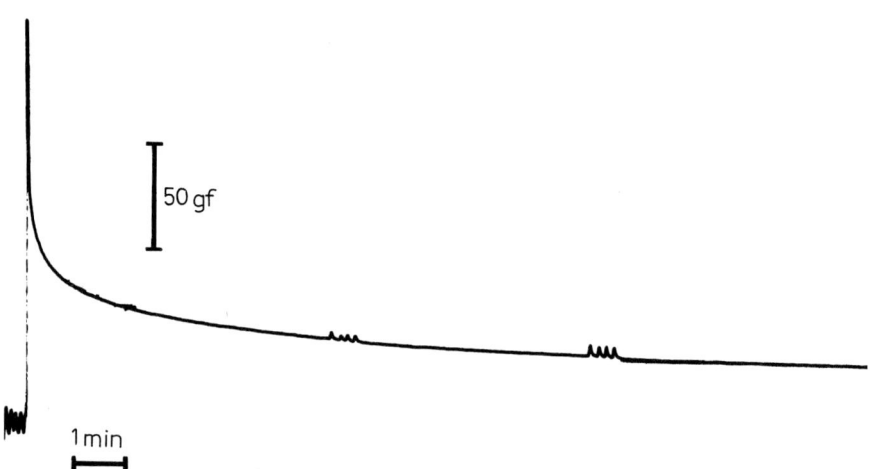

Fig. 6. Measured stress relaxation curve with superimposed spontaneous contractions in bursts. Time runs from left to right

ing strain levels on one set of ureter segments, a significant difference between the segments can nearly always be found. The difference, however, is never very great, so that more than one measurement has to be performed to detect it.

The total stiffness $\bar{E}$ is strongly dependent on strain (Hong et al. 1980). A difference was found between the stiffness-strain relations for transverse and longitudinal sections from the same ureter, the former being steeper. This means that, if measurements are performed at only one strain level, a difference between longitudinal and transverse sections may or may not be found, depending on the strain level. Akimoto et al. (1977) found that, after the application of pressure to segments of a rabbit ureter, the initial increase in diameter was small compared to the initial increase in length, which is consistent with our findings.

A common feature of the segments strained longitudinally and transversely is the relatively small amount of viscosity and the large amount of plasticity exhibited, when compared with for instance bladder wall tissue (van Mastrigt et al. 1978). This means, in the first place, that a ureter segment shows relatively little stress relaxation when strained stepwise, on average about 30% of the evoked stress or force, and in the second place that, when a segment has been strained previously, a subsequent straining yields a much lower force response. The series of measurements performed in different metabolic fluids shows that part of the behaviour which has been described in terms of passive viscoelasticity is at least influenced by active properties, and possibly even caused by them (van Duyl and Glerum 1981). The amount of stress-relaxation is increased significantly in a Ca-free EGTA solution, whereas the total stiffness of the muscle is altered in a non-uniform way. A D 600 solution clearly reduces the total stiffness, while an extra K^+ solution increases the stiffness of longitudinal sections, and decreases that of transverse sections. Directional differences in the contractility of ureteral segments have been reported previously (van Duyl and Coolsaet 1982).

One final aspect of the measurements which should be discussed is the occurrence of spontaneous contractions. When the ureter segments were strained transversely, spontaneous contractions were nearly always detected in some of the segments. An example is shown in Fig. 5, which shows spontaneous contractions, which were almost randomly distributed in time, and superimposed on the measured force relaxation curve. Often, however, the contractions seemed to come in bursts, as demonstrated in Fig. 6. When the ureter segments were strained longitudinally, contractions were hardly ever seen, and if they were detected they were very small.

References

Akimoto M, Biancani P, Weiss RM (1977) Comparative pressure-length-diameter relationships of neonatal and adult rabbit ureters. Inv Urol 14-4:297–300

Coolsaet BLRA, Duyl WA van, Mastrigt R van, Schouten JW (1975) Viscoelastic properties of bladder wall strips. Inv Urol 12-5:351–356

Durben G, Gerlach R (1979) Pressure and velocity of the urine bolus. 1st meeting ISDU, Antwerp

Duyl WA van, Glerum JJ (1981) Spontaneous contractions and micromotion in urinary bladder smooth muscle; viscomotion model. Proc 11th ICS meeting, Lund, pp 26–27

Duyl WA van, Coolsaet BLRA (1982) Potassium-induced contractions in pig ureter strips. Consequences for helical muscle-fiber model of ureter. Urology XX-1:53–58

Griffiths DJ, Notschaele C (1983) The mechanics of urine transport in the upper urinary tract: 1. The dynamics of the isolated bolus. Neurourol Urodyn 2:155–166

Hong KW, Biancani P, Weiss RM (1980) Effect of age on contractility of guinea pig ureter. Inv Urol 17-6:459–461

Mastrigt R van, Coolsaet BLRA, Duyl WA van (1978) Passive properties of the urinary bladder in the collection phase. Med Biol Eng Comp 16:471–482

Mastrigt R van, Glerum JJ, Tauecchio EA (1981) Variation of passive mechanical properties of the ureter along its length. Urol Int 36:145–151

Myogenic Function of Normal and Chronically Dilated Pyeloureters

J. HANNAPPEL[1]

Abstract. The highest pacemaking frequency of spontaneous contractions in the normal pyeloureter occurs in the most proximal parts of the renal pelvis. Therefore, the initiation and organisation of effective orthograde peristaltic contractions are ensured by the spontaneous myogenic activity itself. In vitro investigations on muscle strips show that in the chronically dilated upper tract the hierarchical organisation as well as frequency patterns of spontaneous activity are different. In analogy to the heart these changes might be termed 'heterotopic extrasystolic activity' of the dilated pyeloureter and help to explain the occurence of unorganized, uneffective and retrograde peristalsis in the dilated upper urinary tract.

According to Bozler (1938) two different types of smooth muscle tissue can be differentiated:

"Unitary muscles": These are smooth muscular organs, which are morphologically composed of a large number of individual muscle cells, but behave as a functional syncytium. This applies for the intestinal muscles and the uterus as well as for the ureter.

"Multiunit muscles": e.g. most of the blood vessel musculature and the detrusor are composed of smooth muscles, whereas the single cells or small cell groups are morphologically as well as functionally individual units.

Assuming that the ureteral musculature indeed behaves as a functional syncytium, we have to discuss the question how (neurogenic or myogenic) a peristaltic contraction is initiated and organized. Electromyographic investigations in vivo as well as in vitro studies on muscle strips show that in the normal pyeloureteral system the highest spontaneous frequency is found in the uppermost intrarenal parts. As in a muscular syncytium the cell group with the highest spontaneous frequency takes over the function of the pacemaker, it is obvious that ureteral peristalsis always starts in the uppermost renal parts of the pyeloureteral system and thus, a directed orthograde peristalsis is ensured (Constantinou 1974; Djurhuus et al. 1977; Golenhofen and Hannappel 1973; Hannappel and Golenhofen 1974).

However, in chronically dilated pyeloureters unorganized and retrograde peristalsis has been observed frequently and therefore, we wondered whether the hierarchy of spontaneous myogenic activity in such dilated systems had changed.

Material and Methods

The middle part of the left ureters of 30 adult rats were double ligated with 4–0 silk. Eight weeks later the normal upper tract of the right side as well as the highly dilat-

---

[1] Abteilung Urologie der RWTH Aachen, Pauwelsstr., D-5100 Aachen

ed kidney and ureter of the left side were removed. From both sides we cut off 3 muscle strips as follows: a circular strip from the renal pelvis (RP), a spiral shaped strip from the pyeloureteral junction (PU) and a longitudinal preparation from the proximal ureter (U) (Fig. 1a).

Each muscle strip had a length of 10 to 15 mm and a cross-section of about 1 sqmm. The section was carried out in a cooled preparation solution (Na^+ 144, K^+ 5.9, Ca^{2+} 3.7, Cl^- 157 mmol/l). Then the muscle strips were taken into an organ bath (Na^+ 137, K^+ 5.9, Ca^{2+} 2.5, Mg^{2+} 1.2, Cl^- 124, HCO_3^- 25, $H_2PO_4^-$ 1.2, Glucose 11.5 mmol/l, equilibrated with 95% O_2 and 5% CO_2, pH ca. 7.4) containing modified Krebs solution at a temperature of 37 °C and were then fixed on an isometric force transducer with a pre-tension of about 2–4 mN (Fig. 2). The contraction frequency was determined after a minimum adaptation time of 30 minutes.

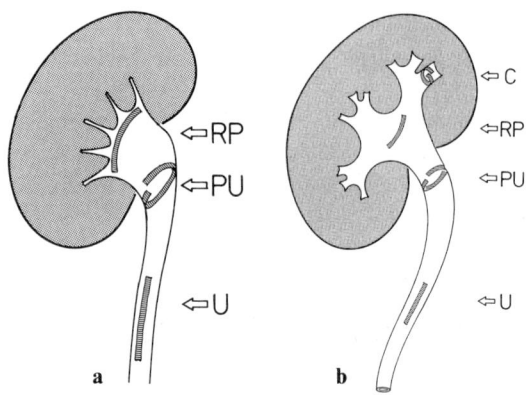

Fig. 1. Section of the pyeloureter preparations in a monocalyceal (**a**) and a multicalyceal (**b**) kidney. *C* calyx, *PU* pyeloureteral junction, *RP* renal pelvis, *U* ureter

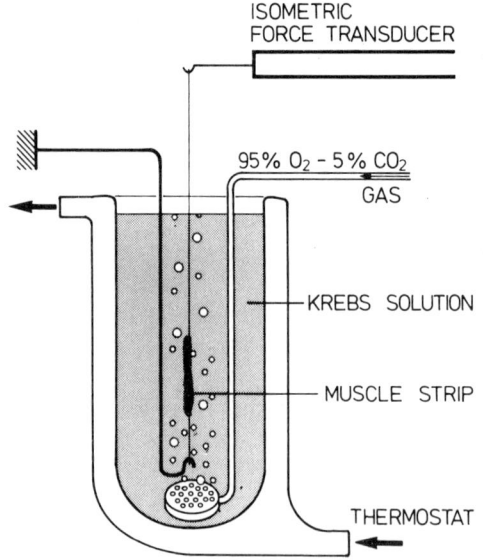

Fig. 2. Assay arrangement for investigation of the spontaneous activity of pyeloureteral muscle strips with the organ bath being kept at a constant temperature of 37 °C

In a second test series we ligated one mid-ureter in 19 guinea-pigs respectively. Three months later the tested animals were killed, the dilated pyeloureter of the ligated side and the contralateral normal organ were removed. We cut off muscle strips as follows: longitudinal strips from the renal pelvis (RP_l), circular strips from the renal calyces (RP_c) and longitudinal strips from the proximal ureter (U_{prox}). Further preparations were taken from the ligated ureters directly distal to the ligature and from the contralateral intact ureters at the corresponding position (U_{dist}). After a minimum adaptation time of 30 min these preparations were also examined in the organ bath for their spontaneous frequency.

In another experiment the mid-ureter of 5 pigs was obstructed by a PVC-tube with an inner diameter of 8 mm and a length of approximately 15 mm. This tube was cut open longitudinally, put around the ureter and closed again with two silk ligatures. Four months later the chronically obstructed and highly hydronephrotic kidney and the normal kidney were used for preparations of muscle strips from the calyx (C), renal pelvis (RP), pyeloureteral junction (PU) and ureter (U) (Fig. 1 b).

In a last series we investigated the spontaneous activity of 179 muscle strips cut off from human pyeloureteral systems in a comparative fashion as in the pigs. The results we received from the normal upper tracts (24 kidneys) are compared with the data we got from chonically dilated organs (8 kidneys).

Results

Within a total of 121 muscle strips from normal pyeloureters of rats we found a definite decrease in the spontaneous frequencies from proximal to distal (Fig. 3). The

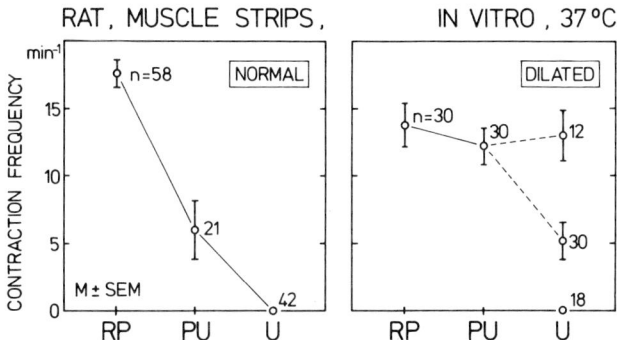

Fig. 3. *Left:* Muscle strips of the non-dilated rat pyeloureter show a spontaneous activity that is decreasing from proximal to distal. None of the 42 tested ureter preparations were spontaneously active. *Right:* Muscle strips of the renal pelvis and the pyeloureteral junction of a dilated pyeloureter show nearly the same spontaneous frequency in the organ bath. Twelve out of 30 tested ureter preparations were spontaneously active. For these spontaneously active ureter preparations we received the same mean contraction frequency as for the RP- and PU-preparations. The *interrupted lines* indicate the two possibilities for calculating the mean frequency: n=12, the mean frequency of all the spontaneously active ureter preparations; n=30, the mean frequency of all the tested ureter preparations including 18 preparations with contraction frequency=0

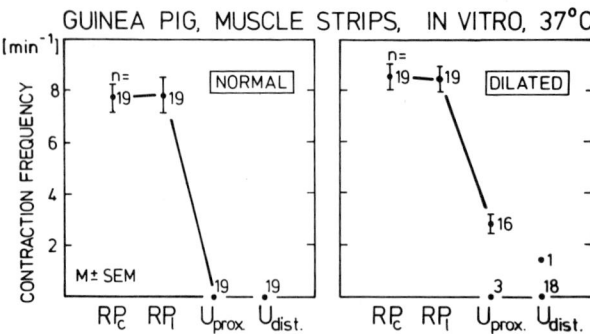

Fig. 4. In the guinea-pig pyeloureter chronic obstruction is also causing a change in the spontaneous activity of isolated muscle strips: Non-dilated isolated ureters are not spontaneously active. After three months of dilatation, however, 16 out of 19 ureter preparations exhibit spontaneous activity

most intrarenal strips of the kidney of the rat – which is a monopapillary kidney – were taken from the proximal renal pelvis. In the organ bath we found a mean isometric contraction frequency of 17.6/min in 58 of such preparations. From the 21 spiral-like strips from the pyeloureteral junctions we obtained a mean activity of 6.0/min. None of the 42 preparations from the ureter of the rat showed any spontaneous activity.

This frequency pattern is completely different in the chronically totally obstructed pyeloureter. The spontaneous frequencies of the dilated renal pelvis and the dilated pyeloureteral junction are almost the same: 13.8/min (RP) and 12.2/min (PU). Twelve out of the 30 chronically dilated ureters now showed spontaneous contractions in the organ bath with the same high frequency as the strips from the renal pelvis and the pyeloureteral junction, but 18 preparations behaved like normal ureters and showed no spontaneous activity. When the mean spontaneous frequency is calculated taking only the active ureteral preparations into account, we find a mean rate of 13.0/min. Of course, if all ureteral preparations are considered including the nonactive ones, then a lower mean value will be calculated, i.e. 5.2/min.

In the pyeloureter of the guinea-pig we could also observe a distinct change in the spontaneous activity of the isolated muscle strips after 3 months of total obstruction (Fig. 4). In the non-dilated system all of the tested preparations were spontaneously active, showing no effect of the longitudinal or circular section on their spontaneous activity or contraction frequency. However, no spontaneous activity could be found in the preparations of the ureter, neither proximal nor distal. Chronic obstruction causes only slight frequency accelerations in the region of the renal pelvis. Quite remarkable is, however, that after three months of obstruction 16 out of 19 ureter preparations showed independent spontaneous activity. This phenomenon can not be found in the ureter distal to the ligature. With one exception all of the U_{dist} preparations were not spontaneously active.

Comparable results could also be found with multicalyceal kidneys: The pyeloureter of the pig shows a pronounced frequency gradient between the calyceal system, the ureter and the renal pelvis (Fig. 5). At the same time the number of non-spontaneously active preparations significantly increases towards the ureter.

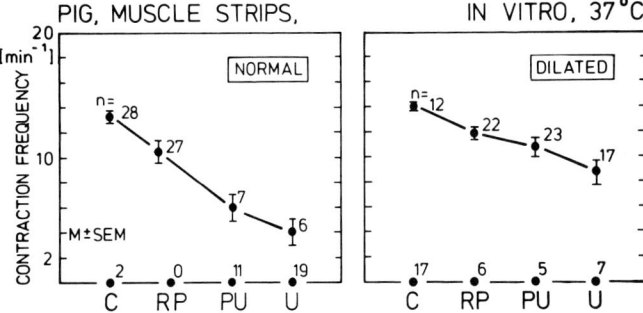

Fig. 5. Comparable results are obtained in the multicalyceal kidney of the pig: The non-dilated system reveals a pronounced frequency gradient from proximal to distal parallel to the increased number of not spontaneously active preparations. This frequency gradient is no longer found in muscle strips of chronically dilated pyeloureters, while at the same time the number of spontaneously active preparations of distal segments of the pyeloureter increases

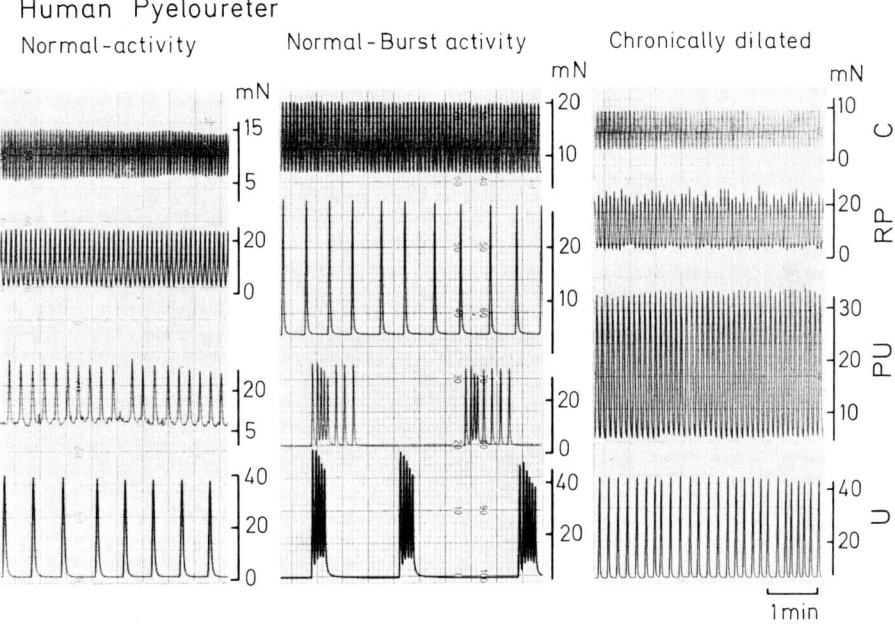

Fig. 6. Spontaneous activity of muscle strips from different parts of the human pyeloureter. Recording of the isometric contractions

In the dilated system the frequency gradient is then markedly levelled out. The mean values of the frequency gradient have been calculated by using only the spontaneously active preparations. Their diminution is even more pronounced if we take into account the number of not spontaneously active preparations. In normal systems most of the PU and U-preparations are not spontaneously active whereas in dilated systems most of the PU- and U-preparations also show rhythmic activity.

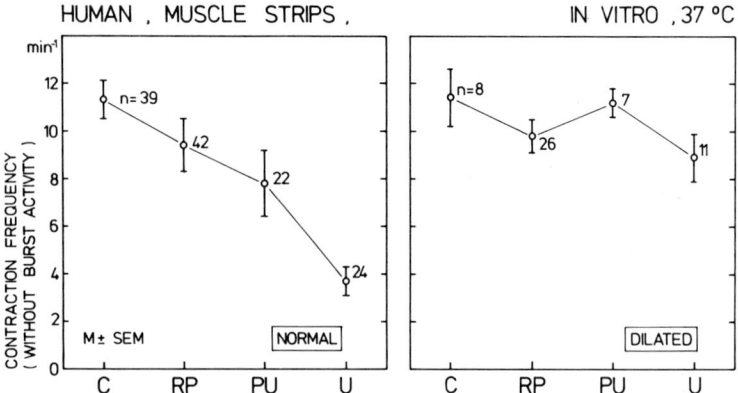

Fig. 7. Eight chronically dilated human pyeloureters showed a pronounced decrease in the frequency gradient from proximal to distal

From 24 human tumor kidneys after nephrectomy the spontaneous activity of muscle strips was investigated in the organ bath. Spontaneously active preparations from the multipapillary human kidney show two distinctly different patterns of activity: continuous regular activity and burst activity (Fig. 6). With burst activity we mean a form of activity where short periods of high frequency contractions alternate with longer periods without any activity (Hannappel et al. 1982). For the determination of the frequency gradient in the human pyeloureter only the continuous activity is considered. Then we also find a definite frequency gradient from the calyces (C) towards the renal pelvis (RP) and the pyeloureteral junction (PU) to the proximal ureter (U) (Fig. 7): C = 11.3/min, RP = 9.4/min, PU = 7.8/min, U = 3.7/min.

Eight chronically obstructed human kidneys could also be analyzed. Three of the cases were idiopathically obstructed kidneys and in five cases the dilatation was caused by a tumor compressing the ureter. In the organ bath we also found almost a complete loss of the physiological frequency gradient in 52 muscle strips which had been cut off from these chronically obstructed upper tracts: C = 11.4/min, RP = 9.8/min, PU = 11.2/min, U = 8.9/min.

Discussion

The frequency gradient in the spontaneous activity of the pyeloureteral musculature, as found by various investigators in different species, is an important factor in the initiation and organisation of a controlled orthograde peristalsis. As the highest frequency is generated in the uppermost intrarenal parts of the muscle system, these muscle cell groups take over the function of a primary pacemaker. All muscle cells with slower spontaneous activity function as latent pacemakers in a myogenically coupled system like this (single unit muscles).

However, when this physiological gradient is lost, as found in the organ bath for muscle strips from chronically dilated kidneys, then virtually all parts of the pyeloureteral system can take over the pacemaker function for a short period of time, and so initiate a contraction wave. Because of the capability of the ureteral musculature to conduct an excitation in both directions, such an accidential pacemaker area can at the same time initiate an orthograde as well as a retrograde peristaltic wave. In analogy to the situation in the heart we may talk about "heterotopic extrasystolic activity" of the pyeloureter.

We conclude confirmed by these in vitro experiments on muscle strips, that some of the functional changes observed in the dilated upper tract are due to the destruction of the physiological hierarchy of spontaneous myogenic activity in the pyeloureter.

In 1982 Djurhuus and Constantinou reported results from in vivo electromyographic investigations of normal and hydronephrotic pyeloureters in pigs. They also found that in the chronically dilated upper tract there was a lack of coordination between the activity of different regions of the pyeloureteral system, which results in an increase of the pressure at rest in the renal pelvis and an absence of effective contractions. The interpretations of their data was based on the assumption that the net effect of chronic obstruction was the loss of electrical conduction through the renal pelvic wall, caused by structural disruption of the pyeloureteral smooth muscles. However, our data show that the pattern and hierarchical distribution of spontaneous myogenic activity itself are also changed by chronic dilatation of the pyeloureteral system.

Our in vitro findings indicate an increased excitability of the chronically dilated pyeloureteral musculature, which then leads to a multicentric and thus uncoordinated peristaltic activity. These changes could also be verified in in vivo electromyographic examinations as a decreased conductivity along with higher contraction rates of the ureter.

References

Bozler E (1938) The action potentials of visceral smooth muscles. Am J Physiol 124:502–510
Constantinou CE (1974) Renal pelvic pacemaker control of ureteral peristaltic rate. Am J Physiol 226:1413–1419
Djurhuus JC, Constantinou CE (1982) Chronic ureteric obstruction and its impact on the coordinating mechanisms of peristalsis (Pyeloureteric pacemaker system). Urol Res 10:267–271
Djurhuus JC, Nerstrom B, Iverson-Hansen R, Gyrd-Hansen N, Rask-Anderson H (1977) Dynamics of upper urinary tract. I. An electrophysiologic in vivo study of renal pelvis in pigs: Method and normal pattern. Inv Urol 14:465–468
Golenhofen K, Hannappel J (1973) Spontaneous generation of excitation in the pyeloureteral system and the effect of adrenergic substances. In: Lutzeyer W, Melchior H (eds) Urodynamics, upper and lower urinary tract. Springer, Berlin Heidelberg New York, pp 46–56
Hannappel J, Golenhofen K (1974) Comparative studies on normal ureteral peristalsis in dogs, guinea-pigs and rats. Pflügers Arch 348:65–76
Hannappel J, Golenhofen K, Hohnsbein J, Lutzeyer W (1982) Pacemaker process of ureteral peristalsis in multicalyceal kidneys. Urol Int 37:240–245

Modelling of the Propagation of an Action Potential Along the Ureter

W. A. VAN DUYL[1]

Abstract. An electrical model of the propagation of the action potential is presented. It consists of an array of reactive cell units. Each unit is stimulated by a signal that is composed of the rising parts of the action potentials generated by the cells in a neighbouring reactive unit. The electrical model used for the reactive unit is based on processes occurring in the cell membranes. By means of the model the reduction in the propagation velocity and the associated changes in the shape of the action potential that are observed under certain conditions can be stimulated. It is concluded that threshold phenomena, in particular refractory behaviour of the ureteral tissue, play an important role in velocity of propagation of peristaltic waves. It seems likely that there is a trend in refractoriness along the ureter, which may cause non-uniformity of the propagation velocity.

Measurement of this non-uniformity is suggested at a means of assessing the quality of conduction in the ureter.

Introduction

The ureter propels urine from the kidney to the bladder by means of peristaltic waves. In the small intestine also peristalsis is the transport mechanism, and many studies have been published concerning the modelling of it. At first sight it seems possible to take advantage of these studies for modelling the peristalsis of the ureter. There is, however, an important difference between ureter and intestine. The small intestine generates wavelike electrical activity spontaneously. Peristaltic waves are accompanied by action potentials which appear to be phase-locked to the slow wave activity; the slow wave activity controls the peristalsis of the small intestine. This spontaneous activity is the basis of a well-known model consisting of an array of coupled oscillators with intrinsic frequencies corresponding to the spontaneous activity of segments of small intestine (Sarna et al. 1971). In contrast to the small intestine the ureter does not exhibit spontaneous electrical activity, so that such a model seems to be unsuitable for the peristalsis of the ureter. Nevertheless a similar model for the ureter has been published. Membrane processes in smooth muscle cells form the common basis of both models (van Duyl et al. 1978).

Normally, peristaltic waves in the ureter are initiated by rhythmic activity in the pelvis of the kidney. A ringlike contraction is produced at the uretero-pelvic junction by a mechanism which couples the ureter to the pelvic activity when the pelvis has reached a certain degree of urine filling. The contraction then propagates, as a contracting ureter segment, at a velocity of about 4 cm/s to the uretero-vesical junction. Although the peristalsis of the ureter is not controlled by electrical activity in

---

[1] Department of Biological and Medical Physics, Erasmus University Rotterdam, P.O. Box 1738, NL-3000 DR Rotterdam

the same way as in the small intestine, it is accompanied by electrical activity generated by depolarizing smooth muscle cells. This activity is measured in the EMG.

In ureter preparations peristalsis can be evoked by electrical stimulation at any point. Hence, after stimulation, peristalsis is an automatic myogenic mechanism. In contrast to the intact ureter, segments of ureter can contract spontaneously and in a more or less rhythmic fashion. There is a trend in the frequency of this spontaneous activity, such that the lowest frequency is observed in the central part of the ureter. This phenomenon of spontaneous activity is an implicit feature of the model. The muscular coat of the ureter consists of a layer of smooth muscle fibers. Ultramicroscopic studies reveal areas of close contact between smooth muscle cells. Depolarizing cell membranes are assumed to initiate depolarization of neighbouring cells via these high-conductance contacts. Following Bozler (1938) ureteral tissue is regarded as a functional syncytium, i.e. a group of many cells electrically coupled together. The action potential propagates from cell to cell via the interconnected membranes of the cells. This propagation is comparable to the propagation of an action potential along an axon, which has been thoroughly studied, in particular by Hodgkin and Huxley (1952). In these studies the cable model has been shown to describe the propagation adequately. The well-known Hodgkin-Huxley equations, which govern the membrane processes leading to action potentials, are included in the model. This yields a rather complicated mathematical model, the features of which are not very transparent. In this paper we give a short description of a model of the ureter which can simulate, and hence account for, certain physiological observations. The model can be regarded as a simplified version of the cable model. A more detailed description is given elsewhere (van Duyl 1984, 1985 a, b).

The Reactive Cell Unit

The cable model of the propagation of an action potential yields the following relation for the propagation velocity v:

$$v = \sqrt{\frac{dK}{R_i C_f}} \tag{1}$$

where d is the diameter of the cable (axon) (m), K is a rate constant (m/s), R_i is the specific resistivity of the intracellular fluid (Ohm · m) and C_f is the capacitance membrane charged during the upstroke of the action potential (F/m²).

According to this theory it is the upstroke of an action potential that stimulates neighbouring membranes to depolarization. The first part of the upstroke rises exponentially; K is the rate constant of this exponential rise. During the upstroke the membrane capacitance C_f is charged via the resistance of the extracellular and intracellular fluids. The resistivity of the extracellular fluid is negligible compared to the resistivity of the intracellular fluid R_i. It follows from (1) that the propagation velocity is proportional with the square root of the diameter of the cable.

Ramon et al. (1976) evaluated relation (1) for smooth muscle. They concluded that the observed velocity of 2–10 cm/s for the propagation of the action potential

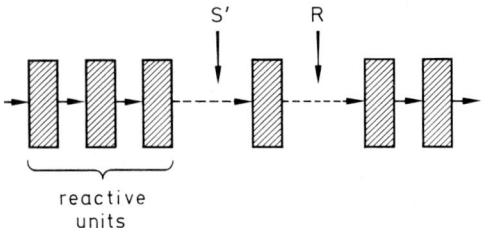

Fig. 1. Model for the propagation of action potentials consisting of an array of reactive units. S' stimulus for a reactive unit, corresponding to the upstrokes of an action potential generated by the cells of the preceding reactive unit; R response of a reactive unit corresponding to action potentials generated by the cells of a reactive unit; S'–R reaction time for a transition of electrical activity from one unit to the next

in smooth muscle is in good agreement with the speed of propagation along a 'cable' of diameter 5 µm. This means that the cable model applies to a fiber with a diameter of one cell. Nagai and Prosser (1963) conclude, however, from their stimulation studies that a minimum diameter of about 100 µm is required for the propagation of action potentials in smooth muscle, and that an electrode with a minimum diameter of 75 µm was required for stimulation. They conclude that functional units comprising the synchronous activity of numbers of cells are required to sustain propagation. About 200–300 individual cells working in synchrony would form a functional unit with a diameter of 100 µm. Such a unit, however, does not behave as a cable with that diameter, because that would imply a propagation velocity of 10–40 cm/s, significantly larger than that observed in smooth muscle. Each cell belonging to one functional unit reacts to its own stimulus. In our model we lump together all simultaneously reacting cells in one reacting unit, represented by a block in Fig. 1. The stimulus for a reactive unit is assumed to be the resultant of the spatially distributed stimuli for the individual cells. Our model, shown in Fig. 1, consists of an array of reactive units. The output of one unit yields the stimulus S' for next unit. The velocity of propagation of the action potential is determined by the length of the units, and the reaction times of units to the stimuli. It is likely that the coupling between cells and its precise structure determines whether a stimulus yields a propagatable action potential or not. In particular the proportion of cells in a reactive unit which do not make contact with cells of next unit is important in this connection (George 1961). Both the size of the reactive units and the reaction time are unknown. Some physiological phenomena connected with the propagation of an action potential, however, can be explained as consequences of two factors determining the reaction time, namely the steepness of the stimulus and the threshold level of the reactive unit. This will be shown by simulation of these phenomena with an electronic model of a reactive unit.

Electronic Model of a Reactive Unit

The features of a reactive unit are determined by the membrane processes of the cells. These processes are governed by voltage- and time-dependent changes in the conductivities of the membrane for certain ions. Pioneer studies on the membrane of the axon by Hodgkin and Huxley (1952) yield a set of so-called H. H.-equations, which describe the processes very well. Several points of correspondence in the behaviour of nerves and smooth muscle indicate that in principle the same equations are valid for smooth muscle. Instead of using mathematical formulas we have built an electronic model which simulates the ionic membrane currents. For the model we use parameter values which are characteristic of smooth muscle. The sodium and potassium conductances of the membrane are simulated by means of field-effect transistors (Fig. 2). Furthermore a conduction path is included corresponding to the membrane leakage current. To simplify the observations on the model the processes are accelerated by a factor 10. The 'action potential' generated by the model is shown in Fig. 3. The rise of the upstroke of the 'action potential' is determined by the rate of activation of the conductance of the Na-path, in agreement with physiological observations. The negative-going flank following the peak is determined by the activation of the conductance of the K-path. Na-activation is followed by a Na-deactivation process, in accordance with standard physiology. Contrary to the original H. H.-model, we include in our model a K-deactivation process as well following in this respect the studies of Beeler and Reuter (1976). The K-deactivation is a slower process than the Na-deactivation. More details of the electronic model are described elsewhere (van Duyl 1983). After an action potential, slow recovery from the deactivation of the sodium conductance, combined with slow recovery from K-activation and K-deactivation, determine a threshold level which has to be exceeded by a stimulus in order to evoke a succeeding action potential. During a short period immediately after an action potential no succeeding action potential can be evoked, regardless of the height of the stimulus. This period is called the absolute refractory period. After this period the threshold for stimulation is higher than normal and gradually falls to its normal level. This is the relative refractory period.

Refractory behaviour is a well-known feature of smooth muscle. The threshold curve of our model is shown in Fig. 4. This graph shows the magnitude of a second block pulse, with a duration of 2 ms, which is just large enough to evoke a second 'action potential', as a function of the time elapsed since a primary pulse of 1 V and 1 ms that evoked a first 'action potential'. By means of this threshold curve of the model we can demonstrate the effect of refractoriness of tissue on the propagation of action potentials.

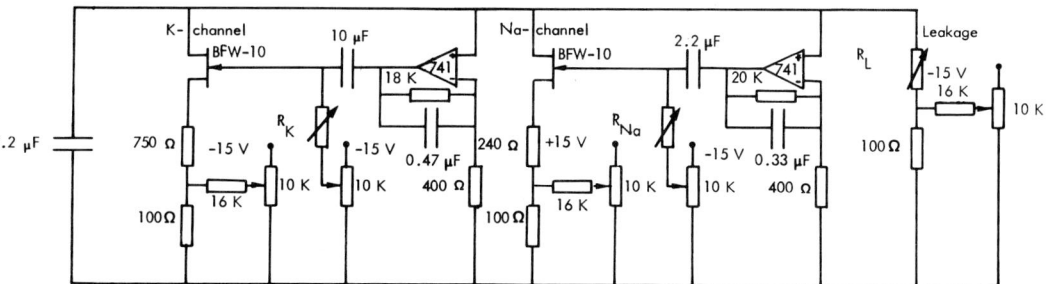

Fig. 2. Electronic model for a reactive unit in which membrane processes leading to action potentials are simulated (van Duyl 1983c)

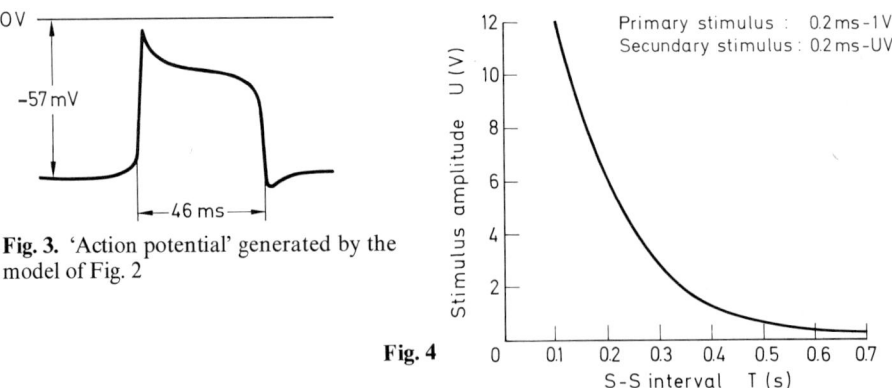

Fig. 3. 'Action potential' generated by the model of Fig. 2

Fig. 4. Threshold curve of the model of Fig. 2 measured by double pulse stimuli with varying interval (*horizontal axis*). The *vertical axis* shows the magnitude of the second pulse required to evoke a second 'action potential'

Effect of Refractoriness on the Reaction Time and the Shape of the Action Potential

Figure 5 shows the threshold curve and two ramp functions representing stimuli S' applied at two different periods after a response R to a previous stimulus S'. This figure makes clear that the reaction time, S'–R, is larger when the stimulus is applied at a shorter period after the previous response. We measured the S'–R time on the model, which was stimulated by a ramp function with a steepness of 15 V/s, for different values of the time between two successive stimuli, the S'–S' interval. It appears that when the S'–S' interval is shorter than 700 ms the S'–R time increases with decreasing S'–S' interval. The reciprocal of the SR reaction time is a measure of local propagation velocity of the action potential. In Fig. 6 the reciprocal of the S'R time, expressed as a percentage of its value when the S'–S' interval is 700 ms, is represented as a function of the S'–S' interval. In this figure are shown also the 'action potential' associated with various values of the S'R-time. It appears that the shape of the 'action potential' is related to the S'–R time. In particular the duration of the plateau is shorter when the S'–R time is shorter. Figure 6 is similar to Fig. 7 which, however, shows experimental data for the dog, obtained using monopolar EMG by Butcher et al. (1957). The similarity between the figures indicates that the reduction in the propagation velocity and the associated changes in the shape of the action potentials are caused by the refractoriness of ureteral tissue. It can be shown that characteristic sequences of SR-intervals that are observed in ureteral peristalsis and which are known as Wenckebach periods, can be explained in a similar way (van Duyl 1984). We conclude from our simulation study that both the normal and the reduced velocities of propagation of action potentials are determined by the steepness of the upstroke of the action potential and the threshold curve, which implies refractoriness of the smooth muscle. The influence of the rate of rise of the action potential on the propagation velocity also follows directly from (1), because of K.

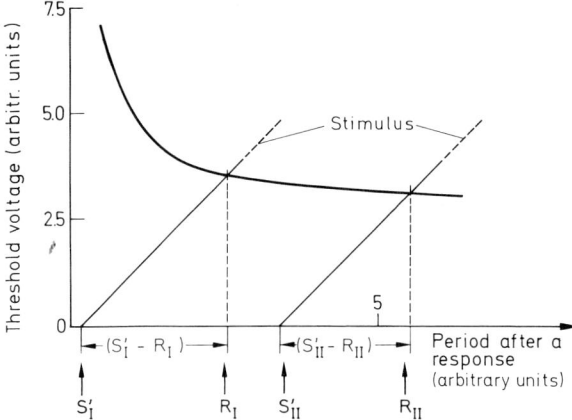

Fig. 5. Illustration of the influences of the interval between stimuli on the reaction time: the horizontal axis represents the time elapsed since the previous response (action potential). Reaction time $(S'-R)_I > (S'-R)_{II}$

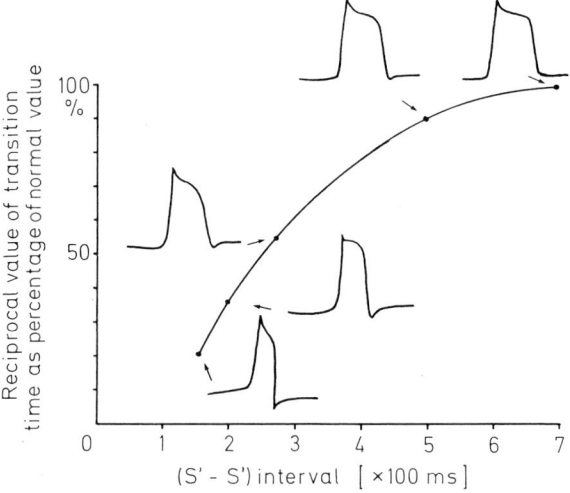

Fig. 6. Locally reduced velocity of propagation of 'action potential', expressed as a percentage of the normal velocity of propagation and plotted as a function of the stimulus interval S'–S'. The curve is derived from the reciprocals of the reaction times measured on the model. The figure also shows that the shape of the 'action potential' is related to the S'–S' interval

The upstroke of the action potential is determined by the activation of the Na-conductance of the membrane. It has been shown that decreasing the extracellular Na-concentration reduces both the steepness of the upstroke and the propagation velocity (Kobayashi and Irisawa 1964). Our conclusion that the threshold curve also is significant in determining the propagation velocity does not follow directly from (1). In a previous publication we expressed the hypothesis that the trend in the frequency of the spontaneous activity of ureter segments corresponds to a trend in the re-

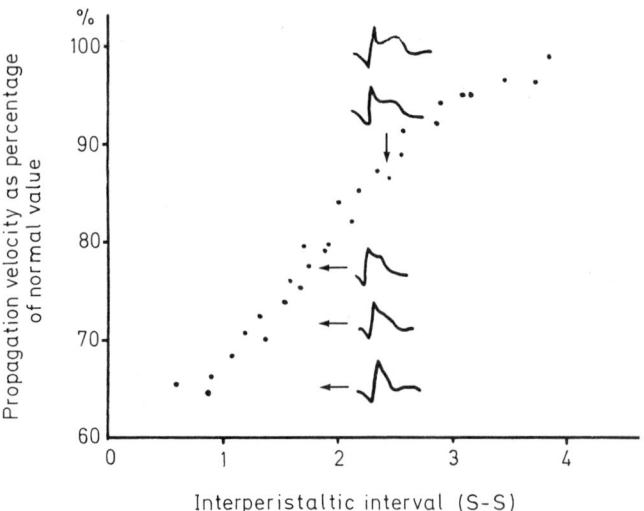

Fig. 7. Reduced velocity of propagation of action potential as a percentage of the normal velocity, plotted as a function of the stimulus interval, observed in the ureter of a dog. The figure also shows that the shape of the action potentials is related to the S–S interval. (After Butcher et al. 1957; compare Fig. 6)

fractory period, so that the tissue of the central part of the ureter has the longest refractory period (van Duyl et al. 1978). In combination with our model this gives an explanation for the observation that a reduced propagation velocity most frequently occurs in the central part of the ureter.

Parameters of the Model Determining the Spontaneous Activity

Because in our model the refractory period is related to the frequency of spontaneous activity, we have measured the effect of the parameters which determine the refractory period of the model when it is passive on the frequency of the 'action potentials' generated when it is active. It appears that, when the leakage resistor R_L in Fig. 2 is increased to about 1150 Ohm, the model generates 'action potentials' spontaneously. When R_L is increased from its normal value of 800 Ohm to 1150 Ohm the resting membrane voltage increases from −58 mV to −57 mV. Hence a membrane voltage of −57 mV appears to correspond to the threshold level in our model; when this level is exceeded the model changes from being passive to active. The larger the value of R_l the higher is the frequency of the spontaneous activity, as shown in Fig. 8. The influence of R_L on the frequency is relatively small. R_K has a much greater influence, as is also shown in Fig. 8. A larger value of R_K means a slower recovery from deactivation of K-conductance after an 'action potential'. The process of recovery from deactivation of the K-conductance is accompanied with increasing K-conductance and hence contributes in keeping the membrane voltage low. When this

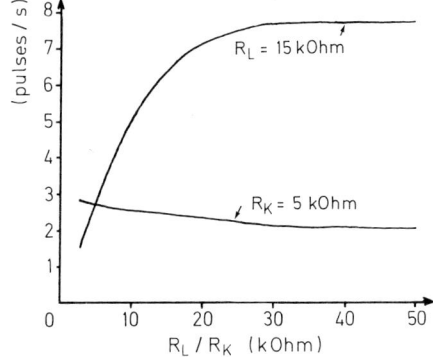

Fig. 8. Frequency of 'action potentials' generated spontaneously by the model of Fig. 2, as a function of the leakage resistor R_L ($R_K = 5$ kOhm), and also as a function of the resistor R_K (with $R_L = 15$ kOhm) that determines the rate of deactivation of the K-conductance

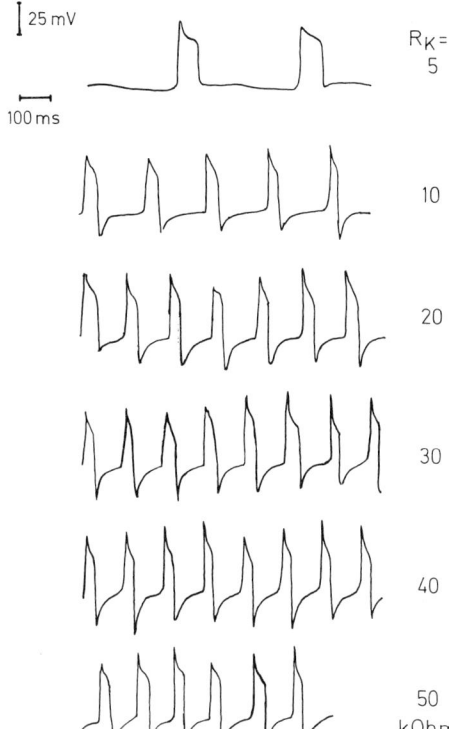

Fig. 9. Recordings of spontaneously generated 'action potentials' for different values of R_K in Fig. 2

process of recovery is delayed, because R_K is large, the initial depolarization is dominated by the processes of recovery from Na-deactivation and K-activation. Recovery from Na-deactivation and from K-activation leads to increasing membrane voltages. Hence, when the influence of recovery from K-deactivation in the initial repolarization is reduced the threshold voltage is reached earlier. This explains the shorter period in spontaneous activity when R_K is larger. Figure 9 shows the 'action potentials' generated at different frequencies. The 'action potentials' are shorter for higher frequencies. Our model indicates that leakage of the membranes, caused for example by sectioning of the ureter, may turn passive ureter tissue into active, although this leakage does not determine the different frequencies of the various ureter segments. It seems likely that these different frequencies reflect differences in the rates of activation and/or deactivation of that K-conductance, which also determine the length of the refractory period when the model is passive.

Conclusion

We have shown how the influence of the interval between peristaltic waves on the velocity of propagation and on the shape of the associated action potentials can be accounted for by combination of a local stimulus, having a certain rate of increase, with refractoriness of the tissue. Our model can be regarded as a simplified, lumped parameter version of the cable model used to describe axons. In this lumped parameter model attention is directed towards individual transitions between cells or cell units. It has been shown that the reaction time of these transitions may play an important role both in normal and in reduced velocities of propagated action potentials. The reaction times are determined by the steepness of local stimuli, which are assumed to correspond to the upstrokes of the action potentials, and the threshold curves of the reactive units. Consequently impaired conduction in the ureter may be caused by abnormal steepness (or magnitude) of the myogenic stimuli and/or abnormal threshold curves of the reactive units. Impaired conduction may be restricted to a very small part of the ureter. Our model indicates that a trend in the frequency of the spontaneous activity of ureter segments reflects a similar trend in the refractory period. According to the model this trend may lead to non-uniformity of the velocity of propagation along the ureter, especially for a wave which appears within a short period of the previous one. It may therefore be possible to assess the quality of conduction in the ureter by determining what interval between two peristaltic waves causes a decrease in the velocity of propagation of the second wave at some point along the ureter.

The size and the shape of the reactive units and the geometric aspects of the stimuli are related to the microanatomic structure of the ureteral wall. Study of these aspects of the structure may throw light on the question of what makes the velocity of propagation of electrical activity in the circumferential direction larger than in the longitudinal direction.

References

Beeler GW, Reuter H (1977) Reconstruction of the action potential of ventricular myocardial fibres. J Biophysics 177

Bozler E (1938) Electric stimulation and conduction of excitation in smooth muscle. Am J Physiol 122:614

Butcher HR, Sleator W, Schmandt KIP (1957) A study of the peristaltic conduction mechanism in the canine ureter. J Urology 78:231

Duyl WA van (1984) Theory of the propagation of peristaltic waves along the ureter and their simulation in an electronic model. Urology XXIV-5:511

Duyl WA van (1985a) Modelling of the electrical activity of the ureter. In: Singh M (ed) Encyclopedea of systems and control. Pergamon Press, New York

Duyl WA van (1985b) An electric analogon of ureter membrane processes. In preparation

Duyl WA van, Brans JM, Coolsaet BLRA, Grashuis JL, Kingma YJ (1978) Provisional model for propagation of electrical activity in upper urinary tract. Urology XII-6:736

George EP (1961) Resistance values in a syncitium. Austr J Exp Biol Med Sci 39:267

Hodgkin AL, Huxley AF (1952) A quantitative description of membrane current and its application to conductance and excitation in nerve. J Physiol 117:500

Kobayashi M, Irisawa H (1964) Effect of sodium deficiency on the action potential of the smooth muscle of ureter. Am J Phys 206:205

Nagai T, Prosser CL (1963) Electrical parameters of smooth muscle cells. Am J Physiol 204(5):915

Ramon F, Anderson NC, Joymer RW, More JWA (1976) A model for propagation of action potentials in smooth muscle. J Theor Biol 59:381

Sarna SK, Daniel EE, Kingma YJ (1971) Simulation of slow wave electrical activity of small intestine. Am J Phys 221:166

Voltage- and Agonist-Induced Activation of Smooth Muscle of the Human Upper Urinary Tract: Different Mechanisms

L. Hertle[1] and H. Nawrath[2]

Smooth muscles are such a remarkably diverse group of tissues that the difference in properties between any two of them may be as great as between a smooth muscle and a striated muscle. With this diversity it is not surprising that the ways in which different stimuli initiate contraction are also extremely varied and interesting although we still know very little about the details of the mechanisms involved. In an attempt to shed some light on the cellular contraction cycle of smooth muscle of the human upper urinary tract, this article will focus on two topics:

1. Previous findings in smooth muscle research will be summarized and discussed briefly as they are pertinent to an understanding of the mechanical activity of the upper urinary tract.
2. Experimental findings from human preparations will be demonstrated as examples for different modes of activation of smooth muscle. Based on findings from other smooth muscle tissues a concept of different activation mechanisms will be presented.

In isolated muscle strips of the human upper urinary tract two general types of mechanical activity can be differentiated: phasic and tonic contractions. For example, in an organ bath segments of the minor calyces exhibit spontaneous, phasic contractions with a frequency between 7 to 10 per minute. This phasic type of activity (Fig. 1) is characterised by regular, rhythmic changes in tension which can be modified in amplitude and frequency. In the purest form of phasic contraction, the baseline is always reached between two contractions. With increasing frequency, however, the baseline seems to rise due to tetanic summation.

Stimulation of a muscle strip by an agonist, e.g. norepinephrine, may induce tonic contraction (Fig. 2), which characteristically remains constant with time under constant conditions; the intensity of contraction can be modified gradually over the whole intensity range by its stimulating control mechanism (Golenhofen 1981).

The exact nature of the processes which link the stimulating and mechanical events (stimulation-contraction coupling) involved in smooth muscle activity in general and in the upper urinary tract in particular is not known, although it is generally agreed that calcium is an important link between these events. Much of the following discussion is derived from information concerning smooth muscle tissues other than from the upper urinary tract but which may still serve as an approach to an understanding of stimulation-contraction coupling in smooth muscle of the human upper urinary tract.

---

1 Abteilung Urologie, Universität Bochum, Marienhospital, Widumer Str. 8, D-4690 Herne 1
2 Abteilung Pharmakologie, Universität Mainz, Obere Zahlbacher Str. 67, D-6500 Mainz

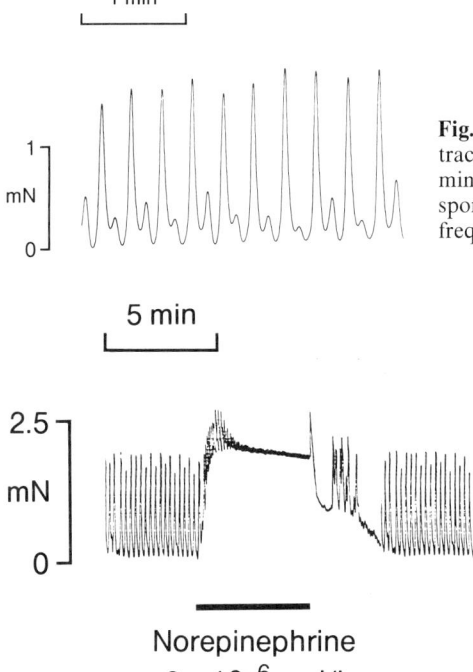

Fig. 1. Example of the phasic type of contraction. Original tracing of an isolated human minor calyx segment. The preparation exhibited spontaneous, rhythmic changes in tension with a frequency of 7 per minute

Fig. 2. Example of an agonist-induced tonic contraction. Original tracing of an isolated, spontaneously contracting human minor calyx segment. The addition of norepinephrine in a concentration of 3×10^{-6} mol/l to the organ bath was followed by a long-lasting 'tonic' contraction accompanied by a slight increase in frequency and a reduction of the amplitude of the spontaneous 'phasic' contractions. After wash-out of norepinephrine the muscle strip immediately returned to its original activity

Calcium and Contraction

Although the actual contractile process has not been studied in the ureter, contraction in muscular tissues in general is related to an interaction between the contractile proteins, actin and myosin, which occurs in the sarcoplasm. In the relaxed state a regulator system, consisting of the proteins troponin and tropomyosin, prevents the interaction of actin and myosin. When calcium binds to troponin, a conformational change occurs which results in the displacement of tropomyosin which thus allows the interaction of actin and myosin and a subsequent contraction.

It is widely believed that the final common step for initiating contraction is an increase in the free ionized calcium within the muscle cell. Typically, the intracellular calcium concentration of unstimulated cells is within the range of 0.05–0.5 µM whereas in extracellular fluids it is 1–10 mM. After electrical or chemical stimulation, the intracellular calcium concentration increases by one or two orders of magnitude. The mobilisation of activator calcium by various stimulating agents can occur by a limited number of mechanisms including uptake of calcium from the extracellular compartment or associated superficial sites as well as release of the ion from the membrane or intracellular binding sites or stores. Thus a number of events in the sequence coupling stimulation to contraction can be termed calcium-dependent steps and clearly, specific actions of a stimulating agent at only one of these points can alter smooth muscle contractility.

Table 1. Modes of activation of smooth muscle

Voltage-induced activation
– pacemaker activity
– high extracellular potassium

Agonist-induced activation
– norepinephrine
– acetylcholine

Stimulation by agonists and by depolarization (Table 1) represent the two most prominent means of activation of smooth muscle; the former acting by binding to specific receptors on the smooth muscle membrane and the latter by depolarization of the cell membrane which is not related to any specific receptor activation. Agonist-induced and voltage-induced activation have been extensively used to study the details of the role of calcium in the activation of smooth muscle. The following discussion will focus on the possible mechanisms of action of these different modes of activation in smooth muscle of the human upper urinary tract. It will also be demonstrated that there are regionally different responses of upper tract muscle strips, particularly to agonist-induced activation.

Voltage-Induced Activation

When a smooth muscle cell is in its resting state, its transmembrane potential (the resting membrane potential) appears to be primarily determined by the distribution of potassium ions across the cell membrane and the permeability of the membrane to potassium. The value of the resting membrane potential in ureteral muscle cells is similar to that of other smooth muscles (average minus 60 mV) but considerably lower than that of skeletal or cardiac muscle, which is in the range of minus 90 mV (for review see Weiss 1978). The process of making the inside of the cell less negative compared to the outside is called depolarization and the opposite change in the transmembrane potential is called repolarization. The resting potential of a non-pacemaker cell is maintained until the cell is excited either by an external stimulus or by conduction of electrical activity (action potential) from an already excited adjacent cell. If a stimulus depolarizes an adequate area of the cell membrane rapidly enough from the resting to the threshold potential, the cell is excited and develops its own action potential.

The action potential is the primary and most important mechanism by which, either directly or indirectly, a rise in free intracellular calcium is produced in those smooth muscles that normally generate and propagate action potentials. It is now generally assumed that voltage-induced calcium influx across the cell membrane is a passive movement of the ion down the electrochemical gradient. Passive movement of calcium across plasma membranes is usually electrogenic, which means that, under favorable conditions, it can be measured as a membrane current. The driving force is the electrochemical gradient of the ion across the membrane, and the likely structures through which the ions permeate are 'pore'- or 'channel'-forming proteins embedded in the lipid bilayer of the membrane. Calcium channels in excitable membranes are controlled by voltage-dependent gating, that is, their opening and closing kinetics are the result of changes in the membrane potential. There is evidence for a 'voltage sensor' in the membrane, for example a protein group with dipole properties, which may be an integral part of an ion channel, and that reacts to the electric field. Any change in membrane potential will cause a reorientation of the charged sensor within the field and, therefore, a change in the ion flow through the channel (for reviews see Katz et al. 1982 and Tsien 1983).

Several types of smooth muscle exhibit rhythmic, spontaneous contractions associated with electrical activity. Two types of electrical activity could be demonstrated, 'slow potentials' of different types, and 'spike' activity. The insensitivity of spike-like action potentials to tetrodotoxin, an inhibitor of the inward sodium current, provided strong evidence that the inward current responsible for the upstroke of a spike is carried predominantly by calcium ions. It is generally accepted that in several types of smooth muscle, including tissue of the upper urinary tract, spike activity is caused by a transmembrane influx of extracellular calcium through voltage-operated calcium channels.

Figure 1 shows a typical tracing of the mechanical activity of an isolated muscle strip from a human minor calyx. Preparations from that region of the human kidney usually show spontaneous, phasic-rhythmic changes in tension. Spontaneous phasic-rhythmic activity of isolated calyceal segments as well as ureteral peristalsis in vivo are both regarded to be induced by action potentials generated by pacemaker cells located in the utmost distal part of the collecting system.

The first direct attempt to examine the role of the action potential in causing contraction was to produce a potassium depolarization. The muscle cell has a resting potential that is close to the potassium equilibrium potential, because the membrane is more permeable to potassium than to any other ion. This intracellular potential is negative compared with the extracellular potential, because potassium is low in the extracellular solution and high in the intracellular solution (Fig. 3). Consequently, raising the extracellular potassium would decrease the potassium concentration gradient and depolarize the cell. This experiment was systematically performed with skeletal muscle by Kuffler (1946), who found that it produced a sustained contraction called a contracture. Potassium depolarizations were used especially in smooth muscle to demonstrate that tension appears to be a graded function of the membrane potential.

Activation by high extracellular potassium concentrations is a method of depolarization different from that occurring in the action potential. Increasing the external potassium concentration results in an increased spike frequency and, at higher potassium values, in a sustained depolarization of the membrane without action potentials (Golenhofen et al. 1973). During the application of high potassium solutions in ureteral muscle strips an increased influx of ^{45}calcium has been demonstrated (L. Hertle and H. Nawrath, unpublished results). This stimulation can be assumed to depend on the opening of voltage-dependent channels through which external calcium can flow into the cell (Casteels and Droogmans 1982).

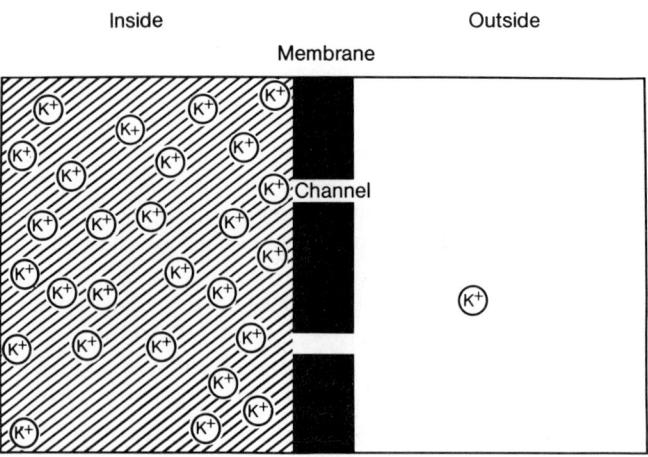

Fig. 3. Schematic illustration of intra- and extracellular distribution of potassium ions in the resting state of a smooth muscle cell. The resting membrane potential is close to the potassium equilibrium potential, because the membrane is more permeable to potassium than to any other ion. This potential is negative intracellularly relative to the outside potential because potassium is low in the extracellular solution and high in the intracellular solution

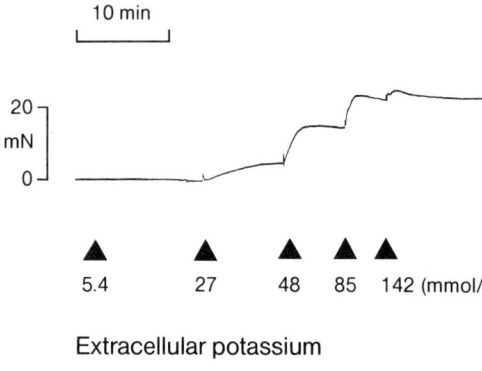

Fig. 4. Effect of increasing extracellular potassium concentrations on tension of an isolated ureteral muscle strip. Increase of the potassium concentration in the Tyrode solution from normal (5.4 mmol/l) to 142 mmol/l in logarithmic increments produced immediate and sustained contractions. Maximal activation was achieved with a potassium concentration of 142 mmol/l

Figure 4 shows the effects of increasing extracellular potassium concentrations on resting tension of an isolated ureteral muscle strip. Increase of the potassium concentrations in the Tyrode solution from normal (5.4 mmol/l) to 142 mmol/l in logarithmic increments produced immediate and sustained contractions. The threshold for induction of contractions was 27 mmol/l, a maximal activation was achieved with a potassium concentration of 142 mmol/l. A potassium concentration of 85 mmol/l produced a submaximal activation of the muscle strips and was therefore chosen to test the response of isolated muscle strips from different regions of the upper urinary tract to depolarization-induced activation. The activation by high extracellular potassium concentration was not affected by 30-minute preincubation with tetrodotoxin (2×10^{-5} mol/l) and phentolamine (10^{-5} mol/l).

Pacemaker-induced contractions are of the phasic type, because the membrane potential changes periodically. Depolarization is followed by repolarization. Potassium-induced contractions are sustained contractions because the membrane is clamped at a certain voltage. But the mechanism common to both types of activation is depolarization of the cell membrane without specific receptor activation.

Agonist-Induced Activation

It is assumed that a number of agonists such as acetylcholine or norepinephrine produce their effects by interacting first with a receptor molecule which is specific to the particular stimulant involved. The evidence for the existence of such receptor molecules is largely inferential because none of them have yet been isolated and characterized; the existence of specific blocking agents and the rather large changes in agonist activity that occur after relatively small changes in the chemical structure are the main indications. For a variety of agonists several features of the actions on smooth muscle can be explained by postulating that interaction with a population of receptors situated in or on the smooth muscle cell increases the intracellular calcium concentration. In support of this idea, we demonstrated an increased uptake of ^{45}calcium in norepinephrine-stimulated human calyceal preparations (L. Hertle and H. Nawrath, unpublished results).

One of the postulated mechanisms is illustrated in Fig. 5. The advent of a nerve signal at the presynaptic nerve terminal leads to a fusion of synaptic vesicles with the presynaptic membrane, which is followed by a release of neurotransmitter molecules into the synaptic gap. The transmitter molecules then bind to the active sites of their specific receptors on the smooth muscle membrane, possibly activating receptor-associated ion channels.

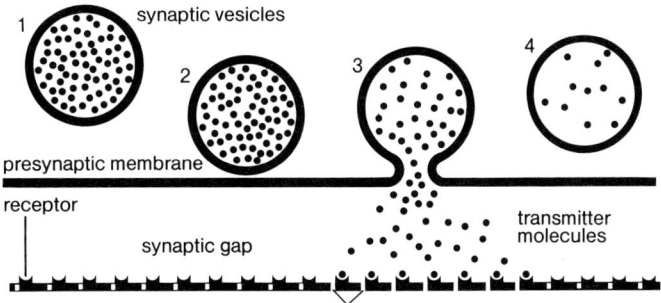

Fig. 5. Schematic illustration of one of the postulated mechanisms of action of a neurotransmitter on smooth muscle membrane. The advent of a nerve signal at the presynaptic nerve terminal leads to a fusion of synaptic vesicles with the presynaptic membrane, which is followed by a release of neurotransmitter molecules into the synaptic gap (*1–3*). The transmitter molecules then bind to their specific receptors possibly activating receptor-associated ion channels

Many research workers found that autonomic neurotransmitter substances influence the basically myogenic activity of the upper urinary tract. In studies of human calyceal preparations norepinephrine increased the resting tension as well as the frequency of spontaneous contractions and caused a reduction in amplitude (Longrigg 1975a; Yano et al. 1981; Hertle 1982). These effects were concentration-dependent and could effectively be blocked by phentolamine, thus indicating the existence of alpha-adrenoceptors. Figure 2 illustrates the effects of norepinephrine on a spontaneously contracting calyceal muscle strip in an original tracing. The addition of the transmitter to the organ bath in a concentration of 3×10^{-6} mol/l was followed by a long-lasting, 'tonic' contraction accompanied by a slight increase in frequency and a reduction of the amplitude of the spontaneous 'phasic' contractions. After the wash-out of norepinephrine the muscle strip immediately returned to its original activity. Similar results were obtained with isolated renal pelvis preparations (Del Tacca et al. 1974; Longrigg 1975b; Kinn and Nergardh 1979). Spontaneously active preparations from that region responded to the addition of norepinephrine by an increase both in frequency and in resting tension. Quiescent preparations responded to the same agonist with an increase in tension with or without occasional, superimposed phasic contractions. In human ureteral preparations (Malin et al. 1968; Malin et al. 1970) norepinephrine increased both the rate and the amplitude of spontaneous, phasic contractions and initiated activity in previously quiescent segments.

The findings concerning the cholinergic agonists are not uniform, some workers have observed an excitatory effect and others no effect at all. When an effect of acetylcholine was observed (Longrigg 1975) the maximum increase in resting tension achieved was only 20% to 30% of that seen with norepinephrine. The fact that the excitatory effects of acetylcholine in human calyceal tissues can be blocked with atropine indicates the presence of muscarinic receptors in this tissue.

Voltage- and Agonist-Induced Activation in Different Tissues of the Upper Urinary Tract

In preparations of the normal human upper urinary tract we compared the responses to depolarization- and agonist-induced activations. The preparations were obtained after tumornephrectomies and were unaffected by the disease. The collecting systems showed no signs of infection or obstruction. The muscle strips were suspended in thermostatically controlled organ baths containing Tyrode solution, equilibrated with 95% O_2 and 5% CO_2, pH 7.4, 37°C. The Tyrode solution had the following composition (mmol/l): NaCl 136.9, KCl 5.4, $MgCl_2$ 1.05, NaH_2PO_4 0.42, $NaHCO_3$ 11.9, $CaCl_2$ 1.8 and glucose 5.5. Tension was recorded isometrically by using inductive force displacement transducers. The stimuli we used were acetylcholine (10^{-4} mol/l), norepinephrine (10^{-4} mol/l) and 85 mmol/l high extracellular potassium. For each stimulus the maximal tension above the baseline was analyzed graphically.

As an example, an original tracing in Fig. 6 shows the different responses of an isolated muscle strip taken from the human renal pelvis to an agonist-induced and

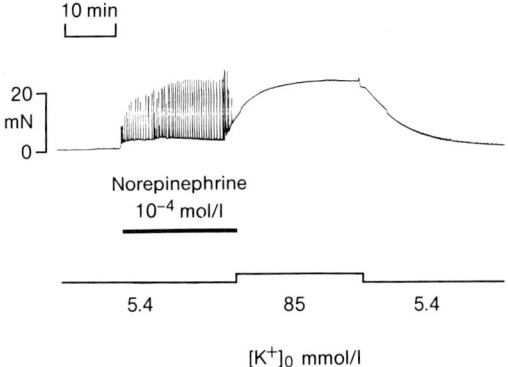

Fig. 6. Different effects of norepinephrine and 85 mmol/l extracellular potassium on mechanical activity of a quiescent renal pelvis preparation (original tracing). Norepinephrine induced spontaneous, phasic contractions together with a slight increase in resting tension. The additional activation with 85 mmol/l extracellular potassium produced a sustained contracture which returned to control values after change to normal tyrode solution

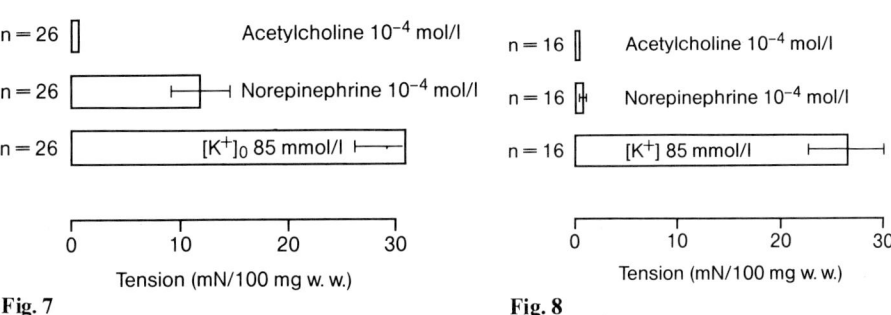

Fig. 7, 8. Comparison of the effects of acetylcholine, norepinephrine and high extracellular potassium contractions on resting tension of calyceal and pelvic in contrast to ureteral muscle strips (means ± SEM, n = 26 and 16, respectively). Acetylcholine had only minor effects on resting tension in all these tissues but occasionally induced phasic contractions. Depolarization with 85 mmol/l extracellular potassium produced sustained contractures of the same order of magnitude in all tissues of the upper urinary tract. Norepinephrine had different effects in different tissues. In usually inactive ureteral muscle stips, norepinephrine induced predominantly phasic contractions, with only minimal effects on resting tension. In contrast, in isolated segments of the renal calyx and pelvis, the same neurotransmitter induced a qualitatively different response, which consisted in a long-lasting 'tonic' contraction

to a voltage-induced activation. The addition of norepinephrine in a concentration of 10^{-4} mol/l to the organ bath containing a normal Tyrode solution with 5.4 mmol/l potassium was followed by the onset of spontaneous, phasic rhythmic contractions together with a slight 'tonic' increase in resting tension. The additional activation with 85 mmol/l extracellular potassium induced a sustained contracture which returned to control values after returning to normal Tyrode solution. Figures 7 and 8 summarize the effects of acetylcholine, norepinephrine and high extracellular potas-

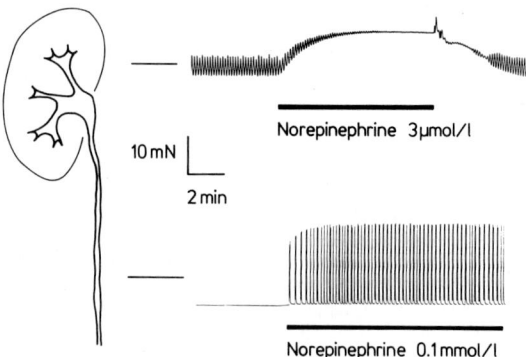

Fig. 9. Illustration of the different effects of norepinephrine on different tissues of the human upper urinary tract. In preparations of the calyceal and pelvic region the drug induces tonic contractions, which are little affected by calcium antagonists. In contrast, in ureteral muscle strips the same agonist induces predominantly phasic contractions, which can be potently suppressed by calcium antagonists. This different pattern of response suggests different and separate coupling mechanisms between the receptors involved and the calcium responsible for contraction

sium concentration on the resting tension of calyceal and pelvic muscle strips in contrast to those from the ureter. Acetylcholine had only minor effects on resting tension in calyceal and pelvic as well as in ureteral muscle strips. In all these tissues acetylcholine occasionally induced only phasic contractions. With respect to the activation by high extracellular potassium there was also no significant difference among the tissues. Depolarization with 85 mmol/l extracellular potassium in the Tyrode solution produced sustained contractures of the same magnitude in all tissues of the upper urinary tract. The main difference was observed in the response to norepinephrine. In usually inactive ureteral muscle strips, norepinephrine induced predominantly phasic contractions, with only minimal effects on the resting tension. In contrast, in isolated segments of the renal calyx and pelvis, the same neurotransmitter induced a qualitatively different response, which consisted of a long-lasting, tonic contraction irrespective of pre-existing spontaneous phasic activity. This different pattern of response is illustrated in Fig. 9.

Concept of Different Activation Mechanisms

The different types of muscle (skeletal, cardiac, and smooth) exhibit fundamental differences in the mechanisms by which their contractile proteins are activated by calcium. Generally, calcium ions can function as messengers in the stimulation-contraction coupling either by entering the cytoplasma across the cell membrane or by being released from stores located within the cell.

The development of large endoplasmic calcium pools is most obvious in skeletal muscle, whereas myocardial fibers and, particularly, smooth muscle cells are less specialized in this respect. Because of these peculiarities excitation-contraction coupling of skeletal muscle is practically insensitive to changes in the extracellular calcium concentration or transmembrane calcium conductivity because the intracellular calcium stores provide sufficient quantities of calcium to induce activation of the contractile system. This is probably the reason why the excitation-contraction coupling of skeletal muscle is also rather resistant to pharmacological interventions.

In contrast, myocardial and smooth muscle contractility is much more susceptible to variations in environmental calcium or to pharmacological agents that affect transmembrane calcium supply, because the intracellular stores have a rather limited capacity and have to be rapidly refilled from extracellular sources during mechanical activity. Thus the degree of contractile activation of these cells is clearly linked to the availability of calcium from extracellular sources or can even appear to be a direct function of the quantity of calcium that enters the cell during stimulation.

Therefore a great interest arose to define the sources of mobilized calcium and their relationship to different stimuli. This proved to be a difficult task for smooth muscle, whose variability does not allow a facile generalisation.

In smooth muscles several sources of calcium appear to be used in stimulation-contraction coupling: (1) free calcium in the extracellular fluid, (2) calcium bound to the surface membrane, and (3) intracellular calcium stored in the sarcoplasmic reticulum and in mitochondria. However, the use of a single source or single translocation route is probably exceptional, and within a given tissue different stimuli may employ different calcium sources. Furthermore, the source of calcium often appears to differ between the individual components (fast and slow) of the response to a single stimulus.

In principle, a combination of procedures can be used to describe calcium mobilization processes, in addition to the classic pharmacologic elucidation of receptor specifity. The four main approaches are: (1) removal of calcium from the extracellular fluid, (2) blockade of transmembrane calcium transport with selective antagonists, (3) measurement of calcium fluxes with radioactive labeled calcium, and (4) electrophysiological studies. Each procédure has its own limitations.

A growing body of evidence suggests that stimulation of smooth muscle by depolarization and by receptor activation use different sources of activator calcium (for review see Bolton 1979). It has long been known that many agonists can initiate contraction independent of the membrane potential. This was first demonstrated by Evans and co-workers (1958), who showed that smooth muscles which were completely depolarized by high extracellular potassium, could be made to contract even further after application of some agonists. This contractile response could be due either to agonist-receptor interaction which would cause a direct opening of the channels with a significant calcium permeability and would therefore allow an increased calcium entry, or to the release of calcium from internal stores. More recently it has become apparent that several tissues *normally* respond to a number of agonists by contraction without any membrane depolarization. This type of activity has been called 'pharmacomechanical coupling' in contrast to 'electromechanical coupling' (Somlyo and Somlyo 1968). Electromechanical coupling means that a given stimulus leads to membrane depolarization by increasing membrane permeability and thus allowing ion flow down electrochemical gradients. In some tis-

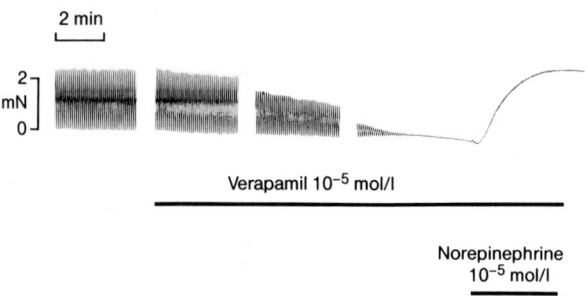

Fig. 10. Effects of the calcium antagonist verapamil on voltage- and on agonist-induced activation. Original tracing from an isolated human minor calyx segments. The drug in a concentration of 10^{-5} mol/l completely antagonized the spontaneous, bioelectrically-induced phasic activity of the muscle strip, whereas the norepinephrine-induced tonic activation was not affected by the drug

sues, stimulation by agonists also increases the rate and size of spike-potentials and induces substantial depolarization of the cell membrane (Bolton 1979).

Further support for the idea of different activation mechanisms in smooth muscle was found by using selective antagonists of transmembrane calcium transport (Golenhofen 1981). These pharmacological tools are a diverse group of drugs called calcium antagonists. The mechanism of action of these substances, typified by verapamil and nifedipine, has been postulated to be a selective blockade of the voltage-dependent influx of extracellular calcium through voltage-operated calcium channels (Triggle and Swamy 1980). These drugs, applied in pharmacological concentrations, seem to have no effects on intracellular mobilization or movements of calcium (Nayler and Poole-Wilson 1981).

For example, Fig. 10 shows the effects of the calcium antagonist verapamil on spontaneous phasic activity and on norepinephrine-induced tonic activation of an isolated human minor calyx. The drug in a concentration of 10^{-5} mol/l completely antagonized the spontaneous (voltage-induced) phasic activity of the muscle strip, whereas the norepinephrine-induced tonic activation was not affected by the drug. By obtaining the concentration-response relationships of norepinephrine on resting tension in calyceal human preparations, we could demonstrate (Hertle and Nawrath 1982) that the maximum response to norepinephrine was reduced only about 35 per cent in the presence of verapamil (10^{-5} mol/l). In contrast, verapamil in the same concentration of 10^{-5} mol/l completely antagonized high potassium-induced activations (Hertle and Nawrath 1982).

Golenhofen and Hannappel (1978) were the first to demonstrate a tonic, nifedipine-resistant response to adrenergic activation in porcine renal pelvis. In their studies, the same agonist in the same concentration range produced nifedipine-sensitive, phasic contractions in ureteral preparations. The authors suggested that the tonic response of renal pelvis musculature may have special functional significance in larger multipapillary kidneys, perhaps due to a reservoir function. Based on selective suppression of phasic activity by calcium antagonists, Golenhofen (1981) presented the concept that in smooth muscle two different calcium activation systems exist which he called the P-system (mainly responsible for phasic activity) and the T-system (mainly responsible for tonic activity). He suggested that the P-system is firmly associated with electrical events of the cell membrane, while the T-system is less under electrical and more under chemical control.

In smooth muscle of the human upper urinary tract phasic contractions induced by pacemaker-activity or by agonists as well as contractures induced by high extracellular potassium are potently inhibited by calcium antagonists, whereas tonic contractions induced by agonists, especially norepinephrine, are partially refractory to these drugs (Hertle and Nawrath 1982). These observations have been explained by the hypothesis that tonic contractions induced by norepinephrine are mediated by releasing an 'intracellular pool' of calcium (Hudgins and Weiss 1968). According to this theory tonic contraction induced by norepinephrine, is not inhibited by calcium antagonists, because no transmembrane calcium influx is required. Therefore we postulate the existence of different pathways of calcium to activate the contractile proteins in the human upper urinary tract (Fig. 11), including voltage-controlled calcium channels, receptor-operated calcium channels and release of a receptor-associated fraction of membrane-bound or intracellular stored calcium. It seems that populations of voltage-controlled calcium channels mediate pacemaker-induced phasic contractions as well as contractures induced by high extracellular potassium. Therefore the potent effects of calcium antagonists on this type of mechanical activity may be due to the blocking of voltage-controlled calcium channels. Receptor-operated calcium channels may be responsible for phasic activity induced by agonists, especially norepinephrine. This type of mechanical activity is also sensitive to calcium antagonists. The lack of effect on agonist-induced tonic contraction may be due to agonist-induced release of membrane-bound or intracellularly stored calcium which is not affected by calcium channel blockers.

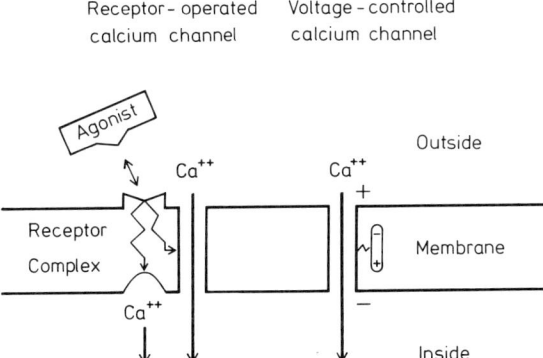

Fig. 11. Schematic representation of the postulated calcium movements in smooth muscle of the upper urinary tract. Calcium entry may occur through voltage-controlled or receptor-operated calcium channels. Voltage-controlled calcium channels seem to mediate pacemaker-induced phasic contractions as well as contractures induced by high extracellular potassium concentrations. Receptor-operated calcium channels may be responsible for phasic activity induced by agonists, especially norepinephrine. These types of mechanical activity are highly sensitive to calcium antagonists. The lack of effect of calcium channel blockers on agonist-induced tonic contraction may be due to agonist-mediated release of a membrane-bound or intracellularly stored fraction of calcium

Systematic investigation of these theories is hampered by the marked difficulties in measuring electrical events and calcium movements in the human upper urinary tract, especially if the calcium involved has an 'activator' role. It should be re-emphasized that the previous discussion of different activation mechanisms is a synthesis of evidence obtained from other smooth muscle tissues and must be considered only as a working hypothesis in understanding the stimulation-contraction interactions in the upper urinary tract.

Conclusion

Under normal conditions an increase in the permeability of the cell membrane to calcium appears to be the primary determinant of tension in the contractile proteins of a smooth muscle cell. Calcium can probably enter the cell via two types of ion channels in the membrane. A population of channels seems to exist that allow calcium to enter after they have been opened by depolarization. Calcium also seems to enter the cell through ion channels associated with receptors for stimulant substances. These receptor-operated channels appear to be a separate and distinct population. Furthermore, there is evidence that calcium is associated with several types of receptors in a bound form (e.g. α-adrenoceptors) and that it can be dislodged by activation of these receptors.

A different pattern of response to agonists, especially to norepinephrine in different tissues of the upper urinary tract, suggests different and separate coupling mechanisms between the receptors involved and the calcium pools responsible for initiation of contraction. We postulate that in the normal ureter activation by depolarization and by agonists, such as acetylcholine or norepinephrine, is predominantly mediated by transmembrane calcium influx via voltage-controlled or receptor-operated calcium channels. Both types of activation are highly sensitive to calcium antagonists. In the normal ureter we did not observe a marked tonic response to these agonists, possibly indicating that in the normal ureter membrane-bound or intracellularly stored calcium is only minimally involved in mediating the response to these stimuli. In tissues of the renal calyx and pelvis, however, we observed a marked tonic response to stimulation with norepinephrine. The insensitivity of this agonist-induced tonic response to calcium antagonists suggests that this type of activity is mediated by a membrane-bound or intracellularly stored fraction of calcium. It can be concluded that the individual smooth muscle cells of the ureter and the renal calyx and pelvis probably differ fundamentally in their ultrastructural organisation of the systems that lead to the activation of the contractile proteins, at least in those systems that mediate α-adrenoceptor stimulation. However, so little is known with certainty about the properties of the calcium activation mechanisms in the human upper urinary tract that at present no substantial proposal can be made, aside from the observation that it does not seem likely that different stimuli interact with calcium in the same ways.

In the upper urinary tract much remains to be learned about the cellular contraction cycle. Our opinion is that most of the problems of altered smooth muscle activity in the upper urinary tract, such as an obstruction of the ureteropelvic junction or idiopathic dilatations and malfunctionings of the ureter, cannot be solved by morphological and in vivo studies alone. Our present perspective and understanding of normal and pathological contractile activity of smooth muscle of the human upper urinary tract is limited by the lack of systematic studies on stimulation-contraction coupling in this tissue.

Acknowledgements. We thank Prof. Dr. R. Hohenfellner, Chairman, Department of Urology, University of Mainz (FRG) for generously supplying human tissues and Prof. Dr. K. Golenhofen, Department of Physiology, University of Marburg (FRG), for helpful discussions and suggestions.

References

Bolton TB (1979) Mechanisms of action of transmitters and other substances on smooth muscle. Physiol Rev 59:606–718
Casteels R, Droogmans G (1982) Membrane potential and excitation-contraction coupling in smooth muscle. Fed Proc 41:2879–2882
Del Tacca M, Lecchini S, Stacchini B, Tonini M, Frig GM, Mazzanti L, Crema A (1974) Pharmacological studies of the rabbit and human renal pelvis. Naunyn-Schmiedeberg's Arch Pharmacol 285:209–272
Evans DHL, Schild HO, Thesleff S (1958) Effects of drugs on depolarized plain muscle. J Physiol 143:474–485
Golenhofen K (1981) Differentiation of calcium activation processes in smooth muscle using selective antagonists. In: Bülbring E, Brading AF, Jones AW, Tomita T (eds) Smooth muscle: an assessment of current knowledge. Arnold, London, pp 157–170
Golenhofen K, Hannappel J (1978) A tonic component in the motility of upper urinary tract (renal pelvis–ureter). Experientia 34:64–65
Golenhofen K, Hermstein N, Lammel E (1973) Membrane potential and contraction of vascular smooth muscle (portal vein) during application of noradrenaline and high potassium, and selective inhibitory effects of iproveratril (verapamil). Microvasc Res 5:73–80
Hertle L (1982) Pharmacological study on the motility of isolated preparations of the human upper urinary tract. Naunyn-Schmiedeberg's Arch Pharmacol [Suppl 319] R 33
Hertle L, Nawrath H (1982) Effects of calcium antagonists on motility of the human upper urinary tract in vitro. Proceedings, 4th Meeting, International Society for Dynamics of the Upper Urinary Tract, Utrecht
Hudgins PM, Weiss GB (1968) Differential effects of calcium removal on vascular smooth muscle contraction induced by norepinephrine, histamine, and potassium. J Pharmacol Exp Ther 159:91–97
Katz AM, Messineo FC, Herbette L (1982) Ion channels in membranes. Circulation [Suppl I] 65:I-2–I-10
Kinn A, Nergardh A (1979) Autonomic receptor functions in the normal and dilated renal pelvis: an in vitro study in man and rabbit. Urol Res 7:261–264
Kuffler SW (1946) The relation of electrical potential changes to contracture in skeletal muscle. J Neurophysiol 9:367–377
Longrigg N (1975a) In vitro studies on the human renal calices. J Urol 114:325–331
Longrigg N (1975b) In vitro studies on smooth muscle of the human renal pelvis. Eur J Pharmacol 34:293–298
Malin JM, Boyarsky S, Labay P, Gerber C (1968) In vitro isometric studies of ureteral smooth muscle. J Urol 99:396–398
Malin JM, Deane RF, Boyarsky S (1970) Characterisation of adrenergic receptors in human ureter. Br J Urol 42:171–174

Nayler WG, Poole-Wilson PH (1981) Calcium antagonists: definition and mode of action. Basic Res Cardiol 76:1–15
Somlyo AV, Somlyo AP (1968) Electromechanical and pharmacomechanical coupling in vascular smooth muscle. J Pharmacol Exp Ther 159:129–145
Triggle DJ, Swamy VC (1980) Pharmacology and agents that affect calcium. Chest [Suppl] 78:174–179
Tsien RW (1983) Calcium channels in excitable cell membranes. Ann Rev Physiol 45:341–358
Weiss RM (1978) Ureteral function. Urology 12:114–133
Yano S, Ueda S, Ikegami K (1981) Effects of some autonomic drugs on the isolated human minor calyx. Urol Int 36:208–215

Effects of β-Adrenergic Agonists on the Action Potentials of Canine Pyeloureter

T. MORITA[1]

Introduction

Pacemaker control of ureteral peristalsis was first suggested by Bozler (1942), who described action potentials with a slow rising phase recorded from the renal end of isolated canine, feline and guinea pig ureters as possibly representing pacemaker potentials. Later, Kobayashi (1965) and Zawalinski et al. (1975) obtained tracings of spontaneous action potentials with constant discharge intervals from isolated feline and guinea pig renal pelvises and advocated the presence of a pacemaker of ureteral peristalsis in the renal pelvis. Cyclic changes in intrapelvic pressure unrelated to urine volume were recorded from dogs in vivo by Constantinou (1974) who thus inferred them to be reflecting activity of a renal pelvic pacemaker.

However, such attempts involve several difficult problems. The isolated tissue preparation is devoid of urine flow which has a profound influence on ureteral peristalsis. Furthermore, recording of intrapelvic pressure in vivo cannot provide information about the mode of propagation of intrapelvic pressure by peristaltic contraction generated by the pacemaker, since the pelvis is extensively covered with the renal parenchyme. Thus, by this method we cannot determine whether the pacemaker is localized in the upper part of the renal pelvis or in the pelviureteral junction (PUJ).

With a view to solution of these problems, Tsuchida et al. (1981) have devised an in vivo-like in vitro experimental model consisting of a canine pelviureteral preparation isolated intact with the pelvis then exposed by resection of the overlying renal parenchyme and kept under conditions corresponding to urinary secretion, i.e. continuous intrapelvic infusion with oxygenated Krebs-Ringer solution at a flow rate equivalent to urinary secretion. It has been demonstrated by observations in this experimental model that the ureteral peristaltic pacemaker exists in the pelvicalyceal border (PC-border), since so-called slow rising potentials were recorded in this region even in the absence of intrapelvic infusion, that is, of urine output, and gradual increase of infusion led to an elevation of the rate of the potential's propagation to the pelvis and ureter. Anatomically, Gosling and Dixon (1974) reported the occurrence of pacemaker cells containing an abundance of cytoplasmic glycogen granules, in the regions of the upper part of the renal pelvis of the dog and the cat.

Those of the β-adrenergic agents, which are classified as β_1-adrenergic agents, increase the heart rate and cardiac contractility whereas β_2-adrenergic agents produce

---

[1] Department of Urology, Akita University School of Medicine, 1-1-1 Hondo, Akita, 010 Japan

relaxation of smooth muscles, e.g. bronchial dilatation. The objective of this study is to explore responses of the renal calyx, the pacemaker of ureteral peristalsis, to β_1- and β_2-adrenergic stimulants in isolated pelvicalyceal preparations.

Materials and Method

Ten mongrel dogs weighing about 10 kg each were used in this study. The animal was laparotomized under anesthesia with intravenous thiamylal sodium, 10 mg/kg, and the kidney was removed by transecting the adjoining ureter about 10 cm distal to the PUJ. The renal parenchyme overlying the renal pelvis was resected in a bath of oxygenated Krebs-Ringer solution with the aid of a stereomicroscope to expose the pelvis up to the PC-border. A 5 Fr. double-lumen polyethylene catheter was then inserted into the renal pelvis through the overlying renal parenchyme using the nephrostomy technique. One end of the catheter was connected to a Harvard infusion pump for continuous intrapelvic infusion of Krebs-Ringer solution at a rate corresponding to physiological urine output, and the other end was attached to a Statham P-50 pressure transducer to permit a recording of the intrapelvic pressure. While the organ preparation was kept in the bath of oxygenated Krebs-Ringer solution at 37 °C, electromyograms (EMG) were recorded from the PC-border, the PUJ and the ureter via suction glass microelectrodes with a diameter of 200 μ (time constant: 0.01 s).

Dobutamine (10^{-5} to 10^{-3} g/ml) and terbutaline (10^{-5} to 10^{-3} g/ml) were used as β_1- and β_2-adrenergic stimulants, respectively. As adrenoceptor blocking agents, metoprolol was used to block dobutamine in equal doses and propranolol to block terbutaline in equal doses. The drugs were administered by adding them to both the intrapelvic perfusate and the bath of Krebs-Ringer solution. Figure 1 is a schematic representation of the experimental procedure.

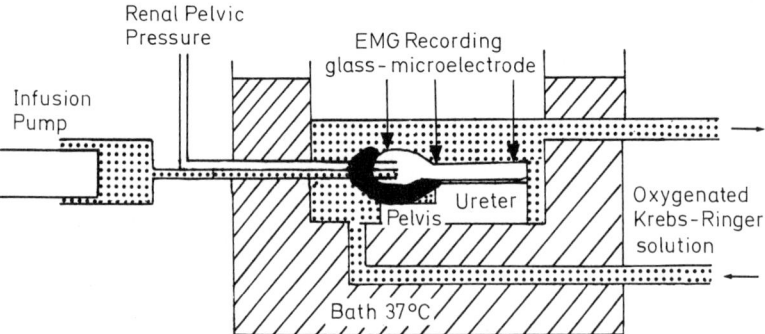

Fig. 1. Schematic illustration of the experimental procedure. EMGs were recorded via electrodes placed on the pelvicalyceal border (pacemaker), pelviureteral junction and ureter, with simultaneous recording of the intrapelvic pressure by continuous infusion of Krebs-Ringer solution into the renal pelvis

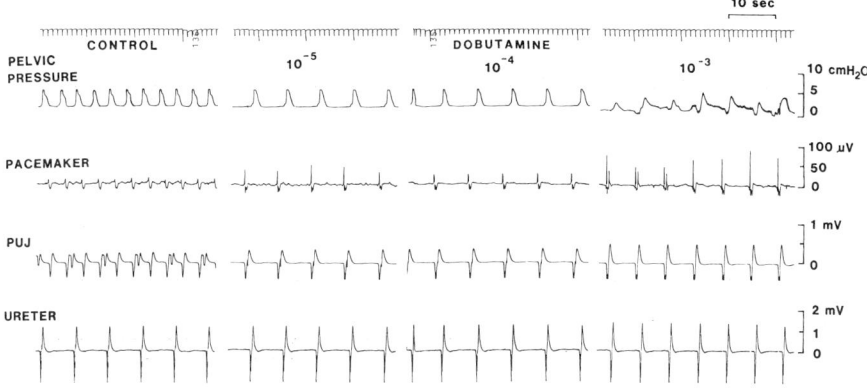

Fig. 2. Representative tracings after administration of dobutamine (organ preparation No. 1). Intrapelvic pressure became slighly inconstant but the contraction pressure remained virtually unaltered at a dose of 10^{-3} g/ml. Pacemaker potential increased markedly and discharge intervals were slightly prolonged with increasing dosage of dobutamine from 10^{-5} to 10^{-4} and to 10^{-3} g/ml. The pelviureteral junction (*PUJ*) and ureter showed no significant change in action-potential

Results

Eight of 20 organ preparations obtained from ten animals, Nos. 1, 3, 4, 6, 8, 11, 12, 13 were subjected to experiments with dobutamine and seven preparations (Nos. 5, 9, 10, 15, 17, 19, 20) were used in experiments with terbutaline. The intrapelvic infusion was carried out at a rate of 0.30–1.00 ml/min, equivalent to the normal urine output of dogs.

Representative tracings of the responses to the administration of dobutamine in organ preparation No. 1 are shown in Fig. 2. The infusion rate was 0.60 ml/min. Minute discharge potentials of about 15 µV with constant discharge intervals of 3.80 ± 0.25 s (n=50) were recorded from the PC-border prior to the administration of dobutamine, and potentials of 500 µV discharged with a matching (1:1) frequency of 3.80 ± 0.32 s (n=50) from the PUJ. In the ureter, slightly increased activities of 1.2 mV with frequencies of 3.80 ± 0.30 s (n=8) and 7.68 ± 0.12 s (n=21), hence at ratios of 1:1 and 1:2 to those at the PC-border, were demonstrated. Intrapelvic pressure waves showed cycles of 3.78 ± 0.10 s (n=50) and were synchronous with those of activities in the PC-border. The contraction pressure of the renal pelvis measured 5 cm H_2O. In response to the administration of dobutamine, the pacemaker potential in the PC-border increased in amplitude two- to threefold (30–50 µV) at a dose of 10^{-4} g/ml and four- to sevenfold (70–100 µV) at 10^{-3} g/ml, compared to the pre-dosing level. The increase of amplitude was accompanied by changes in the wave pattern; the wave pattern became analogous to that of the ureteral potential, which showed an initial small negative deflection, after the drug's administration in a dose of 10^{-3} g/ml. The frequency of discharge became somewhat unstable with prolongation of discharge intervals to 6.8 ± 0.86 s (n=30) at a dosage of 10^{-4} g/ml

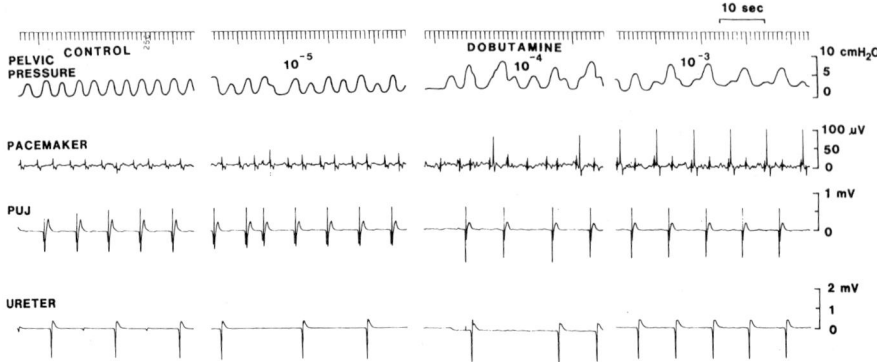

Fig. 3. Representative tracings after administration of dobutamine (organ preparation No. 6). The intrapelvic pressure became slightly inconstant and the contraction pressure elevated slightly. Pacemaker potential increased markedly every second potential, although its discharge interval remained unaltered at a dose of 10^{-3} g/ml. The pelviureteral junction (*PUJ*) and ureter showed no change in action potential and discharge interval

and to 6.0 ± 0.71 s (n = 30) at a dosage of 10^{-3} g/ml. In contrast, the discharges from the ureter and PUJ had interval ratios of 1:1 when compared to those from the PC-border even after administration of dobutamine, which means that it remained controlled by the pacemaker potential. The discharge potential from the PUJ increased slightly but only till it reached the 1.8 fold of its initial potential, even at a dose of 10^{-3} g/ml. No appreciable change occurred in the ureteral discharge potential after the administration of dobutamine. The pelvic contraction pressure did not change at all at a dose between 10^{-5} and 10^{-4} g/ml and became somewhat inconstant, though not conspicuously varying (3–5 cm H_2O), at a dose of 10^{-3} g/ml. The organ preparation exhibited little or no such response to dobutamine when it had been pretreated with an equal dose of metoprolol (Nos. 3, 4). Preparations Nos. 8 and 11 showed exactly the same tendency in response as seen with preparation No. 1, though their pacemaker discharge interval was slightly varying. Other tracings of responses to dobutamine in preparation No. 6 are shown in Fig. 3. The intrapelvic infusion was carried out at a slight oliguric rate of 0.30 ml/min. Before the administration of dobutamine, minute potentials of about 20 µV with constant intervals of 3.82 ± 0.06 s (n = 60) were recorded at the PC-border. At the PUJ, potentials of about 500 µV discharged with an interval of 7.52 ± 0.10 s (n = 24), which is half the frequency of the PC-border. In the ureter, the frequencies of potentials were 15.24 ± 0.12 s (n = 4) (1:4) and 20.24 ± 0.20 s (n = 5) (1:5). Intrapelvic pressure waves were completely synchronous with potentials in the PC-border. The contraction pressure measured 5 cm H_2O. In response to dobutamine (10^{-5}–10^{-3}), every second potential in the PC-border increased in amplitude four- to sixfold, compared to the pre-administration potentials. However, the frequency of discharges changed little in the PC-border by administration of dobutamine. Pelvic pressure waves became unstable and every second wave was much higher than before the drug's administration. No appreciable change was observed in the discharges from the PUJ and the ureter after the administration of dobutamine. The same responses as seen with preparation No. 6 were observed with preparations Nos. 12 and 13.

As seen from the tracings obtained from organ preparation No. 5 shown in Fig. 4, the pacemaker potential in the PC-border had discharge intervals of 2.60 ± 0.18 s (n=48) with an initial amplitude of 20 µV and remained practically unchanged after the administration of terbutaline: 2.28 ± 0.12 s (n=40) with an amplitude of 20 µV at 10^{-5} g/ml and 2.62 ± 0.20 s (n=45) with 30 µV at 10^{-4} g/ml. The interval of the pacemaker discharge still did not vary at all, even after administration of the drug in a dose of 10^{-3} g/ml (2.64 ± 0.16 s, n=40) while the wave pattern changed into an abysmal ravine-like negative deflection, which means that the pretreatment (initial) pacemaker potential wave pattern minus its positive component of deflection. Tracings obtained at the PUJ demonstrated discharges corresponding at 1:1 to the pacemaker potential, with an amplitude of 700 µV, before administration of terbutaline. The discharge interval became prolonged to 2:1 and to 4:1 with increasing dosage of terbutaline and eventually discharge disappeared completely at a dose of 10^{-3} g/ml. Marked discharges of 1.5 mV occurred from the ureter at a ratio of 1:1 compared with the pacemaker potential before drug administration, and the discharge interval was prolonged with increasing dosage of terbutaline and, eventually, the discharges disappeared. Furthermore, the intrapelvic pressure, which was initially 5–8 cm H$_2$O in amplitude, corresponded at 1:1 to the pacemaker potential, but both the contraction pressure and baseline pressure decreased after the administration of terbutaline and disappeared at a dosage of 10^{-3} g/ml. These responses to terbutaline were completely blocked by 10^{-4} g/ml of propranolol. Exactly the same tendency of reactions was observed with organ preparation Nos. 9, 10, 15, 17, 19, 20.

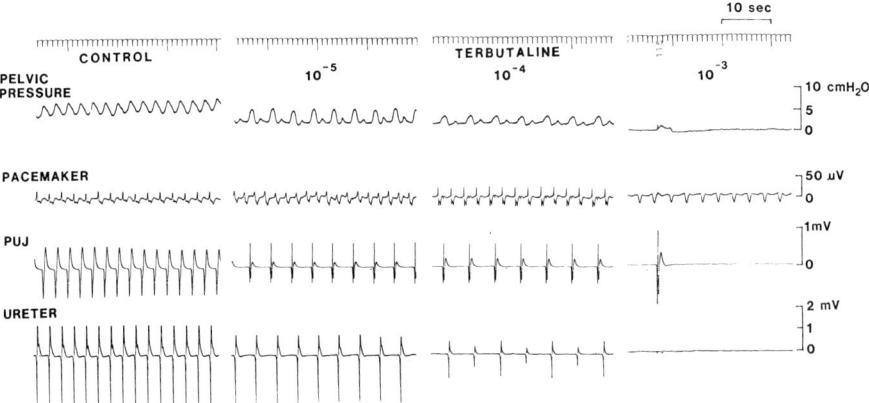

Fig. 4. Representative tracings after administration of terbutaline (organ preparation No. 5). The intrapelvic pressure diminished remarkably with eventual flattening of waves, thus no longer reflecting pacemaker activity. Pacemaker potential showed little or no change in discharge interval after administration of terbutaline, though the wave pattern became altered slightly at 10^{-3} g/ml. Discharges from pelviureteral junction (*PUJ*) and ureter diminished progressively with increasing dosage and eventually disappeared

Discussion

The present data have demonstrated that the β_1-adrenergic stimulant caused a distinct increase in action potential of the pacemaker cells which have been described as existing anatomically in the PC-border of the canine kidney. The drug, however, produced little or no change in discharge potentials from the lower part of the renal pelvis and ureter. These findings seemed to suggest the presence of the cells which respond to β_1-adrenergic stimulation in the canine PC-border with an enhancement of potential, and are therefore somewhat different from the cells of pelviureteral smooth muscles. Moreover, we assumed that it would be impracticable to detect this response by pressure recording or by in vitro observations of muscular tension, in which the intrapelvic pressure remained little changed. Even when the β_2-adrenergic stimulant with a relaxant action on smooth muscles produced flattening of the intrapelvic pressure and vanishment of pelviureteral action potentials, the pacemaker at the PC-border continued to discharge potentials at regular intervals with a rather constant amplitude, though with a slight change in its wave pattern. This fact would indicate that the pacemaker cells are not inhibited by β_2-adrenergic stimulants. The pacemaker potential was no longer reflected in the intrapelvic pressure following administration of the β_2-adrenergic stimulant. Therefore, it seemed to be difficult to detect the pacemaker activity by any other method than the electromyographic technique. It remains uncertain why the alteration in wave pattern of pacemaker activity occurred in response to administration of the β_2-adrenergic stimulant although it seems likely that the smooth muscle which undoubtedly exists in the structure of the calyces might relax to some extent, thereby leading to a modification of the muscular contact with the electrode.

From these results it is suggested that the structure of the pacemaker at the PC-border is somewhat distinct from the pelviureteral smooth muscles, with an electrophysiologic activity resembling that of the heart, in which it exhibits augmented action potential after β_1-adrenergic stimulation and no appreciable inhibition by β_2-adrenergic stimulation. However, unlike the heart, the frequency of the pacemaker discharge was never accelerated by β_1-adrenergic stimulation. In contrast, the frequency became somewhat slower in some preparations. These findings also suggested that the renal pacemaker might be somewhat different from the cardiac pacemaker, whose pace would be accelerated by β_1-agonists.

References

Bozler EA (1942) The activity of the pacemaker previous to the discharge of a muscular impulse. Am J Physiol 136:543–552

Constantinou CE (1974) Renal pelvic pacemaker control of ureteral peristaltic rate. Am J Physiol 226:1413–1419

Gosling JA, Dixon JS (1974) Species variation in the location of upper urinary tract pacemaker cells. Invest Urol 11:418–423

Kobayashi M (1965) Conduction velocity in various regions of the ureter. Tohoku J Exp Med 83:220–224

Tsuchida S et al. (1981) Initiation and propagation of canine renal pelvic peristalsis. Urol Int 36:307–314

Zawalinski VC et al. (1975) Ureteral pacemaker potentials recorded with the sucrose gap technique. Experientia 31:931–933

Effects of Some Directly-Acting Smooth Muscle Relaxant Drugs on Isolated Human Preparations of the Upper Urinary Tract

L. HERTLE[1] and H. NAWRATH[2]

It is generally assumed that drugs which induce relaxation of smooth muscles may be of clinical importance in some urological disorders; such drugs are indeed widely used, for example in the therapy of unstable bladders or to facilitate the passage of ureteral stones. Antispasmodic action may be classified in neurotropic and musculotropic action; the former acting on the autonomic nervous system and the latter directly on smooth muscle cells. Examples for the first type of action are anticholinergic drugs or alpha-adrenoceptor-antagonists, whereas papaverine is a classic drug with the second type of action.

Mechanical activity of smooth muscles is ultimately dependent on the amount of free calcium ions available. Calcium concentration is regulated by transmembrane influx and efflux as well as by release from and sequestration into intracellular stores. Relaxant drugs acting directly on the smooth muscle probably lead to a decrease in activator calcium by different mechanisms; however, the precise mode of action is unknown.

One possible mechanism of smooth muscle relaxation is related to cyclic adenosine 3',5'-monophosphate (cyclic AMP). Pöch et al. (1969) first reported an inhibition of cyclic AMP-breakdown in vitro by a number of spasmolytic drugs. An increase in cyclic AMP is supposed to lead to an enhanced calcium binding to membrane and intracellular storage sites, thereby reducing influx and/or release of calcium. This decrease in calcium in the region of the contractile proteins leads to relaxation of the smooth muscle. A rise in cyclic AMP may be induced by an inhibition of phosphodiesterase, which degrades cyclic AMP to 5'-adenosine monophosphate (5'AMP). Such a mechanism of phosphodiesterase inhibition was proposed for papaverine (Kukovetz and Pöch 1970) and similarly acting drugs like flavoxate (Conti and Setnikar 1975).

An alternative mechanism of smooth muscle relaxation was proposed by Grün et al. (1969) and Fleckenstein et al. (1971) for verapamil and some other drugs with relaxing properties. Inhibition of transmembrane calcium influx, first observed with verapamil and D600 in the heart (Fleckenstein et al. 1968, 1971), was suggested to be the mechanism of action of these drugs. This mechanism of action was described as 'calcium antagonism'. In the past decade nearly a dozen drugs have been described as calcium antagonists. There is probably no other class of drugs that comprises so many chemically diverse structures or has more confusing structure–activity relationships.

---

1 Abteilung Urologie, Universität Bochum, Marienhospital, Widumer Str. 8, D-4690 Herne 1
2 Abteilung Pharmakologie, Universität Mainz, Obere Zahlbacher Str. 67, D-6500 Mainz

The complexity of the regulatory mechanisms controlling the cytoplasmic calcium concentration limits the experimental models which can be designed to assess the site of action, or even the potency of drugs with relaxing properties. Stimulation of smooth muscles by depolarization with high extracellular potassium concentrations and stimulation by receptor activation with norepinephrine represent the two most important means of activation. Depolarization of the cell membrane by high extracellular potassium concentrations is thought to activate voltage-dependent channels through which external calcium enters the cell. In contrast, contractions produced by α-stimulation seem to utilize a receptor-associated fraction of intracellularly bound calcium especially in the case of tonic contractions (Bolton 1979; Golenhofen 1981). These two types of activation are closely related to the concept of electromechanical and pharmacomechanical coupling in smooth muscles (Somlyo and Somlyo 1968).

This article describes the effects of some 'phosphodiesterase inhibitors' and some 'calcium antagonists' on isolated muscle strips of the human upper urinary tract. Two of the compounds used in this study (bencyclane and pitofenone) may be less well known. The pharmacological properties of bencyclane have been described by Komlos and Petöcz (1970) and by Kukovetz et al. (1975) and those of pitofenone by Lindner (1955) and Hertle and Nawrath (1984).

Methods

Human tissues were obtained after tumor nephrectomies and were unaffected by the disease. The collecting systems showed no signs of infection or obstruction. Calyceal and ureteral segments were carefully removed from the specimen, dissected free of connective tissue and then attached to a tissue pillar. The preparations were immediately suspended in 10 ml organ baths containing Tyrode solution (composition in mmol/l: NaCl 136.9, KCl 5.4, $MgCl_2$ 1.05, NaH_2PO_4 0.42, $NaHCO_3$ 11.9, $CaCl_2$ 1.8, glucose 5.5) at 37 °C aerated with 95% O_2 and 5% CO_2. The pH of the solution was 7.2–7.4. The tension was measured under isometric conditions with inductive force displacement transducers and registered on Hellige paper recorders. The preload tension was adjusted to 10 mN. An interval of at least an hour was allowed for equilibration, after which the experiments were performed.

Activation by High Extracellular Potassium Concentrations

For this type of activation only ureteral segments were used. The Tyrode solution for activation contained 85 mmol/l KCl and 57.3 mmol/l NaCl, the other constituents remained unchanged. The effects of the drugs were studied as follows. First, an initial submaximal contraction was produced by exposing the muscle strips to the high potassium Tyrode solution. The change of the potassium concentration was followed by a marked increase in resting tension which remained stable for several hours after equilibration and varied less than approximately 5%. After wash-out of the high potassium Tyrode solution the muscle strip immediately returned to its

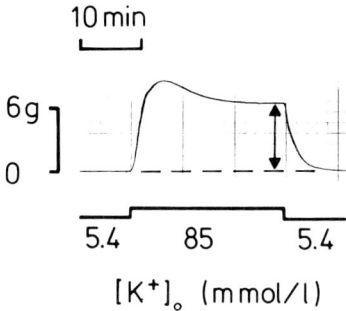

Fig. 1. Effect of 85 mmol/l potassium on tension of an isolated human ureteral muscle strip (original tracing). Depolarization of the muscle strip was followed by a rapid increase in tension, a partial relaxation and a sustained contraction. The equilibrated contracture (*double arrow*) was the reference activation to test the relaxing properties of the drugs. After wash-out of the high potassium Tyrode solution the muscle strip immediately returned to its original resting tension

original resting tension (Fig. 1). Then, a second contraction was produced with a Tyrode solution containing 85 mmol/l KCl. After the contraction had stabilized, a drug was added cumulatively allowing time for stabilisation of the relaxation between each application. The inhibition of the contraction induced by depolarisation was measured as a function of the drug's concentration. There were several reasons for using potassium-induced contractions as a reference to find concentration–response relationships: the responses were stable, reproducible and appeared to provide a good approximation of the amount of smooth muscle present in the ureteral wall. All data are expressed as percentages of the inhibition of equilibrium contraction after depolarization. Only one concentration-response curve was obtained from each muscle strip. The given concentrations were the final concentrations of the drugs in the organ bath in moles/liter. The calculations of the EC_{50} values, which are the concentrations of the drugs eliciting half of the maximum response, were carried out geometrically, based on the printout.

Activation by Norepinephrine

The effects of the drugs on norepinephrine-induced activation were studied in calyceal muscle strips. In this tissue, stimulation by norepinephrine produced a long-lasting 'tonic' contraction. Concentration-response curves for norepinephrine were made cumulatively. The peak tension above the base line was recorded for each concentration. The effects of the drugs on tension induced by norepinephrine were studied as follows. After producing the concentration–response relationship for norepinephrine and washing-out the agonist, a relaxant drug was added to the organ bath in a concentration which completely antagonized contractions induced by high extracellular potassium concentrations. After a pre-incubation period of 30 min the concentration-response curve for norepinephrine was repeated in the presence of the relaxing drug. The results are expressed as percentages of the maximum tension developed.

Drugs

The drugs used were: L-norepinephrine bitartrat (Serva, Heidelberg, FRG), nifedipine (Bayer AG, Wuppertal, FRG), verapamil (Knoll AG, Ludwigshafen, FRG), diltiazem (Gödecke, Berlin, FRG), papaverine hydrochloride (Serva, Heidelberg, FRG), bencyclane (Dr. Thiemann GmbH, Lünen, FRG), flavoxate (Asche, Hamburg, FRG) and pitofenone (Albert-Roussel, Wiesbaden, FRG).

Results

Effects on High Potassium-Induced Activation

Concentration–response relationships of the compounds were obtained by activating ureteral muscle strips with a submaximal concentration of 85 mmol/l potassium in the Tyrode solution. These contractions were not affected in the presence of either tetrodotoxin (2×10^{-5} mol/l) or phentolamine (10^{-5} mol/l). Figure 2 demonstrates an example of the concentration-dependent suppression of tension by the phosphodiesterase inhibitor flavoxate in a ureteral muscle strip previously activated by extracellular potassium in a concentration of 85 mmol/l. The reference activation in this experiment was about 4 g; a concentration of 10^{-7} mol/l was the threshold for relaxing activity, and the potassium-induced activation was completely antagonized at a concentration of 10^{-3} mol/l. The time between each application of the drugs to the organ baths and the stabilization of relaxation ranged between 20 and 30 min for all drugs and concentrations. Eight experiments were performed with each drug. Figure 3 shows the concentration–response relationship of flavoxate while acting on the tension of ureteral muscle strips activated by 85 mmol/l extracellular potassium concentration in the Tyrode solution. The EC_{50} value of the drug in this activation model was about 2×10^{-5} mol/l. A comparison with the concentration-response curve of the calcium antagonist nifedipine (Fig. 4) in the same activation model and the same tissue showed a qualitatively similar action but a marked difference in the concentration range in which the same effects were produced. A concentration of nifedipine of 10^{-6} mol/l completely antagonized the high potassium-induced activation, whereas only a concentration of flavoxate as high as 10^{-3} mol/l produced full relaxation.

Table 1 summarizes all the EC_{50} values (concentrations eliciting half of the maximum response) of the drugs in high potassium-induced activation, each calculated from the results of eight experiments. Further, the table includes the relative potencies of the drugs compared to papaverine. The classical smooth muscle relaxant drug papaverine was chosen as a reference compound and the EC_{50} value of papaverine was defined as one. The data show that the calcium antagonists nifedipine, verapamil and diltiazem were the most potent drugs in this activation model. The EC_{50} value of nifedipine for example was 2.8×10^{-9} mol/l and its relative potency compared with papaverine was about eight thousand times higher. The other compounds, bencyclane, pitofenone and flavoxate showed EC_{50} values similar to papaverine.

Effects on Norepinephrine-Induced Activation

In an original tracing Fig. 5 shows the different effects of the calcium antagonist nifedipine and the phosphodiesterase inhibitor papaverine on the tension of an

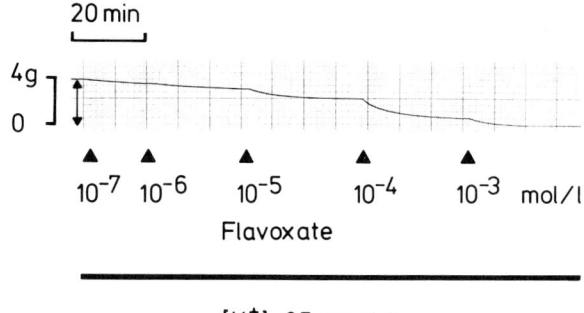

Fig. 2. Effect of flavoxate on tension of a human ureteral muscle strip previously activated by 85 mmol/l potassium. The control activation is marked by the *double arrow*. The drug antagonized the high potassium-induced activation concentration dependently (original tracing)

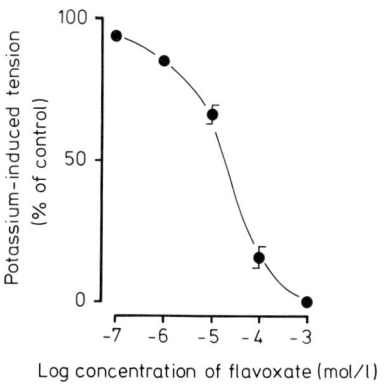

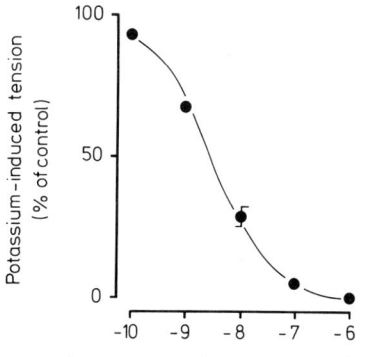

Fig. 3   Fig. 4

Fig. 3. Concentration–response relationship of flavoxate on tension of human ureteral muscle strips activated by high potassium depolarization. *Ordinate* tension induced by 85 mmol/l potassium containing Tyrode solution in percent of control (control was the equilibrated contracture after depolarization); *abscissa* logarithmic concentrations of the drug in mol/l. Means ± SEM (n = 8)

Fig. 4. Concentrations–response relationship of nifedipine. Same conditions as in Fig. 3

Table 1. EC_{50} values of the tested drugs (each calculated from 8 experiments) and the relative potencies with reference to papaverine. The EC_{50} value of papaverine was defined to be 1 to calculate the relative potencies of the drugs

Drug	EC_{50} (mol/l)	Relative potency
Nifedipine	2.8×10^{-9}	8214
Verapamil	6.3×10^{-8}	365
Diltiazem	1.7×10^{-7}	135
Papaverine	2.3×10^{-5}	1
Bencyclane	2.5×10^{-5}	0.9
Flavoxate	2.0×10^{-5}	0.5
Pitofenone	1.7×10^{-4}	0.1

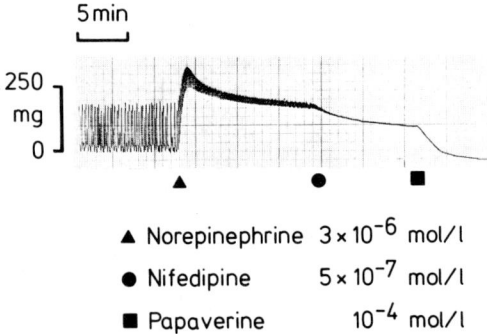

▲ Norepinephrine 3×10^{-6} mol/l
● Nifedipine 5×10^{-7} mol/l
■ Papaverine 10^{-4} mol/l

Fig. 5. Effects of nifedipine and papaverine on tension of a spontaneously contracting isolated human minor calyx additionally activated by norepinephrine. The agonist induced a long-lasting tonic contraction together with an increase in frequency and a reduction of the amplitude of phasic-rhythmic contractions. Nifedipine caused a complete inhibition of the spontaneous phasic-rhythmic activity but only a partial relaxation of the norepinephrine-induced tonic activation, whereas papaverine completely antagonized the residual agonist-induced tension

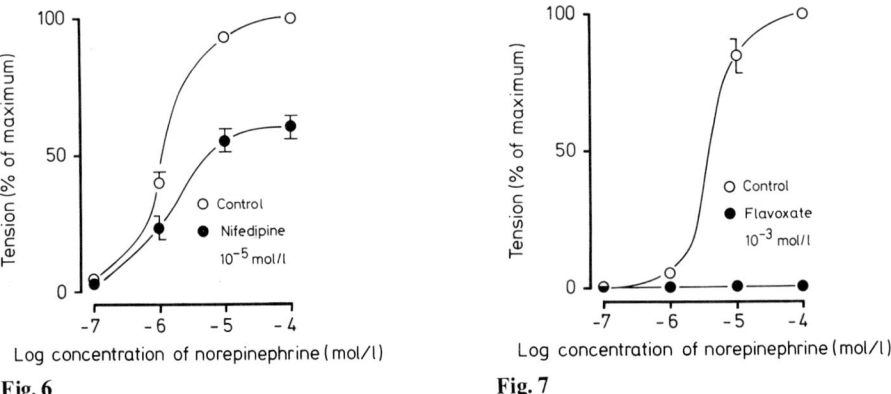

Fig. 6. Concentration–response relationships of norepinephrine acting on human calyceal preparations under control situation and after 30 min preincubation with nifedipine. Maximal induced tension was reduced only about 40% in the presence of nifedipine. Results expressed as a percentage of the maximum response Means ± SEM (n = 8)

Fig. 7. Concentration–response relationship of norepinephrine acting on human calyceal preparations under control situation and after 30 min preincubation with flavoxate. The drug completely suppressed the effects of the agonist. Means ± SEM (n = 8)

isolated human minor calyx activated with norepinephrine. The addition of the agonist in a concentration of 3×10^{-6} mol/l to the organ bath caused a long-lasting tonic contraction together with an increase in frequency and a reduction of the amplitude of the spontaneous phasic-rhythmic contractions. The application of nifedipine in a concentration of 5×10^{-7} mol/l caused a complete inhibition of the phasic-rhythmic activity, but only a partial relaxation of the norepinephrine-induced tonic activation. It should be re-emphasized that in this maximal concentration of 5×10^{-7} mol/l nifedipine completely antagonized the activation by high extracellular potassium concentrations. In contrast, papaverine in a concentration of 10^{-4} mol/l completely antagonized the residual norepinephrine-induced activation in this experiment. Papaverine in the same concentration (10^{-4} mol/l) suppressed both types of activation to the same extent. Similar results obtained with nifedipine and flavoxate are depicted in Figs. 6 and 7. Concentration-response curves of norepinephrine acting on calyceal muscle strips were repeated in the presence of nifedipine or flavoxate. Both drugs were present in concentrations which fully suppressed activations by high extracellular potassium concentrations. The figures show that in the presence of nifedipine the maximum response to norepinephrine was only reduced about 40 per cent, whereas flavoxate in an equi-effective concentration completely antagonized the activation induced by norepinephrine. Like nifedipine, the other calcium antagonists verapamil and diltiazem (both 10^{-5} mol/l) had only little effect on tonic contractions induced by high concentrations of norepinephrine, whereas papaverine (10^{-4} mol/l), bencyclane and pitofenone (both 10^{-3} mol/l) inhibited both types of activation to the same extent.

Discussion

The role of calcium in the mechanism of contraction of smooth muscle is well documented. Evidence has been obtained with skinned smooth muscle fibers, i.e., tissues from which the cell membrane has been chemically removed by a treatment with detergents (Endo et al. 1977; Gordon 1978; Saida and Nonomura 1978). These tissues respond to changes of the calcium concentration in the surrounding medium with a contraction or relaxation. Consequently it can be assumed that in intact smooth muscle tissue contraction and relaxation is also regulated by changes in the cytoplasmic calcium concentration. A contraction is caused by an increase of the sarcoplasmic calcium concentration which may occur by two main mechanisms: an influx of the ions from the extracellular space and a release of the ions from intracellular stores. The influx of extracellular calcium is possible via various types of calcium channels which are controlled by changes in the membrane potential or which are operated by receptors (Bolton 1979). Relaxation of smooth muscle results from a cessation of the transmembrane calcium influx coupled with the uptake and storage of calcium by the intracellular storage sites.

In this study we compared the effects of a number of relaxing drugs on isolated smooth muscle strips of the human upper urinary tract activated by either a depolarizing concentration of potassium in the Tyrode solution or by increasing concentrations of norepinephrine. It is now widely accepted that norepinephrine and a high concentration of potassium differ in the way in which they utilize calcium to elicit contractions in smooth muscles: responses to potassium decline rapidly in a calcium-free medium, whereas those to norepinephrine can persist for extended periods with little reduction (Hinke 1965; Hudgins and Weiss 1968). Similarly, the addition of Na_2EDTA to a calcium-free medium promptly eliminates all the responses to potassium, but those to norepinephrine decline only slowly (Waugh 1962; Hinke 1965; Hudgins and Weiss 1968). These observations suggest that potassium utilizes calcium from a more labile, accessible pool (bound extracellularly and/or loosely and superficially) than does norepinephrine, which may act mainly on an intracellularly bound calcium fraction at least in the tonic type of contraction (for review see Bolton 1979 and Golenhofen 1981).

The present results show marked differences in the effects of the tested compounds on both activation models. The calcium antagonists nifedipine, verapamil and diltiazem were very potent in blocking the activation of ureteral smooth muscles induced by high extracellular potassium concentrations. For example, the relaxing activity of nifedipine was about 8000 times greater than that of papaverine. These findings suggest that the mechanism of an inhibition induced by calcium antagonists in this activation model may be the selective blockade of transmembrane calcium influx through voltage-operated calcium channels, as has been suggested for many other tissues (for review see Bolton 1979). In contrast to this, these drugs in the same maximal concentrations had only little effect on the tonic response to alpha-adrenergic stimulation in calyceal muscle strips. These observations may be explained by the assumption that alpha-adrenergic stimulation in this tissue acts on an intracellularly stored fraction of calcium which is not affected by 'calcium channel blockers'. The partial relaxing effects of these drugs in norepinephrine-induced activation may be due to a blockade of receptor-operated calcium channels which may be partially involved in the response to the agonist.

Papaverine, bencyclane, flavoxate and pitofenone inhibited both types of activations to the same extents but only in very high concentrations. This fact excludes these drugs from the group of 'specific' calcium antagonists and suggests classification of the action of these drugs as non-selective. Relaxation caused by papaverine and flavoxate is associated with a rise in cAMP which is believed to be due to an inhibition of phosphodiesterase (Pöch and Kukovetz 1971; Conti and Setnikar 1975). However, it is not known how a rise in cAMP can relax smooth muscle activated by high extracellular potassium concentrations, for example, when it must be supposed that calcium is continuously entering the cell, unless we suppose that somehow calcium-extrusion or calcium entry blocking mechanisms are considerably accelerated. Calcium binding within the cell cannot continue indefinitely, therefore this can hardly be considered to reduce the intracellular calcium concentration effectively during prolonged high-potassium-induced contractions. Increased intracellular calcium binding without inhibition of its entry into or stimulation of its extrusion from the cell cannot be the cause of relaxation induced by papaverine and related drugs. It is very likely that the inhibitory action of these drugs on contractile activity may be related to other mechanisms of action, unrelated to the effects on phosphodiesterase activity.

Drug treatment of some urological disorders, especially of the unstable bladder, is often disappointing. There is a need for further basic research in this field, especially concerning the smooth muscles of the lower urinary tract; this might lead to the development of drugs which are useful in conditions such as urge-incontinence or prostatic and urethral syndroms.

Acknowledgement. We thank Prof. Dr. R. Hohenfellner, Chairman, Department of Urology, University of Mainz (FRG) for generously supplying us with human tissues.

References

Bolton TB (1979) Mechanism of action of transmitters and other substances on smooth muscle. Physiol Rev 59:606–718

Conti M, Setnikar J (1975) Flavoxate, a potent phosphodiesterase inhibitor. Arch Int Pharmacodyn 213:186–189

Endo M, Kitazawa T, Yaki S, Iino M, Kakuta Y (1977) Some properties of chemically skinned smooth muscle fibers. In: Casteels R, Godfraind T, Rüegg JC (eds) Excitation-contraction coupling in smooth muscle. North-Holland, Amsterdam, pp 199–209

Fleckenstein A, Döring HJ, Kammermeier H (1968) Einfluß von Beta-Rezeptorenblockern und verwandten Substanzen auf Erregung, Kontraktion und Energiestoffwechsel der Myokardfaser. Klin Wochenschr 46:343–351

Fleckenstein A, Grün G, Tritthart H, Byon K, Harding P (1971) Uterus-Relaxation durch hochaktive Ca^{++}-antagonistische Hemmstoffe der elektromechanischen Koppelung wie Isoptin (Verapamil, Iproveratril), Substanz D600 und Segontin (Prenylamin). Klin Wochenschr 49:32–41

Golenhofen K (1981) Differentiation of calcium activation processes in smooth muscle using selective antagonists. In: Bülbring E, Brading AF, Jones AW, Tomita T (eds) Smooth muscle: an assessment of current knowledge. Edward Arnold, London, pp 157–170

Gordon AR (1978) Contraction of detergent-treated smooth muscle. Proc Natl Acad Sci USA 75:3527–3530

Grün G, Fleckenstein A, Tritthart H (1969) Elektromechanische Entkoppelung durch „muskulotrope" Relaxantien der Uterusmuskulatur. Naunyn-Schmiedebergs Arch Pharmacol 264:239–240

Hertle L, Nawrath H (1984) Zur Wirkung von Baralgin^R auf isolierte Präparate des menschlichen oberen Harntraktes. Urol Int 39:84–90

Hinke JAM (1965) Calcium requirements for noradrenaline and high potassium ion contraction in arterial smooth muscle. In: Paul WM, Daniel EE, Kay CM, Monckton G (eds) Muscle. Pergamon Press, New York, pp 269–285

Hudgins PM, Weiss GB (1968) Differential effects of calcium removal upon vascular smooth muscle contraction induced by norepinephrine, histamine and potassium. J Pharmacol Exp Ther 159:91–97

Komlos E, Petöcz LE (1970) Pharmakologische Untersuchungen über die Wirkung von N-3-(1-Benzyl-cycloheptyl-oxy)-propyl-N,N-dimethyl-ammonium-hydrogenfumarat. Arzneimittel-Forsch (Drug Res) 20:1338–1357

Kukovetz WR, Pöch G (1970) Inhibition of cyclic-3'-5'-nucleotide-phosphodiesterase as a possible mode of action of papaverine and similarly acting drugs. Naunyn-Schmiedebergs Arch Pharmacol 267:189–194

Kukovetz WR, Pöch G, Holzmann S, Paietta E (1975) Zum Wirkungsmechanismus von Bencyclan an der glatten Muskulatur. Arzneimittel-Forsch (Drug Res) 25:722–726

Lindner E (1955) Der Einfluß von Derivaten der Diphenylmethanreihe auf acetylcholinvermittelte Wirkungen. Arch Exp Path Pharmak 224:357–367

Pöch G, Kukovetz WR (1971) Papaverine-induced inhibition of phosphodiesterase activity in various mammalian tissues. Life Sci 10:133–144

Pöch G, Juan H, Kukovetz WR (1969) Einfluß von herz- und gefäßwirksamen Substanzen auf die Aktivität der Phosphodiesterase. Naunyn-Schmiedebergs Arch Pharmacol 264:293–294

Saida K, Nonomura Y (1978) Characteristics of Ca^{2+} and Mg^{2+}-induced tension development in chemically skinned smooth muscle. J Gen Physiol 72:1–111

Somlyo AV, Somlyo AP (1968) Elektromechanical and pharmacomechanical coupling in vascular smooth muscle. J Pharmacol Exp Ther 159:129–145

Waugh WH (1962) Role of calcium in contractile excitation of vascular smooth muscle by epinephrine and potassium. Circ Res 11:927–940

Search for Anisotropy in Specific Electrical Conductance of Ureteral Tissue as a Measure of Muscle-Fiber Structure

W. A. van Duyl[1]

Abstract. Electrical conductance is measured in pieces of ureteral tissue in two mutually perpendicular directions by means of a four-electrode technique. No anisotropy in conductance is found. It is concluded that there is no predominant fiber orientation. Passive tissue is a capacitance which, combined with the conductance, yields a value of a time constant which is too short to be a limiting factor in the propagation of peristaltic wave.

Introduction

A prevailing idea is that the annular contraction ring of the ureter and the longitudinal propagation of that ring can be explained in terms of a helical structure of the smooth muscle fibers in the ureteral wall. This helical muscle-fiber model is supported by some anatomic studies (Satani 1919; Dullmann 1967). According to these studies the fibers are intermingled in a braided structure. The pitch of the helices may be 45° or more. Because of helical structure we expect that a contraction will yield components in the transverse and in the longitudinal directions. The ratio between the transverse and the longitudinal contraction components is determined by the pitch of the helix. This theoretical prediction has been used by van Duyl and Coolsaet (1982) to test the validity of the helical model of ureteral tissue. In strips of pig ureter contractions were induced by potassium and measured in the transverse and longitudinal directions. It appeared that the contractions were induced predominantly in the transverse direction. From the measurements it was concluded that, if there is a helical structure, the fibers are oriented predominantly in the transverse direction and not in the longitudinal direction as suggested by earlier investigators.

An alternative method for studying muscle fiber orientation is based on the determination of the electrical conductivity of tissue in different directions. In striated and heart muscle such measurements have revealed an anisotropy in electrical conductance which corresponds with the orientation of the muscle fibers. Cells and fibers have lower specific conductivity than their environment, so that tissue is an electrically heterogeneous medium. When the fibers are oriented predominantly in a certain direction the specific conductance will be highest in that direction and lowest in the transverse direction. This type of anisotropy has been demonstrated for striated muscle e.g. by Geddes and Baker (1967). For skeletal muscle the con-

---

1 Department of Biological and Medical Physics, Erasmus University Rotterdam, P.O. Box 1738, NL-3000 DR Rotterdam

ductivities (σ) reported by different investigators vary considerably. The anisotropy, expressed as the ratio of the conductivities in the transverse (σ_t) and in the longitudinal directions (σ_l), σ_t/σ_l is variable but lies in the range 0.07–0.43. If the helical model of ureteral tissue is valid, we expect to find an anisotropy in conductivity, such that the lowest conductivity is highest along the fiber direction.

Method

The determination of the specific conductivity is based on the measurement of the ratio between the electrical current flowing in the tissue and the associated voltage differential across the tissue. The current can be applied by means of two electrodes and the voltage can be measured between these electrodes. In order to avoid polarization of the electrodes and electrolysis in the tissue the measurements need to be performed with alternating currents. It has been shown in many studies that solutions of NaCl behave as a pure ohmic medium over a wide frequency range (10–100,000 Hz). A physiological solution with a concentration of 0.9% NaCl has a specific conductivity of 0.0139 S/cm (Weast et al. 1978).

Tissue, however, is not a purely ohmic medium. Impedance measurements have shown that tissue has a capacitive component which is manifest in the impedance mainly in the low frequency range. Usually this capacitive component is ascribed to cell membranes (e.g. Nagai and Prosser 1963). In order to take account of the frequency-dependent characteristics of ureteral smooth muscle tissue the complex conductance (or impedance) needs to be determined, which means that the absolute value of the conductance $|\sigma|$ (or of the impedance) together with the phase shift φ between current and voltage, has to be determined at different frequencies. When such measurements are performed via two electrodes in an electrolytic medium such as saline or tissue, e.g. by means of a vectorimpedance meter, the electrical properties of the interfaces between the electrodes and the medium give rise to particular difficulties.

These interfaces have an impedance which may contribute significantly to the relation between the current through and the voltage across the electrodes, especially in the low frequency range. For the determination of the complex conductivity of the tissue the impedance measured between the electrodes needs to be corrected for the contribution of the electrode-medium interfaces. However, an alternative procedure, based on the use of four instead of two electrodes, enables us to reduce this contribution to an almost insignificant level. The crucial point of the four-electrode technique is that the current needed to measure the voltage across two electrodes in the tissue can be very low, so that the voltage drop at the interfaces between these electrodes and the tissue becomes negligible. Figure 1 shows the basic scheme of the four-electrode technique as used in this study. An alternating current smaller than 2.4 µA with a frequency in the range 1000–5000 Hz, is applied to the electrodes numbered 1 and 4. This current is so small that it does not stimulate a smooth muscle preparation to contract. The ensuing voltage distribution in the tissue is measured with the electrodes numbered 2 and 3, which are connected to a

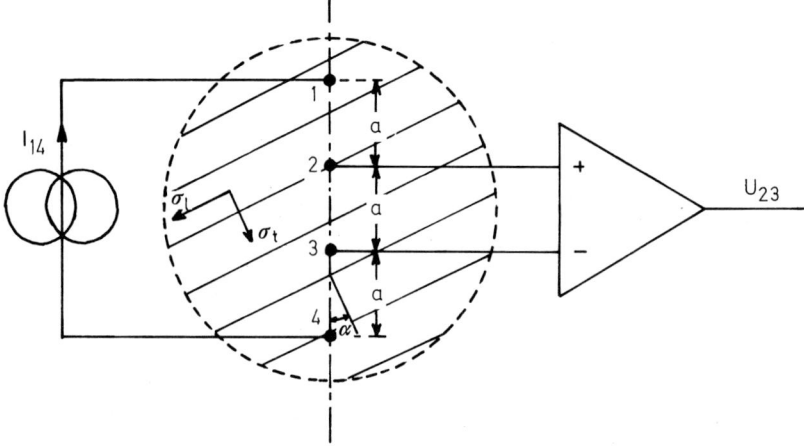

Fig. 1. Measurement of electrical conductance by means of the four-electrode technique in a round piece of muscle tissue (electrode configuration I); σ_l conductance in the direction to the fibers; σ_t conductance transverse to the fibers; I_{14} ac-current from a current source applied to Pt-electrodes 1 and 2; U_{23} differential voltage across the Pt-electrodes 2 and 3 measured via a high input impedance differential amplifier; a interelectrode distance

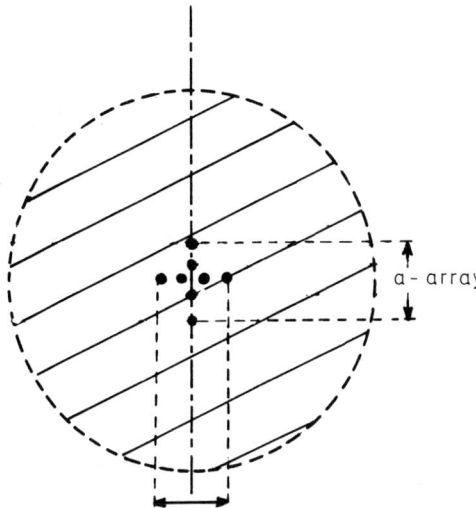

Fig. 2. Arrangement of Pt-electrodes in electrode configuration II; a-array to be placed in axial direction of the ureter, c-array to be placed in circumferential direction

precision lock-in amplifier (E.G. and G., Brookdeal) with an input impedance of 200 MΩ. With this phase-lock amplifier we measure the amplitude of voltage U_{23} and its phase relative to a reference signal. The reference signal is derived from, and in phase with the current applied to the electrodes 1 and 4. Pt electrodes with a diameter of 0.3 mm were used. We used two different electrode configurations. In configuration I, shown in Fig. 1, four electrodes are arranged in a straight-line array with an interelectrode distance $a = 2$ mm. In configuration II, shown in Fig. 2, two

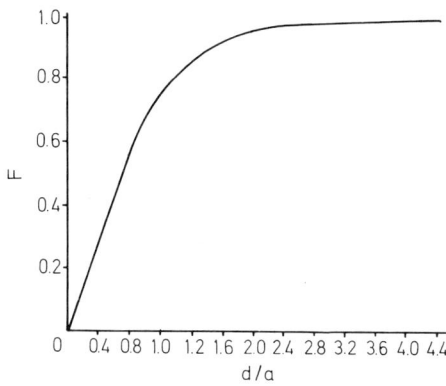

Fig. 3. Correction factor F, to be used in Eq. (1) in text, depending on the ratio of (d) thickness of the preparation and (a) the interelectrode distance (Schnabel 1967)

arrays of four electrodes are arranged in a cross. The interelectrode distance is 0.5 mm. One array, to be placed in the axial direction of the ureter, is denoted by the index a; the other array, denoted by the index c is to be placed in the circumferential direction. The electrode configurations were placed on circular pieces of ureteral tissue with a diameter of 8 mm, taken from different parts of pig ureters. The measurements were done at room temperature. Electrode configuration I was placed at different angles with respect to the axis of the ureter. Repositioning the electrodes on the same piece of tissue has the drawback that extra errors are introduced in the measurements. Replacement is avoided by the use of electrode configuration II. The relation between U_{23} and I_{12} for an anisotropic medium has been derived theoretically for a medium with a semi-infinite geometry by Rush (1962). To take into account the finite thickness of the medium (d), which in our situation is comparable with the interelectrode distances (a), a correction factor F, derived by Schnabel (1967), has to be introduced.

The relation valid in our situation is:

$$U_{23} = \frac{I_{14}}{2\pi a F} \left[\sigma_l \sigma_t \left(\cos^2 \alpha + \frac{\sigma_t}{\sigma_l} \sin^2 \alpha \right) \right]^{-\frac{1}{2}}, \qquad (1)$$

where α is the angle between the direction transverse to the fibers and the direction of the array of the electrodes. F is the correction factor, which depends on d/a in the way illustrated in Fig. 3.

Results

Both electrode configurations were tested initially in a saline solution. The thickness of the layer of saline in which the tests were performed was 1 mm. Hence d/a = 0.5 for configuration I and consequently, according to Fig. 3, F = 0.4. At a frequency of f = 1000 Hz we found with configuration I that U_{23} = 0.358 mV when I_{14} = 2.4 µA and that $\varphi \simeq 0°$. Because the medium is isotropic we can substitute the value $\alpha = 0$ in Eq. (1). Thus we find that $\sigma = I_{14}/2 \pi a F U_{23}$ = 0.0133 S/cm. This value is close to that reported by Weast et al. (1978).

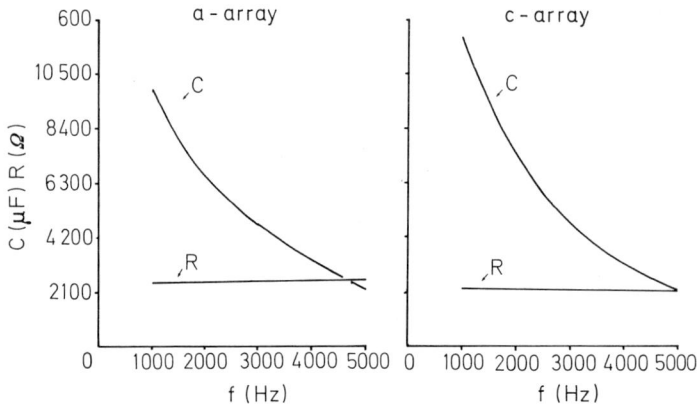

Fig. 4. Capacitance (C) and resistance (R) as a function of the frequency, measured in saline by means of electrode configuration II

With electrode configuration II the measured phase angle was not negligible. We therefore determined both $|Z|$, the absolute value of the ratio U_{23}/I_{14}, and φ, for the two electrode arrays. From these values we derived the ohmic component R and the reactive component X of the impedance Z. The capacitance C was derived from the formula $X = 1/2 \pi f C$. The values of R and C obtained with configuration II in saline are shown graphically in Fig. 4. It is clear that in spite of the use of the four-electrode technique there is a significant capacitive component in the impedance. We estimated that the voltage drop at the interfaces between the electrodes and saline was only 0.1% of voltage U_{23}. Hence the capacitive component is not related to the interface. It might originate, however, in the stray capacitance between the electrodes (Gielen and Boon 1981). At a frequency of $f = 1000$ Hz we find that, for the a-array, $R = 118 \Omega$. Since the value of d/a is larger than 4, F may be taken equal to 1. It follows from Eq. (1) that $\sigma_2 = 1/2 \pi a R = 0.027$ S/cm. For the c-array, $\sigma_t = 0.030$ S/cm.

These conductances are considerably larger than those of saline. This error may be due to the fact that in electrode configuration II the diameter of the electrodes is larger than their minimum separation (0.2 mm). This makes the configuration unsuitable for the measurement of specific conductance. However, it remains suitable for detecting anisotropy, which is based on the ratio of conductances.

Because saline is isotropic we expect to find $R_t/R_l = 1$. The measured ratio differs by about 10% from this theoretical value. This deviation can be ascribed to small geometric differences in the arrangements of the electrodes in the arrays.

We will now report some results relevant to the anisotropy of muscle tissue. A more detailed analysis will be published later.

Table 1 shows the results of measurements on pieces of striated muscle taken from the hind quaters of the pig, which were performed with configuration I at a frequency $f = 1000$ Hz. For a piece of tissue with a thickness of about 3 mm we indeed find an anisotropy; the ratio of the conductances measured in two perpendicular directions is about 2.5. When, however, the measurements are done on a piece of muscle with a thickness of about 10 mm we do not find any anisotropy.

Table 1. Results of measurements of U_{23} in two pieces of striated muscle from the rump of the pig with thickness $d \simeq 3$ mm and $\simeq 10$ mm, with electrode configuration I ($I_{14} = 2.4$ μA, f = 1000 Hz) at two values of the angle (α) between the electrode array and the fiber orientation visible on the surface of the tissue

α	U_{23} (mV)	d
90°	1.92	about 3 mm
0°	2.45	
90°	1.96	
0°	2.44	
90°	1.83	
0°	2.54	
90°	1.45	
0°	2.40	
90°	0.73	about 10 mm
0°	0.72	

Table 2. Results of measurements of U_{23} in three pieces of pig ureter taken from the upper, central and lower parts, measured with electrode configuration I ($I_{12} = 2.4$ μA, f = 1000 and 10,000 Hz) at two values 0° and 90° of the angle (β) between the electrode array and the axis of the ureter. The phase angle between U_{23} and I_{12}, $\varphi \simeq 0°$

f (Hz)	β	U_{23} (mV)	
1,000	0°	1.19	Central part
10,000	0°	1.24	
1,000	90°	1.15	
10,000	90°	1.16	
1,000	0°	1.36	Lower part
10,000	0°	1.37	
1,000	90°	1.40	
10,000	90°	1.37	
1,000	0°	1.00	Upper part
10,000	0°	1.00	
1,000	90°	1.10	
10,000	90°	1.10	

Table 2 gives the results of measurements on pieces of pig ureter taken from the upper, central and lower parts, measured with electrode configuration I at angles (β) of 0° and 90° with respect to the axis of the ureter and at a frequency of f = 1000 Hz and 10.000 Hz. The ratio of the conductivities does not deviate significantly from the value 1 for any part of the ureter. Hence the measurements do not demonstrate any electrical anisotropy. The mean thickness of the pieces of ureter was about 1 mm, so that the conductance estimated according to Eq. (1) is about 0.0034–0.0048 S/cm, which is about three to four times lower than that of saline.

Figure 5 shows the results of measurements performed with electrode configuration II on three pieces of the central part of the pig ureter. From these measure-

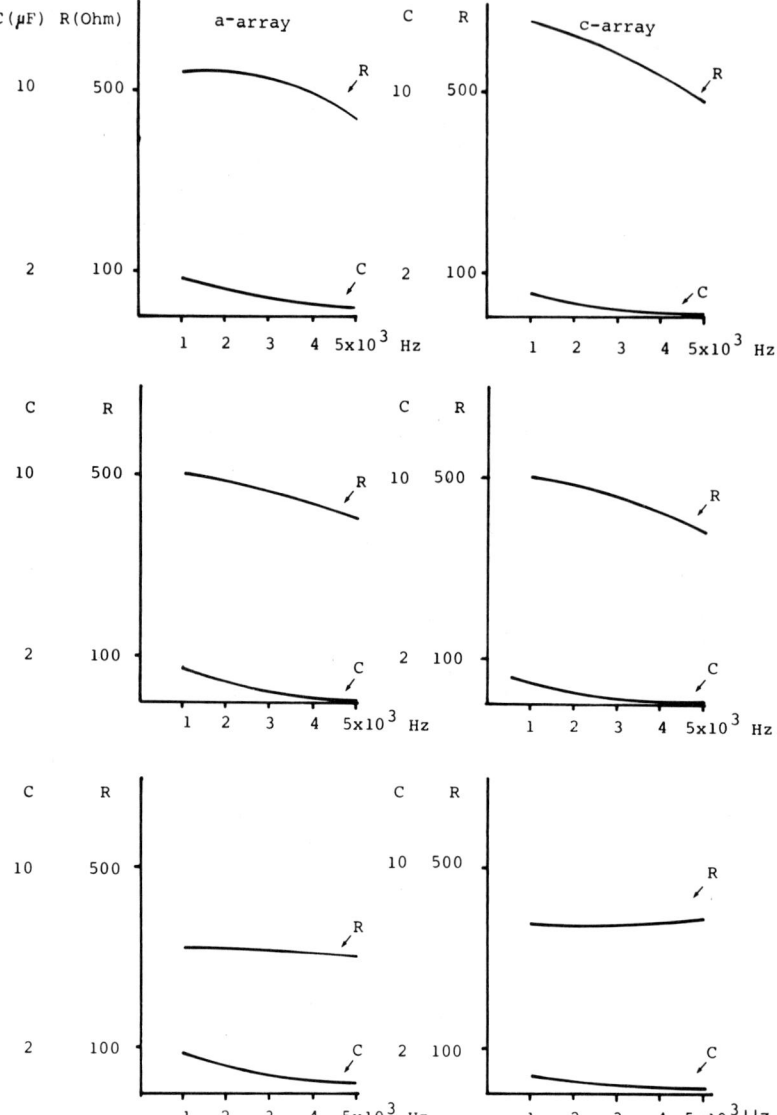

Fig. 5. Capacitance (*C*) and resistance (*R*) as function of the frequency, measured in pieces of the central part of pig ureter by means of electrode configuration II: *a* axial, *c* circumferential direction

ments R and C have been derived in the same way as for the measurements in saline. The graphs show how R and C vary with frequency. It appears that the ohmic component decreases only slightly, while the capacitance decreases considerably with increasing frequency. Furthermore, since the ohmic component found in the longitudinal direction does not deviate systematically from that found in the transverse direction, there is no significant anisotropy. Thus the previous finding that there is no anisotropy with an interelectrode separation of 2 mm is confirmed with an electrode separation of 0.5 mm. Finally we note that the capacitance found for the tissue is considerably smaller than that for saline.

Discussion

We have looked for anisotropy in ureteral tissue by measuring the ratio of the ohmic components of the impedances measured in two mutually perpendicular directions, axial and circumferential.

With an electrode separation of 2 mm no anisotropy is found, although it is detected in a piece of striated muscle. However, anisotropy may exist on a small geometric scale, and yet not be demonstrable on larger scales because of averaging over many regions with different orientations. An indication of this averaging effect is the loss of anisotropy in measurements on a thick piece of striated muscle, in which layers of muscle fibers with different orientations could be distinguished. Measurements on ureteral tissue at a smaller scale with an electrode separation distance of 0.5 mm, did not reveal any anisotropy either. Hence we conclude that a preferred orientation for the muscle fibers in the ureteral wall, as would be expected if the helical muscle fiber model were valid, is not demonstrated by any anisotropy in electrical conductance. We may not conclude from this that there is no muscle fiber orientation at all, because anisotropy associated with a group of fibers with a certain orientation may be cancelled by another group of fibers with a different orientation. In particular, the assumption of a braided fiber structure is not in conflict with our results. Gosling and Dixon (1981) reported, however, that they were unable to distinguish such a fiber structure in their histologic study. On the other hand the conclusion drawn from the contraction measurements referred to in the introduction, that the orientation is predominantly transverse rather than longitudinal, is in conflict with the results obtained here. There is a need for a common explanation for the results of both investigations. The conductance measured in ureteral tissue is about $1/3$–$1/4$ of that measured in saline. If we assume that the passive cells constitute regions of zero conductance in a saline environment, this would imply that the saline content of tissue is about 25–35%.

The fact that the values of the capacitance derived from measurements in tissue are much lower than those obtained for saline, means that the tissue between the electrodes has a capacitance which is in series with the 'stray' capacitance measured in saline. This tissue capacitance is to be found from the obtained value of C by correcting it for the 'stray' capacitance. The tissue capacitance of the tissue between the electrodes with a separation of 0.5 mm lies in the range of 0.2–1.0 µF. Combining this with the value of the resistance between these electrodes of about 400 Ω, we find that the time constant of the tissue between the electrodes is about 0.08–0.4 ms. The propagation velocity of a peristaltic wave is approximately 4 cm/s. Hence it takes 12.5 ms to cover a distance of 0.5 mm. Since the time constant of such a piece of tissue is considerably smaller, it cannot be the factor determining the relatively slow propagation of peristaltic waves. It must be noted, however, that this time constant is a property of passive tissue, while the propagation of the waves is determined by active tissue. In active tissue the electrical currents associated with depolarization of cell membranes are limited by the conductance of the intracellular medium. Because the intracellular conductivity is lower than that of the extracellular medium, it may be imagined that it is another time constant which, among other factors, determines the propagation velocity and which is considerably larger than the time constant concerning passive tissue as it is found here.

References

Dullman J (1967) Konstruktionsanalytische Untersuchung der Ureter und der Glandula vesiculosa. Acta Anat 68:344
Duyl WA van, Coolsaet BLRA (1982) Potassium-induced contractions in pig ureter strips: consequences for helical muscle-fiber model of ureter. Urology XX:53–58
Geddes LA, Baker LE (1967) The specific resistance of biological material. A compendium of data for muscle fibers. Med Biol Eng 5:271–293
Gielen FLH, Boon KL (1981) Measurement of the (complex) electrical conductivity and the anisotropy in skeletal muscle: a new electrode configuration. Proc 5th I.C.E.B.I., Tokyo pp 191–194
Gosling JA, Dixon JS (1981) A three-dimensional analysis of the musculature of the upper urinary tract; abstract. Third Meeting of the Int. Soc. for Dyn. of the Upper Urinary Tract, Aarhus
Nagai T, Prosser CL (1963) Electrical parameters of smooth muscle cells. Am J Physiol 204 (5):915–924
Rush S (1962) Methods of measuring the resistivity of anisotropic conducting media in situ. J Res Nat Bur St Eng Instr 66 C(3):217–222
Satani Y (1919) Histological study of the ureter. J Urol 3:247
Schnabel P (1967) Vierpunktmethode zur Messung der elektrischen Widerstandsanisotropie. Z Angew Phys 22:136–140
Weast RC (1978) CRC Handbook of chemistry and physics, 55th edn. The Chemical Rubber Company, Ohio, USA, D253

Kinetic Urography

L. Ohlson[1]

Introduction

Fluoroscopy of the peristalsis of the upper urinary tract was introduced in 1927 by Legueu et al. The urine was found to be propelled by a peristaltic contraction ring similar to the annular contraction described by Engelmann (1869). The ring could be observed to travel alternately from one of the main branches of the pyelocalyceal system and to spread over the renal pelvis (the confluence of the main branches) and over the entire ureter. Its motion was continuous and its speed close to 3 cm/s. The shortest contraction interval was about 5 s. The morphodynamics in the pyelocalyceal system were complex and rapid, and since kinetic recording was not yet clinically applicable certain morphodynamic processes could not be adequately analyzed, particularly those preceding the appearance of the contraction ring in a main branch. In supplementing fluoroscopy with single exposures as brief as 0.05 s Legueu et al. were able to demonstrate that on its transit over the main branches the contraction ring produced a retrograde injection of the liquid into the calyces, distending each calyx in a rapid sequence terminating within a few seconds. This injection was similar to the injection into the ureter, indicating that the ring might subsequently pass on into the calyces just as it did into the ureter and suggesting the possibility of an antegrade peristaltic contraction preceding the appearance of the ring in a main branch. The morphodynamics of the ureter proved to be far less complex and more conspicuous than those of the pyelocalyceal system, hence more accessible to analysis. The liquid injected by the contraction ring when running in one of the main branches immediately elongated according to the dimensions of the ureter, its forward end running quickly through the lumbar segment and stopping short at the junction between the lumbar and pelvic segments. As the steadily advancing contraction ring approached the junction the bolus grew shorter and thicker, i.e. it distended, and at a certain moment it was injected into the pelvic segment in the same way it had been injected from the renal pelvis.

Leb (1930) found that the contraction interval was much shorter in the upright position than in the recumbent.

Most subsequent investigators confirmed the existence of a peristaltic contraction "wave" in the ureter, travelling at a speed close to 3 cm/s, but the filling of the ureter was considered to be a passive process (Tanagho and Meyers 1971), and it was not clear whether the contractions of the renal pelvis were peristaltic or stationary. Narath (1954) found the urinary conduit to be divided into a series of 5 in-

---

1 Department of Diagnostic Radiology, Karolinska Hospital, Box 60500, S-104 01 Stockholm

dependent units, the calyces, the renal pelvis and 3 compartments in the ureter, each compartment being equipped with a detrusor and sphincter mechanism. No continuous peristaltic wave could be demonstrated. On the contrary, when the renal pelvis contracted the calyces were relaxed but closed off by the sphincters at their bases that protected them from the expulsive pressures of the renal pelvis, and so the renal pelvis had to void into the ureter only. When the renal pelvis relaxed the detrusor voiding of the calyces took place, each calyx voiding in turn in a rapid sequence terminating within a few seconds. Narath concluded that the existence of retrograde injections from the renal pelvis into the calyces was incompatible with the rule that the urine must be transported downward, not backward. Kiil (1957, 1973) confirmed the existence of a continuous peristaltic wave in the ureter but failed to demonstrate any peristaltic injection into the ureter. The peristaltic wave started at the pyeloureteral junction (PUJ) and propagated along the ureter. At the same time as the wave occluded the PUJ the renal pelvis contracted but did this by retracting backwards into the hilum and so keeping the pyelocalyceal liquid from entering the ureter for the duration of its contraction. No further types of contractions in the renal pelvis were demonstrated. There were possible contractions of a sphincter at the base of each calyx, occurring without any obvious coordination with the sphincters of the other calyces or with the renal pelvis, and they were not found to accomplish any unequivocal transport of the liquid. The pressure in the renal pelvis was always low under physiological conditions, and there were no increases in pressure attributable to possible contractions (as occurred in the ureter). The pressure in the calyces could not be distinguished from that in the renal pelvis. Kiil concluded that there were no retrograde expulsive injections from the renal pelvis into the calyces and that, consequently, there was no need for any functional coordination between possible contractions in the renal pelvis and the calyces in order to protect the papillae from too high pressures. Kiil used single radiographs with an exposure time of 0.25–0.32 s and concluded that earlier ideas about the need for rapid recording, such as cineradiography, were based on the erroneous assumption that the muscles of the upper urinary conduit were capable of rapid, strong contractions.

The present technique for kinetic urography started with fluoroscopy in the upright and recumbent positions without kinetic recording and serial radiography during angiography with a frequency of 2–4 images per second at an exposure time of 0.10 s. All the features of the ureteral peristalsis described by Legueu et al. were observed (although independently) and certain further features were recorded, such as the rapid injection of a large column of liquid through the entire ureter and the incomplete closure of the contraction ring in the lumbar segment as distinguished from the complete closure of the ring in the pelvic segment. The morphodynamics in the pyelocalyceal system also proved to agree with those described by Legueu et al. but were considerably more difficult to analyze because of the low image frequency. The retrograde injections into the calyces were usually readily analyzable but contraction rings travelling retrograde could not be conclusively demonstrated. Video recording became available in 1969 but it was not until 1976 that the performance of the equipment reached a level that enabled further details to be studied (Ohlson and Fernström 1981; Ohlson 1982).

Methods

Kinetic Urography. The cooperation of the patient proved essential to the result of the study. Therefore, the purpose and the performance of the examination were explained in some detail, usually when viewing a demonstration recording together with the patient.

Ordinarily a low-osmolality contrast medium with low and rapidly transient diuretic effect was used, and when study at elevated urinary excretion was indicated a high-osmolality contrast medium was injected subsequently. The fluoroscopic image was recorded by 1-inch 180°-wrap two-head video recorders at a frequency of 0.02 s (Oldelft OD-X-40) including time generators with a frequency of 0.01 s (For-A Japan, VTG-33).

Analysis of the video recordings was done at playback in real time and of still frames. Sequences of special interest were manually transferred to transparent plastic film in scales from 1:1 to 1.5:1. The transfers were entered into a topographic coordinate system for measurements and analysis of morphological detail as developing over time (Ohlson 1972). In the present context, the term "antegrade" is defined as the direction of the axis of any segment of the urinary system leading from any fornix toward the ureterovesical junction, thus the direction of the net urinary transport.

Complementary Methods. These included angiography, computer tomography, ultrasound, endoscopy, manometry, cystoscopy and studies at laparotomy.

Results and Comments

Impulse Conduction (Figs. 1, 2, 3, 5, 6)

The progress of the contraction ring, i.e. the impulse conduction, in the urinary system was found to consist in a continuous and uniform motion spreading omnidirectionally from a point of origin outside the fornices. The contraction ring entered the urinary system at the insertion of the wall onto a papilla, the "starting point". Normal unprovoked starts occurred only in the fornices. Starts could take place in any fornix and they alternated over the set of fornices in a given pyelocalyceal system. Once launched on a path the ring pursued its transit as far as the medium reached, the end points being the reciprocal fornices and the vesical orifice of the ureter. The speed of the ring was close to 3 cm/s. The ring was thus never stationary, and the geometric principle for its progress was the same for all starting points and for all segments of any urinary system. Each fornix had a specific refractory period, its module. The actual contraction interval between two consecutive starts in a given fornix was either equal to or a multiple of the module. The shortest module so far detected is 4.25 s. Starts in two or more different fornices could occur at any moment. In the upright position one or several fornices often contracted at module frequency while in the recumbent position the module was usually multiplied by 2 or 3, or more.

Changes in the hydrodynamic parameters, such as the volume, flow and pressure of the liquid, or in the morphodynamic parameters, such as mural stretch and meetings with other rings, proved to be the results of the action of the contraction ring and could in no instance be demonstrated to influence either the triggering of the starts, the location of a starting point or the progress of the ring. Thus, impulse conduction was found to be independent of hydrodynamic and morphodynamic parameters and capable of being analyzed as such whereas these parameters were necessarily dependent upon the contraction ring, firstly in its quality of being an indicator of the impulse conduction, i.e. the determinant of the course of the events developing on a given transit, and secondly, as a morphological element that confers form and quantity to the events.

The motion of the contraction ring seems to be wholly defined by its linearity, being a wave continuum spreading omnidirectionally in concentric waves. Any ring divides into two rings each time it runs into two branches of the urinary system but this behaviour is merely a function of the anatomy of the medium in which it runs and not a manifestation of any intrinsic tendency of the ring to divide. On the contrary, the ring has to divide precisely in order to preserve its integrity and unity as a continuum and so meet the requirements for linearity. With respect to impulse conduction, then, all individual rings deriving from a common start are, whatever their morphodynamic role will be, just generations of the primary ring, the common expression of the impulse flow that makes no distinctions between branches. Thus, under normal conditions there were, among other things, no manifestations of any pacemaker activity within the urinary system from the fornices to the vesical orifice of the ureter.

An adequate analysis of the processes that determine the triggering of the start, as reflected in the alternation of the starts, in the variations in the module of different fornices and in the relations between the module and the actual contraction interval, requires an up-to-date high-performance television system. This is not currently available in our department. Nevertheless, certain observations could be made.

At contraction intervals of 2 or 3 times the module, 2 or more starts in different fornices usually took place in close sequence, typically within 0.50 s, without any starts taking place in the meantime and often extending over a series of 40 or 50 such grouped starts. The order between the starting points often remained invariant for 5–6 grouped starts but then shifted, and even when the order remained invariant the internal delays constantly varied from one grouped start to the next, although the variations in the delays were usually only 0.02–0.40 s. For instance, in the pyelocalyceal system in Fig. 2, starts occurred for several minutes in fornix 6b and fornix 1d at contraction intervals between two paired starts of 9–12 s and with delays between 0.08 and 0.30 s and the first start alternating between the two fornices without any obvious regularity. This pattern then shifted suddenly to another pattern in which the double or triple module of one fornix recurred regularly but in constantly varying combinations with the other fornices, the groups being for instance 4–1d–2c,d; 1a,b,c–4–6b–2c,d; 3d–4–6b–1a,b,c; etc. In this pattern thus only fornix 4 recurs regularly while the variations between the other fornices do not seem to follow any obvious pattern. With the present technique it was usually not possible to distinguish separate starts in compound fornices, such as 1a,b,c, and 2c,d. Separate starts do occur in at least some compound fornices, and so there is a distinct possibility that the variations might prove more regular if all separate starts in compound calyces could be distinguished. The variations seem to be compatible with the presence of one centre that preferentially triggers one fornix and another centre for another fornix while each centre might also induce some secondary cross-triggering. In that case, the constantly present variations in the delays between fornices could be due to interference between impulses from several centres, but at present it seems not to be possible to exclude variations in the speed of the impulse.

These processes could be reproduced to a certain extent by using, for instance, a needle as a stimulus, as a fine-bore needle used before the introduction of catheters into the fornices, especially so when two fornices were punctured, as for perfusion and manometry. For instance, if starts were seen to occur rather regularly in an upper pole fornix, a lower pole fornix that was well distended by the retrograde injections was chosen for the first puncture, which was done when the injection distended the fornix. When the tip of the needle was in the pyramid at a variable distance from the fornix, this fornix typically started to contract and took over the lead. In this situation it proved useful to place the other needle in a middle fornix or an upper pole fornix, both of which distended well at this stage. When the tip of the second needle approached the fornix, this fornix typically started to contract too, establishing a regular high-frequency cross-fire with the opposing fornix while starts in the other fornices generally ceased. When the contraction interval in either of the opposing fornices was fairly long, extra starts could be triggered by a light distinct tap on the needle, enabling a certain degree of control of the alternation of the triggering (and hence of the reciprocal injections used for the puncture). The delay between the excitation and the appearance of the starts was in no instance found to exceed 0.10 s. However, occasionally a start failed to occur with this delay and when the preexisting contraction interval was short it was difficult to distinguish a possible longer delay from the terminal part of the preexisting contraction interval.

In urinary systems with a bifid ureter, the impulse propagated and divided according to the geometric principle for the spread of the contraction ring, the two long branches transmitting the impulses in both reciprocal directions just as any branch in a pyelocalyceal system. In contradistinction, no unequivocal such reciprocity was observed in duplicated ureters with separate orifices in the bladder. In one bifid urinary system one of the ureteral limbs, both of which were about 15 cm long, ended in a blind, concave cul-de-sac lacking a papilla. The absence of renal parenchyma was confirmed by computer tomography. No starts occurred in the blind cul-de-sac, while the contraction rings emanating from the fornices in the pyelocalyceal system of the reciprocal ureteral limb pursued their retrograde transit all the way into the blind end segment just as they did into the ordinary end segments of the pyelocalyceal system.

A necessary condition for the permanence of the geometric principle for the spread of the contraction ring in a biological system such as the urinary system is apparently that two branches originating from the division of a common branch do not connect and establish a closed circuit as do, for instance, the collateral branches of arteries and veins, for in such a circuit a given ring would have to run around indefinitely and hence generate an indefinite number of rings. Closed circuits were also not encountered in any of the urinary systems studied.

Morphodynamics

From the point of view of fluid dynamics, the urinary system may be characterized as a manifold tubular conduit with elastic and compliant walls, hence capable of undergoing variations in shape and volume over time, and even capable of dividing into two or more separate conduits by active complete closure of its lumen. A given patent segment was always filled with liquid and only liquid, the internal shape and volume of that segment being identical with the shape and volume of the liquid; in this sense, thus, a given patent segment was always completely filled irrespective of its actual volume at a given time (its filling) as well as of its maximum volume capacity (its compliance). Since the conduit contained only liquid, the patent segments were subject to the mechanisms of hydrodynamics.

The net displacement of the liquid was from the papillae to the bladder, and over periods of sufficient duration there was an inflow-outflow equilibrium. The overall displacement of liquid generally far exceeded the net displacement. It was achieved (1) by the peristaltic transport, i.e. the propulsive action of the contraction rings, and (2) by the extraperistaltic flow. The inflow consisted of the continuous urinary excretion and the outflow to the bladder made up the net urinary transport. The peristaltic transport was thus always to some extent conditioned by the extraperistaltic flow (ultimately the inflow), whereas in the absence of contraction rings the flow was wholly extraperistaltic.

Non-Peristaltic Factors (Fig. 1)

The Extraperistaltic Flow in Relation to the Compliance of the Conduit

The flow patterns always varied with location as well as with time, thus always being non-uniform as well as unsteady. As a function of the elasticity and compliance of the walls of the conduit both non-uniformity and unsteadiness varied with time. The differences in magnitude of these variations were in many instances so large as to induce categorically different hydrodynamic situations. In the course of the peristaltic transit the variations were always great, and the flow rates within the conduit exceeded those at the inlet and at the outlet by several orders of magnitude. By contrast, the flow rates within the conduit during extraperistaltic flow varied far less, and under certain conditions they were almost equal to those at the inlet and the outlet not only as an average but also for brief distinct periods of time. Under such conditions the walls of the conduit were nearly stable, except for respiratory movements and vascular pulsations, and the flow patterns approximated those in a conduit with rigid walls. These relatively stable conditions were present when at an even inflow rate the compliance of the conduit reached a certain level and remained at that level, and provided certain factors remained unchanged or varied regularly, in the first hand body posture and respiration (q.v.). However, when any of these factors changed, the flow equilibrium was interrupted.

A given rate of inflow (urinary excretion) naturally resulted in far greater hydrodynamic and morphodynamic changes in a small (i.e. slender) urinary conduit, and hence also the duration of the undisturbed inflow, i.e. the contraction interval, affected the small conduit to a proportionally higher degree. At an inflow of, for instance, 0.5 ml/min a slender conduit with a pre-filling at time zero of 1 ml filled up

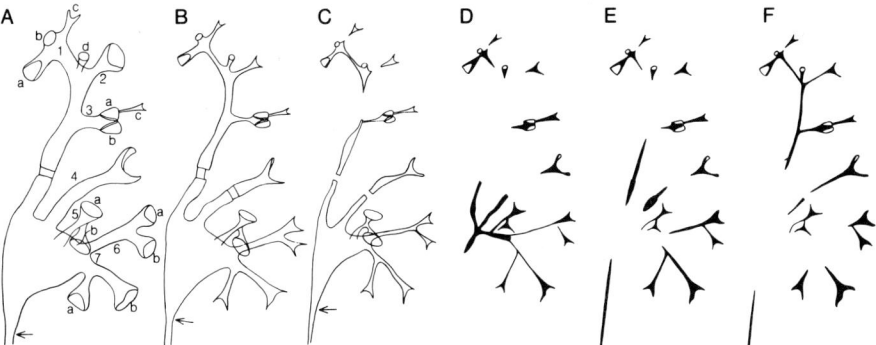

Fig. 1 A–F. Kinetic urography of normal pyelocalyceal system. Left side. Scale 1:2. Apnoea in expiration. **A–C** Supine position. **D–F** Upright position. **A** 'Full distension' at ureteral compression. **B–F** No ureteral compression. Urinary excretion 0.3 ml/min/kidney. Inflow–outflow equilibrium. **A** Volume 18 ml. Relaxation. Contraction interval 12.5 s. Branches identified by Arabic numerals, papillae by small letters. *Arrow* PUJ. **B** Volume 6 ml. Relaxation. Preceding start 55 s before **B**. **C** Volume 2.5 ml. Relaxation. Contraction interval 12.5 s. **D** Volume 0.8 ml. 0.50 s before start in fornix *5a*. Contraction interval 9.60 s. **E** 0.85 s after the start in fornix *5a*. (1.35 s after **D**.) **F** 1.20 s after the start. (1.70 s after **D**.)

Before the start (**D**) parts of the upper and middle branches are empty after the preceding contraction, which started in fornix *1c*. The front end of the liquid lies in the ureter 3 mm below the PUJ. *Ureter:* In **E** the primary ring has emptied the renal pelvis and completed the injection into the ureter. It lies 5 mm below the PUJ and is outlined by the rear end of the liquid column. The column is 10 cm long (extending 7.5 cm below this figure) and has an average diameter of 0.7 mm and a volume of 0.04 ml. In **F** the ring has advanced 8 mm farther. *Upper main branch:* In **E** the ring is 6 mm from the artery crossing the branch; it is outlined by the rear end of the column. The front end of the column has just been injected beyond the artery and runs at a speed of 70 cm/s, while the segment between the ring and the artery distends toward a rounded shape. In **F** the ring has injected the whole column over the artery and is now 2 mm beyond the artery. The injected liquid has merged with the liquid in the calyces. *Branch 4:* In **E** the ring is 5 mm from the artery in that branch, and the front end has crossed the artery. The segment between the ring and the artery is more distended than the corresponding segment in the upper main branch. In **F** the ring has passed the artery but has left a small residual volume behind the artery. The injected liquid has merged with the liquid in the fornix. *Branches 6 and 7:* In **E** the rings inject and distend each of the four calyces. They leave no residual volume. In **F** they are quite close to the fornices, and these cul-de-sacs are so distended that the rings will soon have to open up and let the liquid escape backward. (The time-table for the opening-up, not included in the figure, is *7a* at 1.26 s, *6a* and *b* at 1.34 s, and *7b* at 1.40 s.)

to the double volume within 2 minutes. A contraction ring that started at 1 s thus met a slender conduit that presented a set of hydrodynamic factors typical of a relatively small volume and that led to a typical hydrodynamic pattern as the ring subsequently evolved over the manifold conduit. A ring that started after 2 min of extraperistaltic flow met another conduit, much more well-filled and so presenting a different set of hydrodynamic factors. This gradual quantitative change thus proved to lead to categorically distinct qualitative hydrodynamic conditions. If the inflow was raised to 2 ml/min the 1 s ring met the same conduit as before (total volume 1 ml), while a 30 s ring met the same conduit as did the 2 min ring at the lower inflow rate (total volume 2 ml), and the 2 min ring met a conduit filled to 5 ml and so

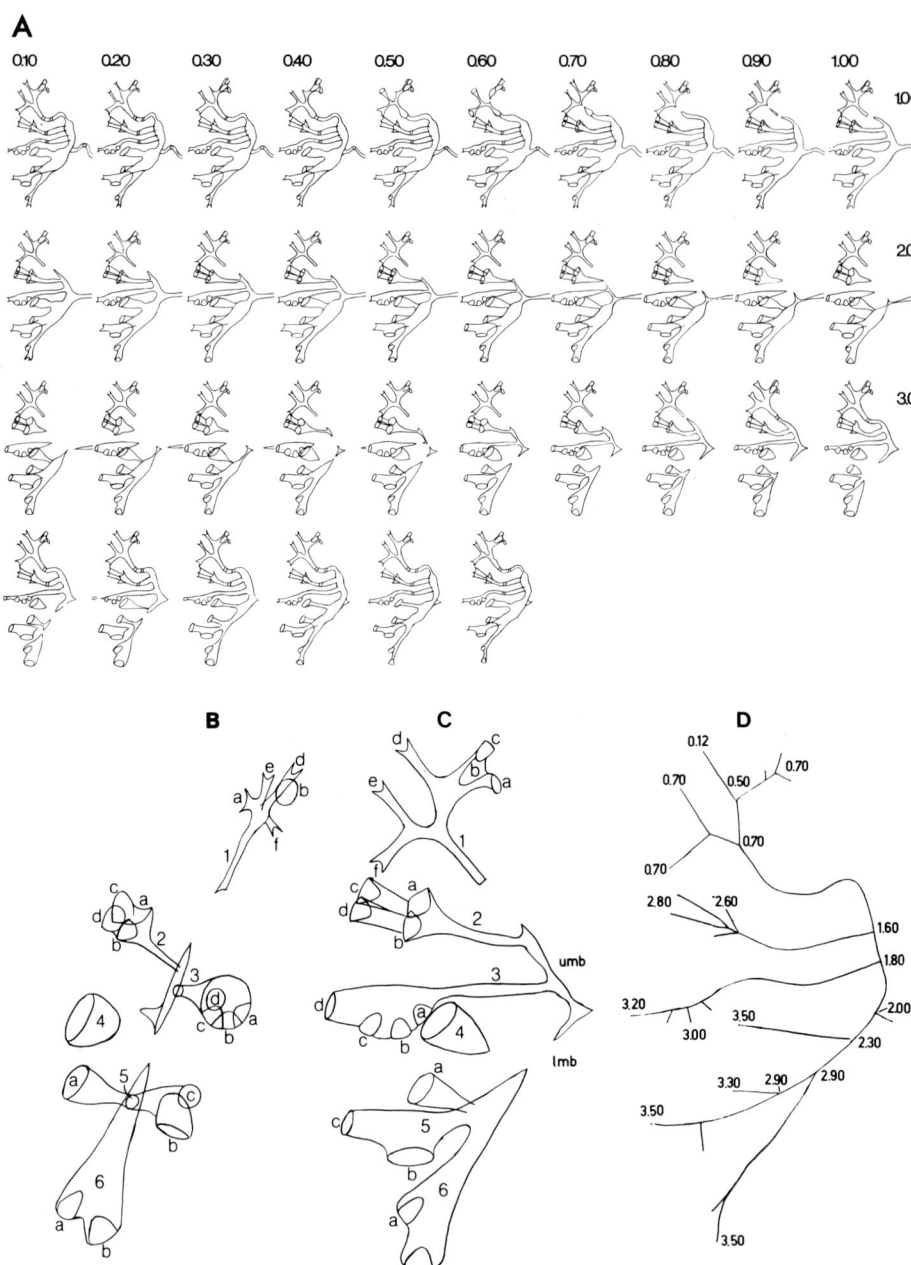

Fig. 2A–D. Kinetic urography of normal pyelocalyceal system. Right side. Upright position. Contraction interval 8.5 s. Urinary excretion 0.3 ml/min/kidney. Inflow–outflow equilibrium. Pyelocalyceal volume before start 7 ml. Apnoea in expiration. **A** Sequence of entire transit. Frontal projection. Scale 1:4. Time in seconds. Interval between reproduced pictures 0.10 s. **B** lateral projection. Scale 1:1. Recorded 2 min after **A** at 2.60 s after a start in fornix *1d*. Branches identified by Arabic numerals, papillae by small letters. Branches *2* and *4*, PUJ and calyx *5a* directed anteriorly. **C** Picture at 2.60 s in **A** in scale 1:1. Same stage of transit as in **B**.

presenting it with a third kind of hydrodynamic conditions. On the other hand, an inflow of 0.5 ml into a conduit with a pre-filling of 10 ml increased its volume by a mere 10 per cent, and the morphodynamic effects of this increment were negligible. Further increments had proportionally small effects.

These types of filling were frequently encountered in the recumbent position. When the subject was upright, the shape and filling of the conduit at time zero were usually essentially unchanged, and so the 1 s ring met the same conduit as it did in the recumbent position. As the filling proceeded it emerged that certain conduits never did dilate beyond a small total volume, such as 2 ml. All further inflow went on by displacement to the bladder, and the walls of the conduit were nearly stable (with the usual exception of the regular movements due to respiration and vascular pulsations). Thus, a conduit with a compliance limit of, for instance, 5 ml in the recumbent position typically had a compliance limit of 2 ml in the upright position. At

◀───

Branches and papillae designated as in **B**. **D** Road map and time-table for transit in **A**. Time in seconds. (The detailed anatomy of papilla *1c* in **B** could not be determined.)
Start in fornix *1d* at 0.12 s. The primary ring is completely closed on its passage over the papilla and on its transit in calyx *1d* (0.20–0.40 s), injecting all the liquid contained in this calyx into the adjoining calyces and the upper part of branch *1*. When it enters the confluence of the calyces it opens up and lets calyx *1d* fill again (at 0.70 s). At 0.70 s it enters branch *1*. When it enters the confluence of the calyces it opens up and lets calyx *1d* fill again (at O.70 s). At 0.70 s it enters branch *1* and distends the segment above the artery crossing that branch. Just before 0.90 s it opens up and lets a small bolus of liquid escape backward. At 1.00 s the bolus merges with the liquid in the calyceal system. Compare also Fig. 5, lower row.
At 1.20 s the ring begins to extend into branch *2* and at 1.30 s into branch *3*. At 1.70 s branch *2* has shortened from a precontraction length of 35 mm to 27 mm and branch *3* from 42 mm to 33 mm. These two branches pull the upper main branch laterally, making its medial border run 3 mm lateral to its lateral border in relaxation. See also Fig. 3 D. At 1.70 s the volume in branches *2* and *3* has grown from a precontraction value of about 0.20 ml to about 0.85 ml, and the pressure is about 18 mm Hg. At 1.76 s the ring closes off branch *3*, and during the ensuing isovolumetric phase it reduces the patent segment of the branch to half the precontraction length. The ring meets the growing resistance from the cul-de-sac and so it flares out, but it does not open yet and goes on distending the cul-de-sac. The liquid penetrates into the space between the wall and the base of each papilla that was closed before the start (0.10 s), and goes on unfolding the wall about its insertion onto the pyramid. See also Figs. 2 B and 3 D. Finally (at 2.40 s) the evaginated wall fits snugly around the juxtapapillary region of the pyramid, and the papilla and this region project into the space as one structure. The top of the pyramid is also flattened out and displaced 3–4 mm into the parenchyma, and the liquid fills the terminal portions of the excretory ducts. – At 2.48 s the ring opens up and lets the cul-de-sac expel its liquid in an injection that reaches the upper main branch within 0.02 s. The opening pressure in the cul-de-sac is 22–23 mm Hg, and the front end of the liquid travels at 75 cm/s. The cul-de-sac empties rapidly, and when the ring reaches fornix *3d* (at 3.20 s) it manages to close completely a second time.
At 2.40 s the five completely closed rings in branch *2,* branch *3,* the ureter, the lower main branch and branch *4* divide the system into no less than seven non-communicating hydrodynamic compartments. At this stage the overall redistribution reaches its peak. Branch *1* is still drained to a volume of about 0.4 ml, and the upper main branch is empty (except the minute incipient injection from branch *2*), while the remaining volume of about 6 ml (the injection into the ureter was 0.4 ml) has been driven into the opposite branches in the lower pole and, to a lesser extent, into branches *2–4*. See also Fig. 3C. From 2.50 s on, the return of the liquid to its precontraction distribution proceeds quickly and is completed at 3.60 s

an inflow of 2 ml/min, then, the 30 s ring met the same conduit as in the recumbent position but the 2 min ring did not meet the 5 ml conduit but instead the same 2 ml conduit as did the 30 s ring. In one situation, though, the filling in the upright position did of course exceed the ordinary (2 ml) volume capacity, thus exceeding the ordinary compliance limit, namely when the patient rose from the recumbent position while the conduit was filled to 5 ml. This filling represented a considerable "overfilling" of the upright conduit, presenting a challenge to its emptying capacity comparable to that achieved by perfusion. At this pre-equilibrium stage the morphodynamics of both the extraperistaltic flow and the contraction rings were characteristic.

After the passage of a contraction ring the extraperistaltic flow filled the pyelocalyceal system and the lumbar segment fairly evenly. The first constant point of resistance encountered by the liquid was the lumbopelvic junction. All other points of resistance consisted in arteries crossing the branches (Fig. 1), and their obstructive effect was variable and always far inferior to that of the lumbopelvic junction. All other portions of the wall offered even less resistance. The resistance of the bases of the branches, including the PUJ, was the same as for the other portions. Thus, the liquid invariably passed readily across the PUJ just as it passed across the entrance of any other branch, whereas it invariably accumulated above the lumbopelvic junction. When the lumbar segment had become distended to its ordinary compliance limit, the pyelocalyceal system continued to fill while still no liquid passed across the lumbopelvic junction, and only when all parts of the conduit above the lumbopelvic junction had reached their compliance limit did the pelvic segment begin to fill. In the lumbar segment no constant points of resistance were encountered. In the pelvic segment the internal iliac artery, the entry of the ureter into the bladder wall and the vesical orifice were in most cases distinct physiologic thresholds but invariably less marked than the lumbopelvic junction.

The extraperistaltic flow was often the predominant type of urinary transport in the recumbent position, capable of continuing for 15–20 min, or more, with perfect equilibrium between inflow and outflow and, by definition, in the complete absence

Fig. 3A–D. Kinetic urography of same pyelocalyceal system as in Fig. 2, showing the subsequent transit, starting in the same period of apnoea 8.66 s after the start in Fig. 2A. **A** Sequence of entire transit recorded as in Fig. 2A. **B** Road map and time-table for transit in **A**. **C** Superposition in topographical coordinate system of pictures at 2.60 s in Fig. 2A (*solid lines*) and Fig. 3A (*dotted lines*). Scale 1:1. **D** Superposition in topographical coordinate system of picture at 2.60 s in Fig. 2A (*solid lines*) and 0.10 s in Fig. 3A (*dotted lines*). Scale 1:1.

Start in fornix 6b at 0.20 s. The primary ring remains completely closed on its transit in branch 6, injecting all the liquid contained in that branch into the lower main branch and branches 4 and 5. At 0.70–0.80 s the ring enters these branches and at 0.80–0.90 s each ring closes off the branch in which it runs. At 1.20 s the ring in branch 5 opens up and the liquid released from that branch rapidly fills the lower main branch up to the primary ring and runs back into branch 6. At 1.50 s the primary ring closes off the PUJ, and the derived ring in the upper main branch closes off that branch and so transforms the upper part of the conduit into a manifold isovolumetric compartment that contains almost all the liquid (6 ml out of the total 7 ml) and which the ring goes on to distend. At 1.80 s the ring closes off branch 3 to a separate isovolumetric compartment, and at 2.10 s the analogous process takes place in branches 2 and 1.

Kinetic Urography

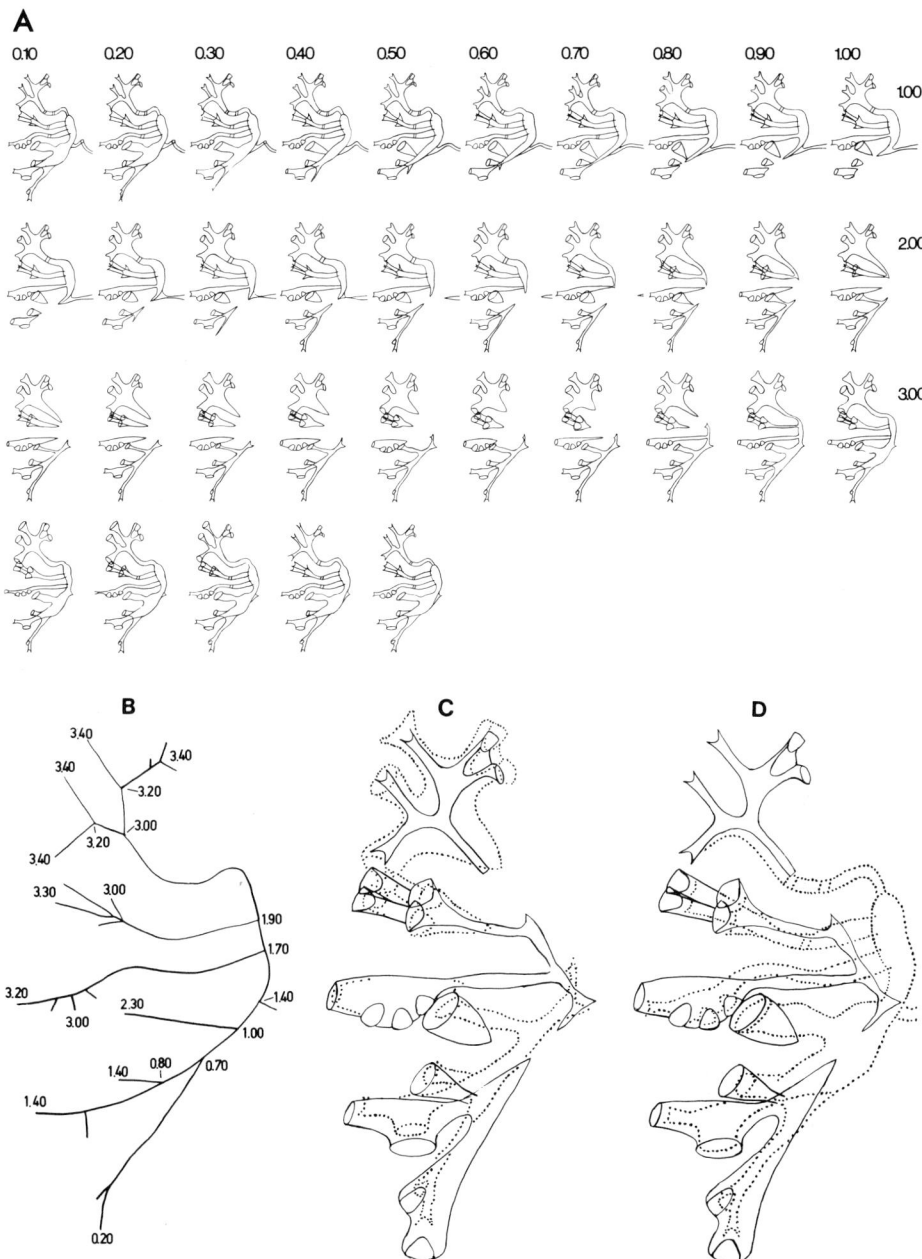

Compare the configuration of branch *1* at this stage with its configuration at the corresponding stage of a transit starting in the opposite pole, i.e. the transit in Fig. 2A, as shown in Fig. 3C. – At 2.60 s the overall redistribution reaches its peak, and at 2.70 s the ring in branch *3* opens up and so initiates the return of the liquid. At 2.90 s the same process takes place in branches *2* and *1*. The return to the precontraction distribution proceeds quickly and is completed at 3.50 s

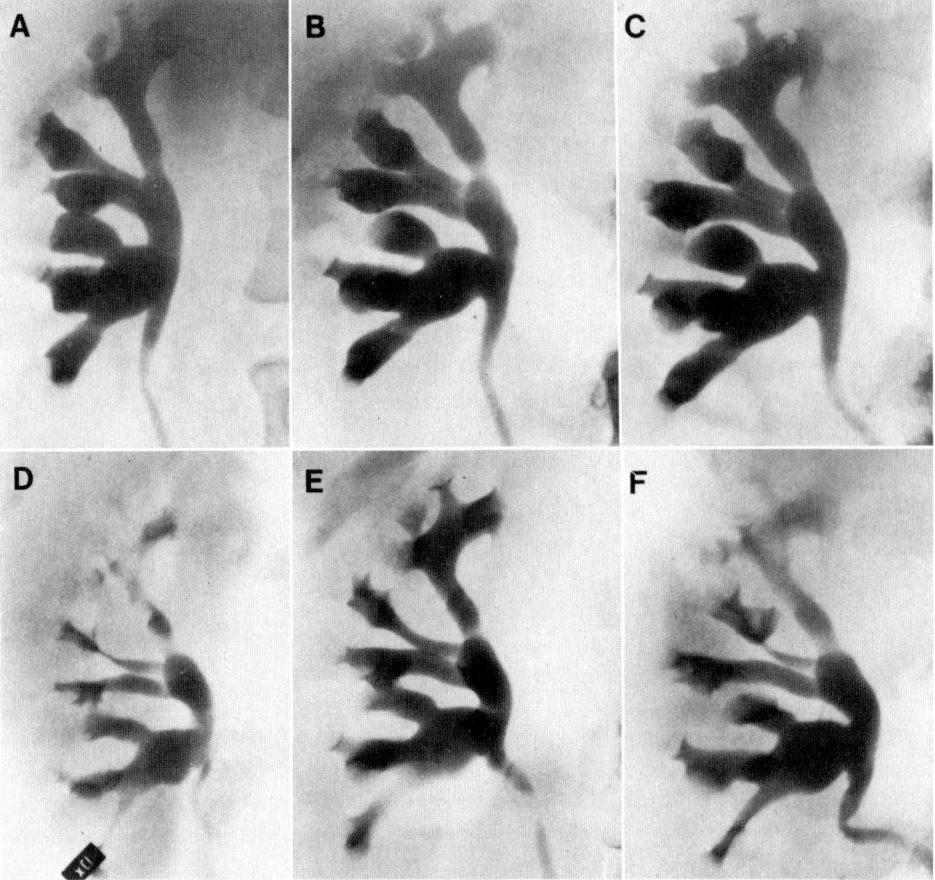

Fig. 4 A–F. Urography of same pyelocalyceal system as in Figs. 2 and 3. Scale 0.65. **A–C** 'Full distension' at ureteral compression. Pyelocalyceal volume 22 ml. **D–F** No ureteral compression. **A** Left anterior oblique projection (about 35°). **B** Frontal projection. **C** Right anterior oblique projection (about 35°). **D** Frontal projection. Volume 7 ml. **E, F** Frontal projection. Volume 11 ml

of contractions in all parts of the urinary system. The contraction ring that put an end to a period of extraperistaltic transport had the same characteristics as any other normal ring.

Morphologic and Physiologic Factors

(1) In the pelvic segment of the ureter the normal contraction ring always remained completely closed for its entire transit. In all the other segments the aperture of the ring proved to vary between complete closure and different degrees of patency. Thus, a completely closed ring running into a cul-de-sac always had to open up at some stage and let the liquid in the cul-de-sac escape; in this situation the contractile force of the ring, i.e. the muscle layer in the segment in question, was cor-

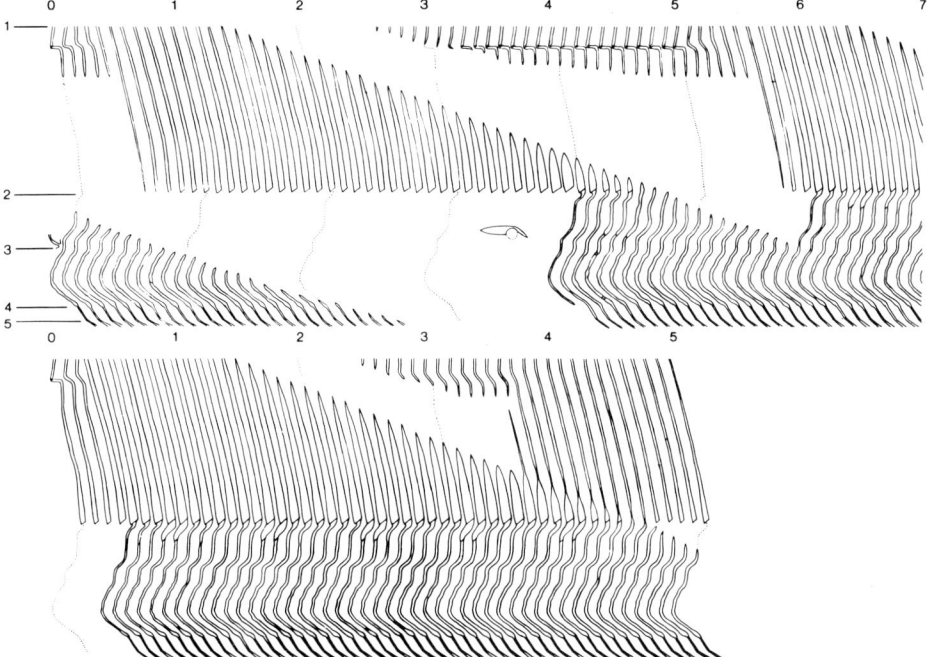

Fig. 5. Kinetic urography of normal ureter. Right side. Scale 1:6. Time in seconds. Interval between reproduced pictures 0.10 s. Upright position. Urinary excretion 1 ml/min/kidney. *1* PUJ; *2* lumbopelvic junction; *3* lower border of right sacroiliac joint; *4* entry of ureter into bladder wall; *5* vesical orifice of ureter.

Upper row: At 0.00 s a contraction ring has just emptied the lumbar segment and advances in the pelvic segment. It injects all the liquid as a jet into the bladder. It leaves the ureter at 2.40 s. – At 0.00 s the front end of the consecutive extraperistaltic column lies 4 cm below the PUJ. At 0.44 s, when the ring is 3 cm above the PUJ, it produces an injection into the ureter. The front end of the column travels at a speed of 90–100 cm/s, opening up the lumbar segment to a circular column with a sharply pointed apex. At 0.50 s it reaches the lumbopelvic junction and stops short. From this moment on the lumen grows only by radial expansion. The front end broadens and adapts to the convexity of the artery. – The ring passes the PUJ at 1.50 s and so initiates the isovolumetric phase in the ureter. It shortens the closed-off segment from 13 cm to 2.6 cm and distends it into a rounded compartment with a maximum diameter of 6.5 mm. At 3.94 s the injection into the pelvic segment sets in. It has the same characteristics as the injection into the lumbar segment. The ring enters the pelvic segment at 4.70 s and proceeds in this segment in the same manner as the preceding ring.

At 5.60 s a new injection from the pyelocalyceal system sets in. It is larger than the preceding one, and the halt at the lumbopelvic junction is merely 0.25 s while the preceding halt lasted for 3.44 s. The new injection into the pelvic segment opens up the preceding ring from behind and merges with the preceding column.

Lower row: 0.00 s corresponds to 17.44 s in the upper row. The entire length of the lumbar segment has been filled by the residual volume and the extraperistaltic flow. At 0.30 s the injection from the pyelocalyceal system produces a displacement pressure wave in the liquid, distending the lumbar segment to its compliance limit and injecting the pelvic segment after a halt of only 0.10 s. The contraction ring passes the PUJ at 1.50 s. It stays completely closed on its transit in the upper portion of the lumbar segment but suddenly it gives way (at 3.60 s) and lets a column of liquid escape backward. The front end of this column runs 6 cm in 0.60 s and merges with the consecutive extraperistaltic column to form a continuous filling in the lumbar segment. Compare Fig. 2 branch *1* 0.30–1.00 s

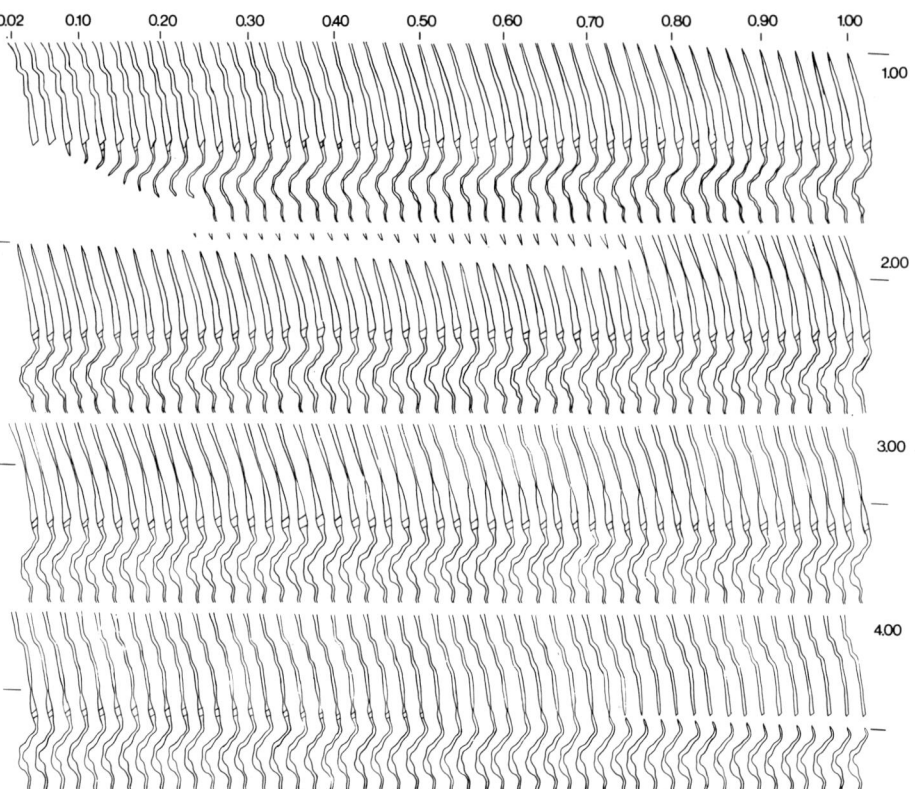

Fig. 6. Kinetic urography of normal ureter. Right side. Scale 1:8. Time in seconds. Interval between reproduced pictures 0.02 s. Supine position. Urinary excretion 3.5 ml/min/kidney. Contraction interval variable; present interval 47 s. Volume in lumbar segment at 0.02 s 3.5 ml. – At 0.06 s injection into pelvic segment. At 0.24 s the liquid enters bladder as a jet. The jet continues until ring leaves ureter at 7.62 s. At 0.74 s contraction ring passes PUJ. Further progress of contraction ring indicated by extensions of its slope in right and left margins. At 1.72 s ring opens up. Refluxing liquid is injected into pyelocalyceal liquid at 1.76 s. Contraction ring passes lumbopelvic junction at 3.72 s. It remains completely closed for its entire transit in pelvic segment. Peak pressure pulse distension of right common iliac artery at 0.64 s, 1.50 s, 2.34 s, and 3.10 s

related with the liquid pressure in the upstream segment. However, the ring in these segments also proved to open up in situations in which the upstream pressure was far lower than in the pelvic segment and yet the ring in that segment remained completely closed. This might indicate that the contractile force of the ring in the pelvic segment, i.e. the force of the muscle layer in that segment, would be greater than in the other segments. As a result of the constantly complete closure of the contraction ring the flow in the pelvic segment lacked the complex properties present in the other segments.

(2) In about 15 per cent of cases the entire lumbar segment of the ureter was filled already in relaxation, communicating freely with the renal pelvis. In conduits of this type the lumbar segment was thus integrated with the pyelocalyceal system

just as the other branches, and the lumbopelvic junction was equivalent to the pyeloureteral junction in conduits lacking this anatomy. The outflow to the pelvic segment was too small in comparison with the volume of liquid remaining in the branch to be capable of exerting any distinctive hydrodynamic effects. In an additional group of about 15 per cent, the communication was lost in the beginning of a period in the upright position but was rapidly reestablished by the extraperistaltic flow. This was also frequently the case for the other branches (Fig. 1). The incorporation of the lumbar segment into the pyelocalyceal system was thus a common and entirely normal anatomical variant. See also Fig. 5 and 6.

(3) The anatomy of the base of the ureter could not be demonstrated to exhibit any anatomical features distinguishing it from the base of any other branch connected to the renal pelvis, nor could any anatomical landmark for the PUJ be found. In default of anatomical landmarks, the complete closure of the contraction ring on its passage across some point in the base of the ureter was used as a provisional landmark, demonstrable only at kinetic urography. In many situations, though, this criterion could not be used, as when the contraction ring stayed completely closed both before and after passing the supposed location of the PUJ at all physiological levels of filling. In contradistinction, the lumbopelvic junction proved to be an anatomical landmark, and one present in all conduits under all conditions. The contraction ring began to close when it was 3–4 mm above the upper (craniolateral) convexity of the artery upon which the ureter rested, and it completed its closure before the convexity turned into the lower (mediocaudal) aspect of the artery. Both the upper and lower aspects of the artery bulging into the ureter were distinct in all situations. The pulsations from the artery were the same as in the other branches but the excursions were much greater than in the pyelocalyceal branches, the ureter bouncing forward and the impression broadening by 2–3 mm, i.e. to occlusion or near-occlusion, each time the artery was injected and distended by the systolic pressure pulse. When the ureter was injected and distended the impression diminished but was never completely levelled out (Figs. 5 and 6), as was usually the case for the arteries crossing the pyelocalyceal branches (Figs. 1, 2 and 3).

The anatomy of the lumbopelvic junction was further examined at laparotomy, at autopsy and in specimens obtained at autopsy, kept in 37° physiological saline and injected with contrast medium. The anatomy was well demarcated under all these conditions. In the specimens the shape remained for several days. In no instance were any narrowings due to stenosis or valves present.

Respiration

The mechanical effects of respiration usually predominated markedly over the mechanical effects of posture, tonus and vascular pulsations, transforming the conduit not only in relaxation but also during a transit. They were much more marked in the recumbent position than in the upright. Already at ordinary calm respiration in the absence of talking, inspiration compressed the parenchyma over the upper and middle calyces and squeezed the liquid out of these into the main branches and the renal pelvis proper and further into the lower main branch and its calyces and the lumbar segment. The upper and middle calyces were often almost completely evacuated and so the injection into the other branches often amounted to 3–4 ml.

During each expiration the liquid returned to the distribution before the onset of the inspiration. The pressure variations were parallel with the displacements and ranged between 2 and 5 mm Hg. When the apex of the liquid lay in the lumbar segment of a ureter of ordinary width (compliance) it moved regularly with the respiration, typical excursions being 2–3 cm. When the filling was continuous from the calyces to the lumbopelvic junction and the lumbar segment contained typically 1.5 ml at expiration, the filling on inspiration increased to 2.5–3 ml, and the lower main branch filled in analogous manner. The pressure in the lumbar segment was the same as in the other branches and varied according to the same pattern.

When a subject held his breath without straining the displacements stopped and the entire urinary conduit remained immobile with the exception of the vascular pulsations. When apnoea was induced in full expiration the shape and dimensions of each segment and hence of the entire conduit were thus very different from those at apnoea in full inspiration. These anatomical differences were often so extensive and so radical that from a hydrodynamic point of view there was actually one branched conduit in expiration and a categorically different branched conduit in inspiration. When a start took place the progress of the contraction ring was of course identical in expiration and inspiration. In contradistinction, the hydrodynamic development of all the phases was radically different.

During a period of extraperistaltic flow the filling of the lumbar segment grew evenly and so the distension at the lumbopelvic junction increased for each inspiration. At a certain point the inspiratory distension drove a small portion of liquid across the artery. The pressure rise just above the artery was the usual rise in relaxation, thus 2–5 mm Hg, whereas the corresponding rise in the peristaltic injection across the artery was 15–20 mm Hg. Subsequently the filling of the pelvic segment proceeded at a regular slow pace, quite distinct from the peristaltic injection but with the characteristic halts of the apex at the usual physiologic thresholds in the pelvic segment, i.e. the internal iliac artery and the entry of the ureter into the bladder wall. During extraperistaltic flow the liquid flowed into the bladder at a low pressure and not as the jet produced by the peristaltic contraction ring.

When straining, particularly in inspiration, most normal subjects readily raised the pressure in the urinary conduit to 50–60 mm Hg. The compression of the kidney and the evacuation were analogous to those at ordinary inspiration. In certain conduits the extent of the evacuation was the same as on ordinary inspiration but usually it comprised all the pyelocalyceal branches and occurred as a rapid and voluminous injection into the lumbar segment. If the pyelocalyceal filling was sufficiently large a similar period of straining produced a large injection into the pelvic segment and into the bladder. This was thus one of the normal types of urinary transport to the bladder in the absence of contractions. Still larger emptying to the bladder was first observed accidentally during unrestrained laughter and subsequently reproduced in normal subjects during repeated coughs and/or laughter. In certain conduits (but not in all) these manoeuvres resulted in an explosive evacuation, the apex of the liquid travelling from the upper portion of the lumbar segment to the bladder in 0.08–0.10 s (=about 200 cm/s), thus faster than so far observed for the ordinary peristaltic injection, and reducing the pyelocalyceal volume from 15 ml to 2 or 3 ml in 10–15 s. It will be obvious that the patient's control of his (her) respiration is essential to the performance of the examination.

Posture

The impulse conduction was the same in the upright and recumbent positions while the morphodynamics displayed a number of characteristic and consistent differences. When a subject stood up the kidneys took part in the general rearrangement and changes in shape that accompanied the descent of the abdominal organs and structures. The respiratory excursions of the kidneys were always far smaller in the upright than in the recumbent position, with correspondingly smaller respiratory variations in shape. As a function of the more slender dimensions of all the branches in the upright position the inspiratory displacement into the lower main branch and its polar branches was reduced.

Tonus

The tonus consisted of a longitudinal component and a component involving circular and oblique muscle fibres. When a subject rose from the recumbent position tonus increased and remained at the higher level until the subject lay down, and at that moment it returned to the lower level. The transitions occurred within 5–6 s. An increase in the tonus from the upright to the recumbent position was not observed in any segment in any situation. The degree of tonus in the recumbent position could thus not be directly determined with kinetic urography only. In 100 subjects with normal urinary conduits on both sides the tonic contraction occurred on the right side in 72 per cent and on the left side in 82 per cent.

The longitudinal tonic contraction produced a shortening of segments that were sinuous in relaxation in the recumbent position. The shortening was usually proportional to the degree of preexisting sinuosity. The curves were generally shortened to a nearly straight configuration. Unlike the peristaltic longitudinal contraction (q.v.) the tonic contraction was not observed to shorten already straight segments. The most extensive shortening occurred in conduits with marked sinuosity of the upper half of the lumbar segment of the ureter, a 10 cm long sinuous portion being capable of shortening to a nearly straight length of 6 cm. The shortening of the pyelocalyceal branches typically amounted to 25–30 per cent of the precontraction length.

In the manifold junctions of the pyelocalyceal system and of bifid ureters the circular and oblique contractions proved to achieve an extensive transformation of the anatomy, identical with that developing over time through the action of the contraction ring. In Fig. 1, the circular and oblique fibres as well as the longitudinal participate in the contraction of the renal pelvis that takes place when the subject rises from the recumbent position (A–C) to the upright position (D), but some longitudinal and oblique fibres contract the lateral portion of the triangular renal pelvis to such an extent that they turn into transverse circular fibres in the newly formed lower main branch. The existence of this branch is apparent in the upright position only (Fig. 1 A–F).

The contribution of the circular and oblique tonic contraction to the reduction of the circumference of unbranched segments was usually difficult to determine with kinetic urography alone because the reduction was almost evenly distributed over the whole length of the segment. Thus, when the diameter of the ureter and the pyelocalyceal branches diminished from, say, 3 mm to 1 mm in a urinary conduit that emptied from 6 ml to 1 ml after a shift from the recumbent to the upright position, as occurs in Fig. 1 from B to D, the adaptation of the wall to the reduced volume might also involve the compliance and elasticity of other elements than the muscle layer. However, in an ordinary slender urinary conduit, such as the one in Fig. 1, an isolated column of liquid of 0.06 ml driven ahead by the peristaltic contraction ring in the ureter in the recumbent position extended over a length of 3 cm and expanded the wall to a luminal diameter of 1.6 mm whereas in the upright position the column was 10 cm long and had a diameter of 0.9 mm. This great change in the compliance of the wall to radial expansion indicates a significant participation of the muscle layer. Compare also the contractile force of the peristaltic ring in relation to the passively distended segment.

Peristalsis

The Longitudinal Contraction (Figs. 2, 3, 5)

The longitudinal contraction occurred as part of the tonus (q.v.) and as a peristaltic contraction coupled to the progress of the ring. It was present in all urinary conduits but its magnitude varied greatly with the anatomy of the conduit, being directly proportional to the degree of sinuosity and inversely proportional to the degree of fixation of the extremities of a given segment. It preceded the contraction ring by 0.2–1.5 s, usually by 0.5–1.0 s, and remained after the passage of the ring for 0.5–0.8 s.

The typical pattern for the longitudinal contraction can be followed in Figs. 2 and 3. In Fig. 2 all the branches that can be straightened out are indeed straightened out, the greatest shortening involving the branches that are most sinuous in relaxation, i.e. branches 1, 2 and 3 and the uppermost segment of the ureter. At 1.20 s branches 2 and 3 are straight but from this moment on the straight branches continue to shorten further, pulling the upper main branch toward their fornices. At 2.60 s branch 2 has shortened from a precontraction length of 35 mm to 27 mm and branch 3 from 42 to 33 mm. As can be seen (Fig. 3D) the shortening involved displacement only of the medial end, attached to the highly mobile upper main branch whereas the lateral end, attached to the parenchyma, was not pulled medially. (It is actually displaced laterally with the papillae but this is due to a different mechanism, the peristaltic injection.) Shortening of an already straight segment occurred mainly in the pyelocalyceal branches, and when these were nearly straight in relaxation it was the main manifestation of the longitudinal contraction.

When the longitudinal contraction engaged a segment with one end comparatively firmly fixed, as a calyceal branch attached to the papilla, the shortening involved the entire segment simultaneously and uniformly. This would imply that the impulse conduction of the longitudinal contraction might involve each segment as a unit, thus proceeding stepwise from one segment to the next in a fashion quite different from the stepless progression of the contraction ring. However, in the sinuous upper portion of the lumbar segment of the ureter the progress of the longitudinal contraction could be directly observed to be continuous. When this portion was markedly sinuous it typically displayed 3 or 4 large U-shaped curves with a transverse crest-trough distance of 1–2 cm, with a total length of 11–12 cm and winding in the sagittal plane as well as in the frontal. When the longitudinal contraction entered at the upper end of this portion it began by taking up the slack of the first curve and did not proceed to the second curve until the first one had been almost straightened out, the same procedure being repeated for the ensuing curves. Finally the whole segment was nearly straight and only 6 cm long. The same mechanism can be seen to apply to long segments in the pyelocalyceal system. For instance, the segment in Fig. 2 extending from branch 1 to fornix 5c is equipped with connecting branches that serve as markers for the longitudinal contraction, namely branches 2 and 3, the ureter, and branches 4, 5a and 6. As can be seen, there is a considerable time overlap between the shortenings of the successive subsegments.

The sinuosities in the upper portion of the lumbar segment of the ureter gradually lead over to the nearly straight lower portion. In this portion no unequivocal longitudinal contractions were observed. In the pelvic segment local sinuosities were present only in the portion of the ureter coursing in front of the internal iliac artery. The longitudinal contraction straightened these curves, although to a far lesser extent than it straightened the curves in the lumbar segment.

The longitudinal contraction gave rise to a small antegrade and retrograde displacement of the liquid but there was no evidence that it might participate in the peristaltic transport. The onset of the longitudinal contraction at any given level occurred at an exactly fixed moment on the schedule of the contraction ring whereas the onset of the injection varied in accordance with the morphodynamic parameters of the peristalsis. Consequently, the onset of the injection was perfectly capable to occur long before as well as long after the onset of the longitudinal contraction.

Ureteral Reptations. The upper part of the lumbar segment of the ureter displayed a type of movements that involved longitudinal contractions but longitudinal contractions which were not concomitant with the transit of the contraction ring but which went on precisely between the transits and also seemed to be confined precisely to the upper part of the lumbar segment. The contractions gave rise to regular periodic reptatory movements of the sinuosities of this part of the ureter. The movements reached their greatest excursions in conduits with U-curves of a high transverse amplitude but sometimes shallow curves made greater excursions. In nearly straight segments the reptations were quite small yet they were quite distinct. Usually the rhythmic pattern was characteristic for each conduit. Thus, in one conduit an outward U-curve with a transverse amplitude of 1 cm would turn at a constant velocity into the corresponding inward curve in the course of 4 s while in another conduit this period would be 3 s. In a third conduit a similar curve would remain stationary for 3 s and then move over to the reciprocal position within one second, the acceleration and deceleration being rapid but invariably gradual. In many cases one pattern would go on for 2 or 3 min and then shift suddenly to a quite different but equally regular pattern, but sometimes the shifts were gradual and consequently more complex. After a period of 4 to 5 min the reptations were usually interrupted by a quiescent period of approximately equal length.

So far no interdependence between the transit of the contraction ring and the reptations has been found. Thus, the reptations occurred with equal temporal distribution in periods of regular transits at a short contraction interval and at long and irregular contraction intervals, and the same pattern went on before and after the passage of a contraction ring. When the precursory longitudinal contraction arrived the reptating curves were successively straightened out in the fashion described for the longitudinal contraction. The reptations were absent while the longitudinal contraction and the ring passed and then resumed.

The Contraction Ring (Figs. 1, 2, 3, 5, 6)

The Principle for Peristaltic Transport. The contraction ring was the prime mover of the peristaltic morphodynamics. It worked in constant interaction with the non-contracted parts of the wall, the liquid serving to transmit reciprocally the variations in pressure developed by the interaction. In the urinary conduit as in other elastic and compliant tubes the volume of the liquid proved to be an important parameter. The development of the morphodynamic events was determined by the principle for the progress of the contraction ring as applied to the anatomy of the individual urinary conduit.

Thus, in the course of its progress over the conduit the ring displaced the liquid in its own direction of travel, leaving the segments traversed more or less drained of liquid while injecting the liquid from these segments into the segments lying ahead of it. The farther the ring travelled the more it built up the forward accumulation (injection). The accumulation induced distension of the wall (mural stretch) and the response of the wall to the distension was to impart immediately a reciprocal pressure rise in the liquid, acting back on the ring. The ring thus had to meet the gradually increasing resistance created by its own action. The distension of the wall was accompanied by a simultaneous parallel rise in the liquid pressure. The liquid pressure within a segment in muscular contraction was lower than that in a passively distended segment. In other words, the liquid reacted only to the shape of the conduit and not to the state of muscular contraction of its wall, so the liquid pressure did not in itself give any indication about the presence or absence of a muscular contraction, although the peristaltic contraction always formed a narrow segment.

The Aperture of the Contraction Ring. The contraction ring could close completely in any part of the urinary conduit, thus dividing one communicating vessel into two or several non-communicating hydrodynamic conduits. The completely closed ring drove all the liquid before it ahead and so it had a forward propulsive effect of 100 per cent.

When the ring was not completely closed its aperture could vary between almost complete closure and different degrees of patency. The hydrodynamic function of the patent ring was that of a stenosis, its propulsive effect being synonymous with the obstructive effect of a stenosis and so directly proportional to the degree of its reduction of the cross-sectional area of a given segment. The segment lying ahead of a patent ring and which the ring injects and distends was thus the high-pressure hydrodynamic upstream segment whereas in the narrow segment, i.e. the patent ring, the pressure was at its lowest level and in the downstream segment behind the ring it was intermediate.

The faculty of the contraction ring to close completely in any segment does not mean that it could in all situations close completely for the entire transit in a given segment. For instance, a contraction ring travelling toward the cul-de-sac of a calyx always had to open up at a certain stage. This is of course a necessity: if the ring could remain completely closed all the way out to the papilla the fornix would have to rupture. On the other hand, while the "same" ring travelled the same segment in the opposite direction, i.e. travelling antegrade after having been emitted in a fornix of that segment, it proved perfectly capable of remaining completely closed from the start and on the entire transit in that segment. In one further situation the contraction ring sometimes but not invariably had to open up in this way, namely while running toward the lumbopelvic junction and working against the pressure in the liquid trapped between the artery and itself. This mechanism was present in all situations in certain conduits while in other conduits it proved to be absent in certain situations.

The completely closed ring could be forced to open up at different distances from a given cul-de-sac under different conditions, not only in the end segments but also in intermediate segments. All intermediate segments in the pyelocalyceal system are potential end segments and the lumbar segment of the ureter functions as a hydrodynamic end segment in many situations, the only intermediate segment always provided with an outlet at its far end thus being the pelvic segment of the ureter.

In the absence of an overtaking injection from behind, the flow within the patent ring was always directed from the upstream segment downstream. Thus, the forward propulsive effect of the patent ring was always lower than that of the corresponding completely closed ring. When the aperture was small the effect was close to 100 per cent, decreasing with increasing aperture but remaining positive from the opening point to the point where the backward flow equalled the speed of the ring. At this point the net flow reversed and below this point the ring instead exerted a backward propulsive effect.

The opening point represents a distinct turning point, transforming two closed-off conduits into one. In contrast, the net flow reversal point is merely a level of the gradually increasing or decreasing flow. It does not exert any local effects, yet it exerts distinct effects on the upstream and downstream segments of the communicating vessel, evolving over time.

The Contractile Force. When the precontraction filling of a given segment was the same throughout a series of transits with the same starting point, all the morphodynamic factors proved nearly identical throughout that period. This regularity indicates that the muscle layer in a given segment may always apply the same contractile force at a given filling. When the filling was increased, as by perfusion, and was subsequently kept constant, the aperture of the ring widened and subsequently remained constant at the new level. This indicates that the contractile force applied did not increase parallel with the increased resistance and that it might not increase at all but might instead remain constant for all degrees of resistance. In our experience the regularity of these morphodynamic parameters, in the first place the shape of the contraction ring and the distension of the upstream segment as developing over time, have proven useful and sensitive indicators of the pressure variations in the urinary conduit.

The morphodynamic parameters displayed this constancy during periods of regular short contraction intervals, such as 4.25 s, as well as at long contraction intervals, such as 25 s. Thus there were no signs that the higher frequency of neurogenous stimulation induced alterations in the contractile force.

A ring resulting from a meeting of two rings could be expected to display morphological characteristics due to a possible summation of the neurogenous stimulation. Rings were not observed to meet head-on at exactly the same point for repeated transits, and even shifts in the meeting point as small as 2–3 mm transformed the morphodynamic development to such an extent that no two transits were strictly comparable with regard to the shape of the combined ring at a head-on meeting. In contrast, the shape of each ring after a head-on meeting proved not to differ from the shape of the same ring running the same segment without having gone through a meeting. There were thus no signs of any alteration of the force of contraction attributable to a possible refractory state that might have been induced by the reciprocal ring running the same segment in the opposite direction before the meeting, i.e. well within the shortest refractory period as yet observed for consecutive starts in a given fornix, viz. 4.25 s.

The shape of two rings that run convergent courses and coincide at the junction of two branches might also be expected to be different from that of either ring travelling the same segments as a single ring. Such meetings were frequent in all branches, including the ureter. No alteration was observed.

The Injection of a Segment as a Function of Its Distance from the Starting Point. The amount of liquid displaced by the ring was directly proportional to the distance travelled by the ring. Since the starts alternated over the set of fornices in a given pyelocalyceal system, the distance travelled by the ring was different for starts at different locations, and the development of the hydrodynamic events at a given location varied accordingly. Thus, when the ring started in a fornix close to a given cul-de-sac it gathered only a small amount of liquid on its way and the injection into the cul-de-sac was small, as it is in branch 5 in Fig. 3 after a start in the nearby fornix 6 b (Fig. 3 A–D). On the other hand, when the ring started in a fornix at a greater distance from the same cul-de-sac, as in Fig. 2, it gathered a larger amount of liquid on its way. Accordingly, the injection into the end segment and its cul-de-sac began at an earlier stage of the transit and the amount interposed between the two opposing forces, the ring and the cul-de-sac, occupied much longer segments of the conduit. At a great starting-point–cul-de-sac distance, thus, the injection and its effects, the wall distension and the pressure rise, were more marked and more long-lasting than at a short distance.

(a) Starts in reciprocal polar fornices: In a pyelocalyceal system of ordinary anatomy the upper, middle and lower main branch and their tributary branches each constitutes a more or less separate manifold conduit, and usually the upper and lower systems are anatomically similar and approximately symmetrical, forming two functionally analogous and reciprocal but topographically opposite counterparts. The intermediate branches, on the other hand, are not arranged as equivalent counterparts but rather the relatively large middle main branch faces the more slender ureter. In accordance with the increase of the distension as a function of the distance travelled by the ring, a start in the upper pole brings about a peak filling of the lower pole branches, as occurs in Fig. 2, while a start in the lower pole brings about a peak filling of the upper pole branches, as occurs in Fig. 3. The geometric principle for the progress of the ring is the same in both instances and the hydrodynamic events developing by the application of this principle are the same as well but they are also the reverse of each other as a function of the opposite location of the starting point. The filling of the polar branches, which lie at the greatest distances from each other, was thus the opposite for starts in the opposite poles, being either maximum or minimum, while the filling of the intermediate branches, including the ureter, was intermediate for starts in either pole, with correspondingly smaller variations. (Needless to say, the effects were never perfectly symmetrical but varied with the type and extent of the asymmetry of a given system.) The location of the starting point thus proved to be the main determinant of the volume injected into the ureter as well as into any other branch at any given transit, hence the main factor in the regulation of the urinary transport.

(b) Starts in intermediate branches: When a start occurred in a fornix belonging to an intermediate branch, in the pyelocalyceal system in Fig. 2 thus any of branches 2, 3 or 4 (a common middle main branch is not present), the ring propelled only a small amount of liquid from the emitting branch into the confluence of the main branches and further into the branches opening from the confluence. The ureter then received a very large part of that amount, whereas the injection into each of the upper and lower main branches was approximately equal and thus smaller than after a start in either of the polar regions. In this instance the polar systems were thus exposed to the same conditions not only with regard to impulse conduction but with regard to hydrodynamics as well, and the derived ring in each one of the symmetrical polar systems propelled the same comparatively small amount into a manifold whose preexisting filling was the same as that of the opposite one, the anatomy, the impulse conduction and the hydrodynamic development in each being the mirror image of the other one.

(c) Subintrant starts: A second instance of symmetry occurred when two starts took place simultaneously in both opposite poles. (The starts were not observed to be exactly simultaneous but a time lag below 0.5 s generally gave rise to the development described below. This time lag applied, for instance, to the pyelocalyceal system in Fig. 2 when the first start took place in the upper pole as well as vice versa.) When the two approaching rings were approximately in the upper part of each main branch, as in Fig. 2 at 1.00 s and in Fig. 3 at the same point in time, the portions of liquid propelled from the polar regions met in the main branches and distended these but at this stage each of the opposing rings managed to keep completely closed or nearly so, and so it prevented the liquid from being injected into the polar branches behind it. Rather than entering the blocked polar branches the liquid filled the open branches between the opposing rings in proportionally larger amounts. In this situation the intermediate branches received the largest injections observed in them, nearly as large as the maximum filling of the polar branches on one-way transits. The receptive capacity of the intermediate end segments being limited, the greatest outflow developed in the ureter, leading to the largest ureteral injections so far observed. When the opposing rings came closer together the liquid that had not yet been injected into the ureter still had enough resistance to force each one of the rings to open up, and this occurred at a much earlier stage than at the corresponding one-way transit. When the rings opened up some liquid escaped across their aperture into the drained polar regions but the filling of these was, at this stage, much less than on one-way transits. The two primary rings subsequently coincided at the PUJ and coalesced. They closed completely at the passage across the PUJ, but did not manage to do this in the intermediate end branches which were already filled to capacity when the rings entered their base. After the meeting each ring continued its transit in the reciprocal polar branches according to the impulse conduction.

The mechanism for the peristaltic injections and the progressive accumulation as a function of the distance travelled by the ring was tested by exchanging one of the ordinary catheters used in transparenchymal manometry for a larger catheter with its tip placed in the cul-de-sac of a calyx. For instance, a catheter with an outer diameter of 2.10 mm and an inner diameter of 1.70 mm and inserted via the papilla of fornix 5c filled nearly the entire width of the lumen of branch 5 in Fig. 2 in relaxation. When the catheter was kept closed the extraperistaltic flow slowly accumulated between the wall and the catheter but when the catether was left open the wall fitted snugly around it and the extraperistaltic flow passed freely from the calyx into the catheter and exited at its open end at relaxation pressure. When a start occurred in fornix 5c there was no distension of branch 5 whether the catheter was closed or open, i.e. the morphodynamics were as usual. When a start occurred in a reciprocal fornix, as in fornix 1d in Fig. 2, and the catheter was kept closed the calyx and its cul-de-sac were injected and distended as usual, as they do for instance in Fig. 2 from 1.80 s to 3.25 s. When the catheter was opened before the injection set in, as when the contraction ring travelled in branch 1 in Fig. 2, calyx 5 was injected but the distension did not come about. Instead the injected liquid passed on into the catheter and exited at its open end as a jet reaching 18–20 mm H_2O. In this way the end segment was thus transformed into an intermediate segment, the catheter being the extension of the intermediate segment and similar to the pelvic segment of the ureter.

(d) Asymmetrical pyelocalyceal systems: When the branches of either polar region were small and those of the opposite pole were large, starts in the smaller polar system resulted in a small accumulation in the main branches and a proportionally small injection into the opposite polar system as well as into the ureter, whereas starts in the larger polar system resulted in a small injection into the opposite polar system and a proportionally large injection into the ureter. In pyelocalyceal systems with this asymmetrical anatomy, therefore, the variations in the volume injected into the ureter with the starting point were greater than in the common symmetrical type. A catheter introduced into a polar branch, as described above for the conduit in Fig. 2, transforms a symmetrical pyelocalyceal system into an asymmetrical system by establishing a steal from the branches of the pole in question, as is also the case for ordinary nephrostomies applied to a lower or upper pole branch.

The Injection of a Segment as a Function of the Pyelocalyceal Volume. The pyelocalyceal volume of about 7 ml in Figs. 2 and 3 was the ordinary pyelocalyceal volume at upright equilibrium for this conduit. It was also its smallest volume under physiological conditions. The corresponding moderate pyelocalyceal volume was between 12 ml (in the recumbent position at regular short contraction intervals) and 14 ml (in the recumbent position at contraction intervals of 3 min or more). At a moderate volume the distribution of the liquid between the different segments in relaxation was similar to that at a small volume (branch 1 is an exception, being relatively more voluminous at a moderate pyelocalyceal volume), the filling of each branch thus being about twice the small volume. The contraction ring thus met a relatively large amount of liquid at a shorter distance from its starting point and injected a proportionally larger amount into farther branches that were already relatively well-filled. The cul-de-sacs were injected and distended to their compliance limit at an earlier stage and responded by a backward resistance that met the ring at a correspondingly earlier stage. After a start in fornix 1 d, as in Fig. 2, branches 5 and 6 reached their peak distension at about 1.80 s, i.e. one second earlier than at the small volume present in Fig. 2. The ring managed to stay completely closed on its transit in the upper main branch but it could do so only because the adjoining branches could still accommodate some of the liquid. The larger precontraction filling of branches 2 and 3 made them rapidly fill to capacity. At that stage, therefore, the ureter was the only branch offering a free outlet. Consequently the injection into the ureter started earlier than at a small volume (at 1.00 instead of 1.20 s) and reached a higher flow rate and a larger volume. When the primary ring had continued into the ureter at 2.10 s the ring in the lower main branch rapidly met the resistance from the end segments of branches 4, 5 and 6 and had to flare out far more than in Fig. 2. It had to open up already at 2.50 s (cf. Fig. 2 at a small volume), and subsequently did not manage to close completely again at any stage, and the net flow reversal point occurred already at about 2.80–2.90 s. At a moderate pyelocalyceal volume the relative displacement of the liquid was thus smaller and the distension of all the branches was more marked and more protracted than at a small volume, and it stayed at peak level for a much longer time. These effects increased markedly with the starting-point–cul-de-sac distance.

The pyelocalyceal volume of normal conduits did not under physiological conditions exceed the moderate amount present in the recumbent position. However, during perfusion normal conduits reached the same volume and shape as during the "full distension" at urography with ureteral compression (Fig. 4A–C), i.e. a large pyelocalyceal volume obtained without blocking the ureter. In the pyelocalyceal system in Fig. 2 a volume of about 22 ml and the same shape as in Fig. 4A–C was maintained at inflow-outflow equilibrium for about 30 s at an inflow of 0.3 ml/s (= 18 ml/min). During repeated periods the starts occurred regularly in fornix 1 d at a contraction interval of 8.5 s for several minutes of moderate filling as well as during the subsequent perfusion. The timetable for the transit of the contraction ring at a moderate as well as a large filling is that in Fig. 2. At a moderate filling the precontraction pressure in the cul-de-sac of branch 3 was about 5–6 mm Hg and the peak pressure during the peristaltic retrograde injections varied between 15 and 20 mm Hg for different transits. During perfusion the precontraction pressure in the same cul-de-sac was about 24 mm Hg. At the large pyelocalyceal volume the contraction ring remained completely closed in the emitting calyx 1 d and it also closed completely just below the confluence of the calyces of branch 1, as in Fig. 2 at 0.80 s. However, it had to open up already at 0.90 s or 1.00 s. At that stage there was a small additional distension of the already "fully distended" segments lying before the ring and the pressure in the cul-de-sac of branch 3 was about 38–39 mm Hg. Subsequently, the primary ring and the derived rings did not close completely at any stage of the pyelocalyceal transit. The primary ring opened to about 50 per cent of the lumen already in the lower part of branch 1, at about 1.30 s. At that stage it did not have any forward propulsive effect and the redistribution of the liquid within the pyelocalyceal branches was only a small fraction of that at a moderate (or small) volume. However, the injection into the ureter was still larger and faster than at a moderate volume. It set in already at 0.40 to 0.60 s, varying from one transit to another, and the volume injected was regularly close to 2.5 ml. Also, when the primary ring came close to the PUJ it rapidly narrowed and was on all transits completely closed on its passage across the PUJ. At about 1.30 s the pressure in the cul-de-sac of branch 3 reached its peak of about 35 mm Hg. When the ring entered branch 3 it again narrowed to about 50 per cent of the lumen but it soon opened up to 70–80 per cent and achieved only a very small redistribution. The pressure began to drop while the ring opened up and when the ring reached fornix 3 d it had returned to the precontraction level. The further transit in the lower main branch and its tributaries was similar to that in branch 3, the aperture of the rings being about 70–80 per cent of the lumen and the redistribution being minimal.

At a small pyelocalyceal volume, then, the redistribution of the liquid was marked. In the pyelocalyceal system in Fig. 2, the overall displacement was about twice the volume of 7 ml, and during the period 0.50–3.50 s the overall flow was about 3 ml/s. The pyelocalyceal system in Fig. 1 displayed similar values in the recumbent position (B and C), whereas at the still smaller filling in the upright position (D–F) the overall flow was about 6 ml/s.

At a moderate volume of 12 ml the overall displacement was approximately equal to that volume, corresponding to an overall flow of about 1.5 ml/s. The only exception to the relative reduction in flow was the ureter.

At a large volume, finally, the overall displacement was only a few per cent and the peristaltic transport in the pyelocalyceal branches was inefficient, but this did not compromise the injection into the ureter or the peristaltic transport in the ureter.

Segmental Physiologic Characteristics of the Ureter. The chief effects on the peristaltic transport in the ureter caused by its division into the lumbar and pelvic segments are accounted for in Figs. 5 and 6.

References

Engelmann TW (1869) Zur Physiologie des Ureter. Pflügers Arch Ges Physiol 2:243–293
Kiil F (1957) The Function of the ureter and renal pelvis. Saunders, Philadelphia London, vol 43, pp 80–94
Kiil F (1973) Urinary flow and ureteral peristalsis. In: Lutzeyer W, Melchior H (eds) Urodynamics. Upper and lower urinary tract. Springer, Berlin Heidelberg New York, pp 57–68
Leb A (1930) Die Röntgenpyeloskopie. Fortschr Röntgenstr 42:291–311
Legueu F, Fey B, Truchot P (1927) La pyéloscopie. Maloine, Paris
Narath PA (1954) The physiology of the renal pelvis and the ureter. In: Campbell MF (ed) Urology. Saunders, Philadelphia, pp 61–79
Ohlson L (1972) The Expansion of the uterus in pregnancy analyzed by a topographical coordinate system. Radiographic, anatomical, and statistical studies of the ovarian vessels, the ureters, and associated structures. Medical Thesis, Stockholm
Ohlson L (1982) The principles of impulse conduction in the normal upper urinary tract. 4th Meeting of the International Society for Dynamics of the Upper Urinary Tract, Utrecht
Ohlson L, Fernström I (1981) Le péristaltisme normal des voies urinaires supérieures. XVth International Congress of Radiology, Brussels, Abstracts, Section 1, p 591
Tanagho EA, Meyers FH (1971) Ureteral peristaltic activity. In: Boyarsky S, Gottschalk CW, Tanagho EA, Zimskind PD (eds) Urodynamics. Hydrodynamics of the ureter and renal pelvis. Academic Press, New York London, pp 119–124

The Reproducibility of the Pressure-Flow Relationship in the Normal Upper Urinary Tract of the Pig*

J. MORTENSEN, J. C. DJURHUUS, S. BISBALLE, and H. LAURSEN[1]

The widespread use of reconstructive surgery in the management of upper urinary tract dilatations has created a need for diagnostic procedures by which it will be possible to discriminate between a stable and a progressive dilatation. In 1965 clinical use of urodynamics in the upper urinary tract was introduced (Bäcklund et al. 1965). The theory of the investigation was that an obstructed system would show a high pressure response to a given flow rate in contrast to a non-obstructed system. Later the method was standardized with regard to flow rate and normal ranges were outlined (Whitaker 1973). In the following years several reports in favour of using this urodynamic test were published (Pfister 1982; Whitaker 1978, 1982). Unfortunately documentation of the predictive value of this method is still not available. On the contrary several reports question its value. Clinical investigations have shown that a low pressure response system may exist in spite of progressive disease (Coolsaet et al. 1980; Djurhuus et al. 1982) and that a high pressure response may be present in spite of stable kidney function (Kinn 1981). Experimental investigations have shown that the normal range of pressures in the multicalyceal system of the pig clearly exceeds the clinically accepted normal range (Mortensen et al. 1983), and furthermore do partial experimental obstructions not always exhibit an obstructive pressure flow response in spite of progressive disease (Koff and Thrall 1981).

The reason for the discrepancy between the results of these investigations and the interpretation of the pressure flow test might be inconsistency of intraindividual measurements. In order to elucidate this question we performed a study of the reproducibility of the pressure flow relationship in a pig model.

Material and Methods

Nine upper urinary tract systems of 9 female pigs of Danish Landrace breed comprised the material. They weighed 32–45 kg at the first investigation and showed a weight gain of 0–3 kg at the second investigation two weeks later. All pigs were preoperatively fasted for the last 24 hours, but had access to 2 litres of water. All investigations were performed under general anaesthesia induced by Ketalar (ketamin NFN) 10 mg/kg i.m. and maintained with Halothane 1.5–2% in oxygen in a semiclosed system which allowed spontaneous respiration of the pig. Core tem-

---

* Supported by a grant from the Danish Medical Research Council No. 12-0727.
[1] Institute of Experimental Clinical Research, University of Aarhus, Aarhus County Hospital, DK-8000 Aarhus C

perature was continuously measured transrectally. By a midline incision from the symphysis pubis to the xiphoid process the kidney and the proximal part of the ureter were exposed retroperitoneally. Urine samples for culture were aspirated by puncture of the bladder which then was opened in the midline and kept open throughout the investigation. Through the uretero-vesical orifice two 6-F catheters were guided one by one up into the renal pelvis so that the proximal tip penetrated the renal parenchyma. They were then withdrawn until the distal tip with side and end holes lay in the renal pelvis. One of the catheters was connected to a Siemens 746 strain gauge transducer and amplifier keeping the transducer at the level of the kidney and the other to a roller pump. One 8-F catheter with side and end holes for urine collection was placed in the distal part of the ureter. After a resting period of 30 min measurements were performed.

Measurement Procedure

After measurements of the baseline pressure and diuresis for 10 minutes the urine collection catheter was removed. During continuous registration of the pressure the pelvis was perfused with 2, 4, 6, 8, 10 and 20 ml/min. Isotonic saline heated to 37 °C was used as perfusion fluid and the perfusion rate was increased when the pelvic pressure had been stable for 5 min.

At the conclusion of the investigation the catheters were removed, the bladder was closed in two layers with continuous 3-0 catgut and finally the abdominal wall was closed in three layers. During the first postoperative week the animals were treated with ampicillin 1 g i. m. daily.

Two weeks later the second investigation was performed. The same anaesthesia and surgical technique as in the first investigation were undertaken.

Urine for culture was aspirated from the bladder by puncture. During the second operation the pressure flow measurements were repeated three times with an interval of ½ hour between measurements. Each time the baseline diuresis was measured together with the baseline pressure. The first measurement during the second investigation was used for the long-term reproducibility study. The material thus comprises 9 units which are to elucidate the long-term reproducibility of the pressure flow relationship as well as 9 units for the short-term reproducibility.

For analysis the lowest pressure between peristaltic contractions at stable level was used. The baseline pressure as well as the mean of the pressures during perfusion were used for the analysis.

Results

All urine cultures were sterile and the animals showed macroscopically normal upper urinary tracts in both investigations. The baseline diuresis varied between 0.15 and 1.0 ml/ureter/min. The differences in baseline diuresis between the two investi-

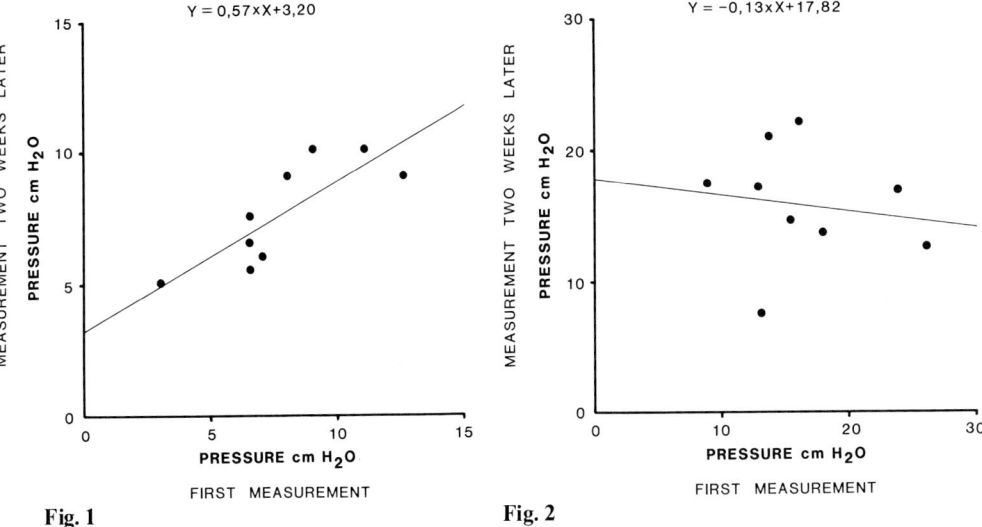

Fig. 1. The correlation (R=0.81) between renal pelvic baseline pressures with a time interval of 2 weeks in 9 renal pelvis units of the pig

Fig. 2. The relationship between pressures during perfusion with a time interval of 2 weeks in 9 renal pelvis units of the pig. The correlation factor was 0.16

gations of the long-term reproducibility were up to 0.60 ml/ureter/min and of the short-term reproducibility up to 0.50 ml/ureter/min, but these differences did not have any correlation to the level of the baseline pressure. The temperature varied initially between 36 and 37.5 °C and showed a decrease during the investigation of maximally 1 °C.

In the first investigation the baseline pressure in the pelvis varied between 3.0 and 12.5 cm H_2O (mean 7.8 cm H_2O) and in the second investigation two weeks later between 5.0 and 10 cm H_2O (mean 7.6 cm H_2O). Figure 1 shows that a good correlation was found between the baseline pressure of the two investigations (R=0.81). The correlation between the mean perfusion pressures at the two investigations was 0.16 (Fig. 2). Furthermore, the mean low flow correlation (2–4 ml/min) was 0.35 and the mean high flow correlation (10–20 ml/min) was 0.04.

In the investigations on the same day the baseline pressure in pelvis varied from 5.0 to 10.0 cm H_2O (mean 7.6 cm H_2O), from 5.0 to 11.0 cm H_2O (mean 7.8 cm H_2O) and from 4.5 to 12.0 cm H_2O (mean 7.8 cm H_2O), respectively. Figure 3 shows the relationship between the baseline pressures in the first and the second investigation on the same day where the correlation coefficient was 0.94, and Fig. 4 shows the relationship between the first and the third investigation where the correlation coefficient was 0.96. Figure 5 shows the relationship between mean perfusion pressures at the first and the second investigation where the correlation coefficient was 0.88 and Fig. 6 the relationship between the first and third investigation where the correlation coefficient was 0.84.

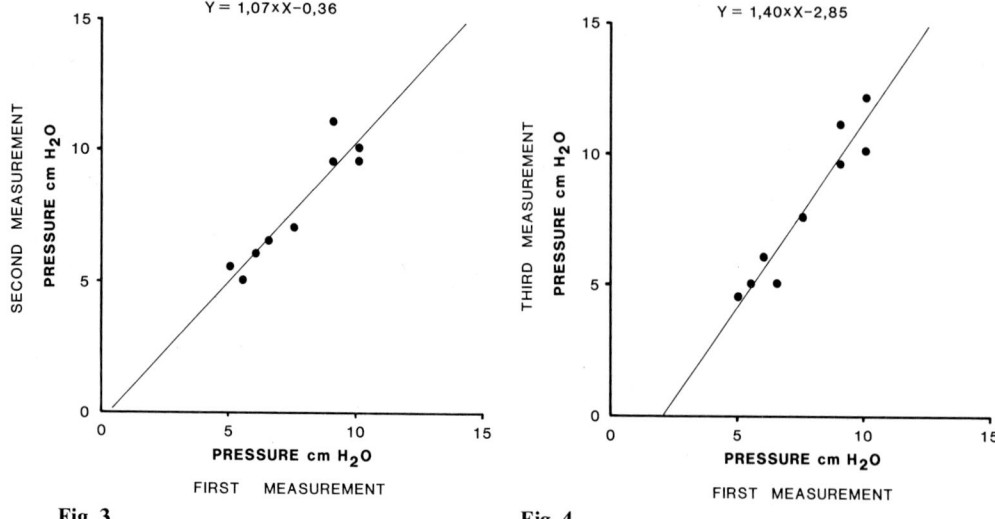

Fig. 3. The relationship between renal pelvic baseline pressures at the first and the second examination on the same day with a time interval of approximately 1.5 hours. The correlation factor was 0.94

Fig. 4. The relationship between resting pressures in renal pelvis at the first and the third examination on the same day. Time interval was approximately 3 hours. The correlation factor was 0.96

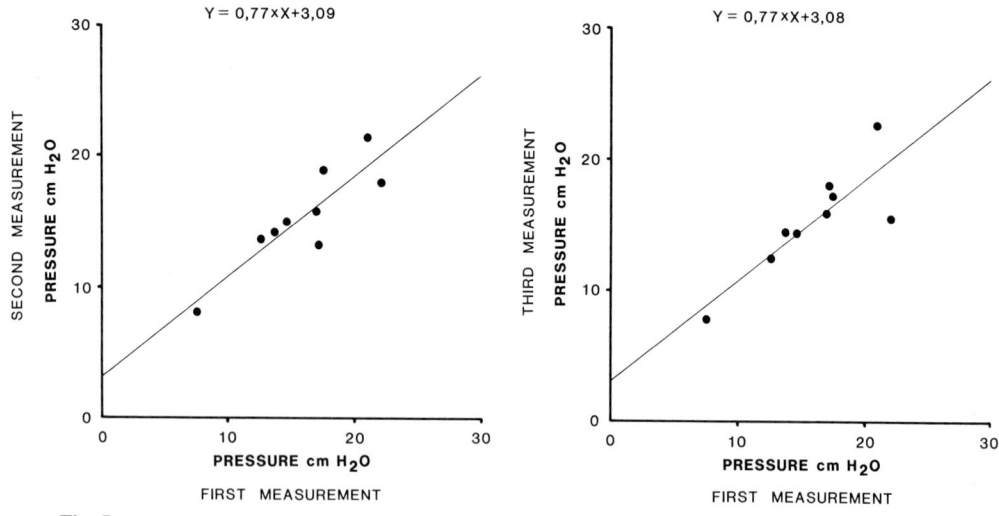

Fig. 5. The relationship between mean perfusion pressures at the first and the second examination with a time interval of 1.5 hours. The R-factor was 0.88

Fig. 6. The relationship between mean perfusion pressures at the first and the third examination on the same day with a time interval of approximately 3 hours. The R-factor was 0.84

Discussion

In order to make sure that the two sets of observations obtained with an interval of two weeks are comparable a few conditions must be fulfilled. Firstly the measuring equipment and the pump used must be identical in both investigations. Secondly artefacts induced by the surgical intervention in the first investigation must not influence the second investigation in any measurable way. Thirdly, any possible influence on the investigation by increase in weight and age of the animals must be minimal, and fourthly, all animals must be subjected to the same preoperative preparation.

The measuring equipment and the calibration was identical in both investigations. The possible artefacts induced by the first operation are obstruction and infection. Bacterial infection is known to cause alterations of the normal peristaltic activity (Boyarsky et al. 1978; Weiss and Biancani 1981). Both obstruction and infection might therefore change the transport mechanism of the upper urinary tract and thereby change the results from the first investigation to the second. Apart from the normal healing procedure, which made it more difficult to expose the kidney a second time, all cases showed normal macroscopic appearance, and the urine was sterile in all cases. Therefore, the surgical intervention in the first investigation seems to be of only minor importance. The weight of the animals was almost stable between the investigations and should therefore be of little importance to the outcome of the investigation. Finally the preparation of the animals made the systems comparable in both investigations showing only minor differences in baseline urine production. Based on these facts this study of the reproducibility of the pressure flow test should be acceptable.

The immediate reproducibility of the pressure flow relationship was good. This means that within 3 hours one can expect nearly the same result of a pressure flow investigation. In contrast to our findings, Ripley and Somerville (1982) found a very low degree of reproducibility in patients and dogs with pressure differences of up to 300% at the same flow rate. Consequently they suggested a change in methodology so that the infusion pressure was constant whereas the infusion rate varied. The infusion would then cease when the pelvic pressure was equal to the infusion pressure and start again when the pelvic pressure decreased. By this methodology they gained a reproducibility of the same degree as in this study. They suggested the change because they assumed that the low degree of reproducibility during constant perfusion could be explained by excessive stimulation of the stretch reflex in the upper urinary tract. This was underlined by the fact that the lowest degree of reproducibility was found at high flow rates. In our investigations a gradual increase in flow rate from 0 to 20 ml/min (Mortensen and Djurhuus 1985) did not cause any significant change in mean pelvic pressure at a given flow rate compared to an abrupt increase in flow rate from 0 to 8 ml/min (Mortensen et al. 1983). The modest difference found may be explained by the possibility that an abrupt increase in flow rate demands a longer perfusion time before a stable pressure value is reached. In a dog model, Thachil and Struthers (1983) measured the pelvic pressure at flow rates from 1.0 to 10 ml/min furnished either by perfusion or increase in diuresis. Both methods showed a high degree of reproducibility. However, they found that the pelvic pressure was significantly lower at flow rates induced by diuresis compared to the perfusion rates. They concluded that an unknown substance in the urine facilitates transport through the upper urinary tract during diuresis. When diuresis was induced they measured the flow over a period of 5 min and when they obtained the desired average flow value they measured the pressure. Therefore there was a risk that they might not obtain steady state in the system.

The investigation performed with an interval of 2 weeks showed reproducible baseline pressure in the pelvis and no reproducibility of the perfusion pressure. Therefore it is likely that the pressure flow relationship in the normal multicalyceal system of the pig is a non-stable parameter from time to time. It is evident that based on the differences between animals and humans, although small concerning the chosen animal, one cannot without precaution apply these findings to the clinical situation, but this investigation certainly raises the question whether the pressure flow relationship is a constant parameter in the clinical situation. We have already shown that the flow resistance in the normal system is mainly situated in the ureter (Mortensen et al. 1984). The explanation of the change in the pressure flow relationship could be differences in tonus of the musculature and thereby differences in ureteral transport capacity at different times. According to the law of Poiseuille the cross-sectional area of the narrowest point is decisive for the resistance in the system. Gosling and Dixon (1978) found that the ureter is normal distal to the dilatation both in idiopathic hydronephrosis and in the megaureter. In both diseases the normal part is supposed to be the narrowest part of the system and should therefore be decisive for the transport capacity. According to our findings this suggests that there is a great risk of finding the same low degree of reproducibility especially in the case of hydronephrosis.

The good immediate reproducibility of the pressure flow relationship suggests that pressure flow investigations may be of major value in investigations of pharmacological activity and influence of drugs on the upper urinary tract. This is a matter for further research.

References

Bäcklund L, Grotte G, Reuterskjöld A (1965) Functional stenosis as a cause of pelviureteric obstruction and hydronephrosis. Arch Dis Childh 40:203–206

Boyarsky S, Labay P, Teague N (1978) Aperistaltic ureter in upper urinary tract infection – cause or effect. Urology 12:134–138

Coolsaet BLRA, Griffiths DJ, Mastrigt R van, Duyl WA van (1980) Urodynamic investigation of the wide ureter. J Urol 124:666–672

Djurhuus JC, Jørgensen TM, Nørgaard JP, Nerstrøm B, Hvid-Hansen H (1982) Constant perfusion provocation in idiopathic hydronephrosis. Urology 19:611–616

Gosling JA, Dixon JS (1978) Functional obstruction of the ureter and renal pelvis. A histological and electron microscopic study. Br J Urol 50:145–152

Kinn AC (1981) Pressure flow studies in hydronephrosis. Scand J Urol Nephrol 15:249–255

Koff SA, Thrall JH (1981) Diagnosis of obstruction in experimental hydroureteronephrosis. Urology 17:570–577

Mortensen J, Djurhuus JC (1985) Hydrodynamics of the normal multicalyceal pyeloureter in pigs. The pelvic pressure response to increasing flow rates, its normal ranges and intraindividual variations. Invest Urol (to be published)

Mortensen J, Djurhuus JC, Laursen H, Bisballe S (1983) The relationship between pressure and flow in the normal pig renal pelvis. An experimental study of the range of normal pressures. Scand J Urol Nephrol 17:369–372
Mortensen J, Frøkiær J, Tofft HP, Djurhuus JC (1984) Renal pelvis pressure flow relationship in pigs after transsections of the ureter. Scand J Urol Nephrol 18:329–333
Pfister RC (1982) Pressure flow studies II. In: O'Reilly PH, Gosling JA (eds) Idiopathic hydronephrosis. Springer, Berlin Heidelberg New York, pp 68–78
Ripley SH, Somerville JYF (1982) Whitaker revisited. Br J Urol 54:594–598
Thachil JV, Struthers NW (1983) Does perfusion equal diuresis in the upper urinary tract. Br J Urol 55:133–135
Weiss RM, Biancani P (1981) Clinical implications of ureteral physiology. In: Susset J (ed) Female incontinence. Alan R Liss, New York, pp 399–403
Whitaker RH (1973) Methods of assessing obstruction in dilated ureters. Br J Urol 45:15–22
Whitaker RH (1978) Clinical assessment of pelvic and ureteral function. Urology 12:146–150
Whitaker RH (1982) Pressure flow studies I. In: O'Reilly PH, Gosling JA (eds) Idiopathic hydronephrosis. Springer, Berlin Heidelberg New York, pp 62–67

The Time-Distance Diagram of the Ureteral Transport

R. Gerlach[1]

Introduction

In many cases an assessment of the function of the upper urinary tract by using merely the excretion urogram is very difficult. The excretion urogram represents an instantaneous documentation, thus allowing an exact registration of the dynamics to a limited degree only. Even monitor recordings of the peristalsis are difficult to objectify in cases of disturbed motility, as we then have to deal with partially very fast flow processes. This is the reason why in the past decades a great number of invasive and non-invasive measuring procedures have been developed all over the world. Due to the differences in the applied measuring techniques and the large physiological variation range among patients and experimental animals we now find various, even contradictory interpretations of the peristaltic transport. This dissension can partly be explained by the fact, that in most of the research works only a few parameters have been measured, while the influence of all the important parameters has been neglected (Lutzeyer 1963). Beside the multitude of X-ray examination and documentation methods, nuclearmedical measurement and ultrasound examination are also available as further non-invasive procedures. By means of measuring probes installed in the ureter lumen the flow velocity, the ureter's cross section and the electrical muscle potential can be measured. The propelled volume is determined by the drop-counting-method and indirectly by a pressure measuring procedure.

Methods

All the experiments dealing with the kinematics and dynamics of the ureteral transport were performed on animals. Non-invasive methods of investigation were applied to human beings as well. For that purpose we arranged a standardized experiment (Fig. 1). All the parameters were measured simultaneously and recorded by a plotter.

After the injection of an X-ray contrast medium, fluoroscopy allowed a direct observation of the urinary transport. A documentation of this process was achieved by kinematographic record (with an 35 mm X-ray camera, 25 frames/s), followed by single frame observation. At the same time the camera functioned as a trigger for

---

[1] Abteilung Urologie der RWTH Aachen, Pauwelsstr., D-5100 Aachen

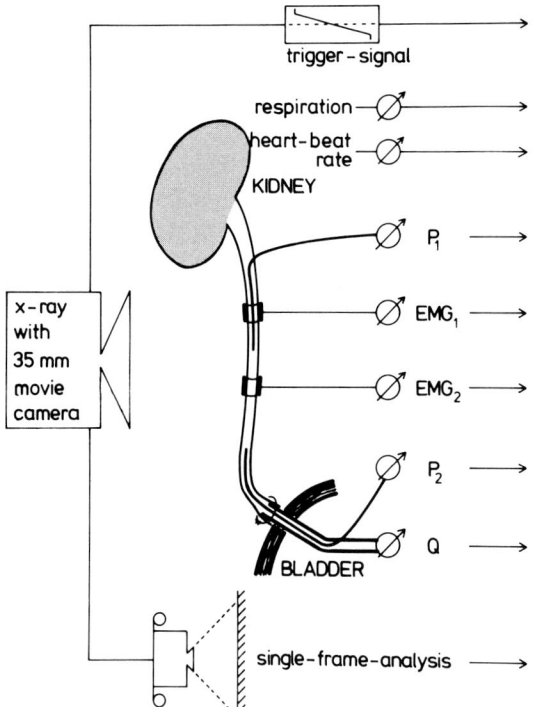

Fig. 1. Assay arrangement for the investigation of the peristaltic urine transport

the plotter, which allowed an exact temporal coordination of X-ray film and electrical signal.

The pressure within the urinary tract was measured by inserted catheters (2.4 Chrr.) at different locations of the ureter. One of the catheters was inserted via the ostium of the bladder, the other in a prograde direction through the ureteral wall. In both cases we received the same results. In principle we only used catheters with a central drainage hole, as a lateral aperture for the pressure would falsify the measuring signals.

The urine volume propelled by the bolus was conducted to an electric weighing device or to a flowmeter via a catheter which had been installed at the ostium. The accuracy of both techniques is almost the same. A manipulation of the catheter can simulate alterations of the intravesical pressure. The electric potential of the musculature is measured by bipolar electrodes attached to the ureteral wall. According to the method of investigation the electrodes are installed intra- or extraluminal.

In order to avoid false interpretations of the measured values caused by respiratory interferences a record of the breathing is necessary. The heart frequence was measured also to avoid additional artefacts.

Results

Explanation of the Time-Distance Diagram

Length and position of the bolus in the urinary tract can be described precisely for any moment of time by single frame analysis (Fig. 2). At the moment of t_1 the level of the X-ray contrast medium is still reaching the renal pelvis. After the formation of an active contractile ring of the muscles (t_2) the bolus is displaced more distad. At the time of t_3 the bolus is located approximately in the middle of the ureter. It is then shorter, its diameter, however, is wider due to the constancy of its volume. At the moment of t_4 the ejaculation into the bladder occurs. The bolus front and rear end was plotted in a diagram as a function of time. Thus we received the Time-Distance Diagram of the urinary transport (Durben et al. 1980). The quantitative analysis of the ureteral peristalsis from the kidney towards the bladder is illustrated in Fig. 3. The shaded area describes the position and length of the bolus at any moment of time. The two limiting graphs indicate the temporal alterations of the parameters. We have to differentiate the filling-time in which the renal pelvis and the proximal segment of the ureter are filled passively by the renal filtration pressure, and the transport-time in which the urine is propelled actively, whereas the electric potential of the muscle moves towards the bladder with a constant velocity. The active contractile ring (proximal graph in the diagram) propels the urine towards the bladder. The distal graph is steplike, which means that the urine passively flows distad. External and possible internal resistances produce changes of velocity of the rear end of the bolus, which cause – due to the constancy of its volume – permanent changes in the bolus length and diameter.

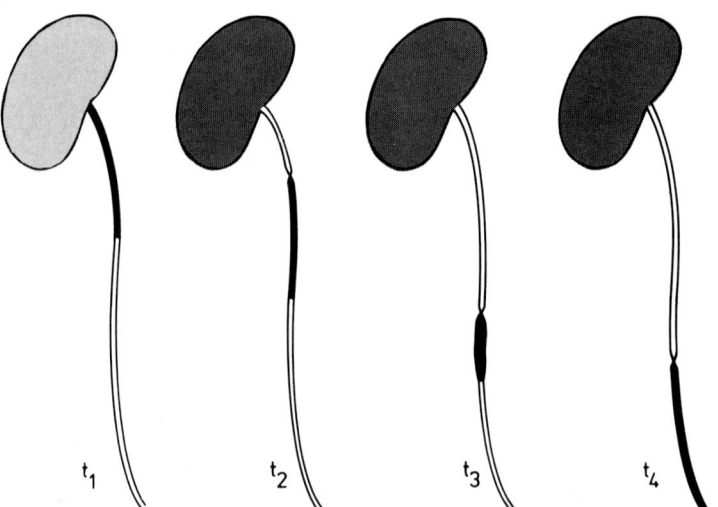

Fig. 2. Schematic demonstration of single boli within the ureter

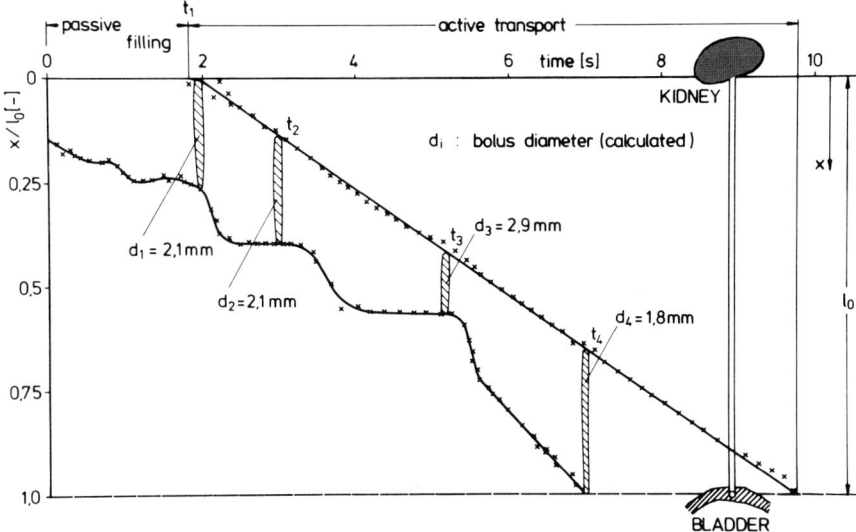

Fig. 3. Time-Distance Diagram of the ureter

Time-Distance Diagram Compared with Other Parameters

Pressure measurement within the ureter only allows a local analysis of the temporal changes of pressure. An interpretation of the entire ureter is not possible with this technique. However, comparing the time-pressure course with the Time-Distance Diagram (Fig. 4) we find locally an obvious correlation between the ureteral transport and the pressure occuring thereby. The catheter for the pressure measurement was inserted about 5 cm into the ureter via the surgically exposed bladder. Naturally this part of the ureter can not be demonstrated in the Time-Distance Diagram.

For the contractile ring we find a typical linear course of the time-distance graph. The inserted catheter proves to be an internal hindrance for the urinary transport leading to an additional step of the rear end of the bolus.

In the state of rest – no bolus or contractile ring near the catheter's tip – we measured the ureteral resting pressure, which is identical with the pressure of the abdomen. When the end of the bolus facing the bladder reaches the catheter's tip (at about $t = 3.5$ s or $t = 13$ s) the pressure increases. This time-pressure course corresponds to the pressure within the urine bolus. This pressure is mainly composed of the unsticking pressure and to a smaller degree of the loss of flow due to friction (Griffiths and Notschaele 1983). The bolus is then obstructed slightly by the catheter. The muscular contractile ring which follows the end of the bolus facing the kidney, causes another distinct increase in pressure (at about $t = 5$ s and $t = 15.5$ s). Behind the contractile ring the pressure drops to the initial value.

Comparing several measured parameters along the ureter (Fig. 5) we find locally a good correspondance with the radiological interpretation. In the Time-Distance Diagram only the linear graph of the muscular contractile ring is represented. Both

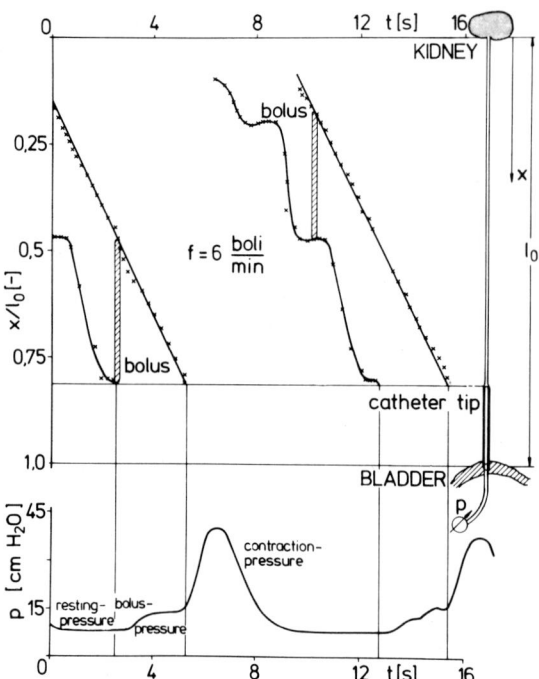

Fig. 4. Time-Distance Diagram including the local time-pressure course (Gerlach 1980)

electromyograms (EMG_1 and EMG_2) show that at the same time as the contractile ring is reached, an electric signal is sent from the measuring spot. The reason for the difference in the graphs of the two electromyograms are superposed longitudinal shifted potentials of the ureter. In the pressure course p_1 we again have to discriminate the pressure within the bolus from the distinctly higher contraction pressure. The interior pressure of the bolus (p_1) shows an artefact caused by respiration during the period of $t = 11$ s to $t = 14$ s.

The pressure of the prosthesis inserted in the ostium (p_2) depends on the flow resistance distal to the prosthesis and is therefore physiologically irrelevant.

In order to receive an accurate interpretation of the graphs a sufficient plotter velocity is very important. In Fig. 6 it starts with 50 mm/min. For example, an analysis of the pressure p_1 at this velocity would not allow a differentiation between the interior pressure of the bolus and the contraction pressure. It seems that the maximal contraction pressure is the only factor which has a decisive influence on the peristaltic transport. Only after raising the paper's velocity (for example to 50 mm/s) can the measured values be recorded and interpreted distinctly.

In this experiment the flow was registered by an electromagnetic measuring system (Fig. 6 below). The integral of the area below the flow curve is a parameter for the volume propelled by the urine bolus which in this case was 0.16 ml.

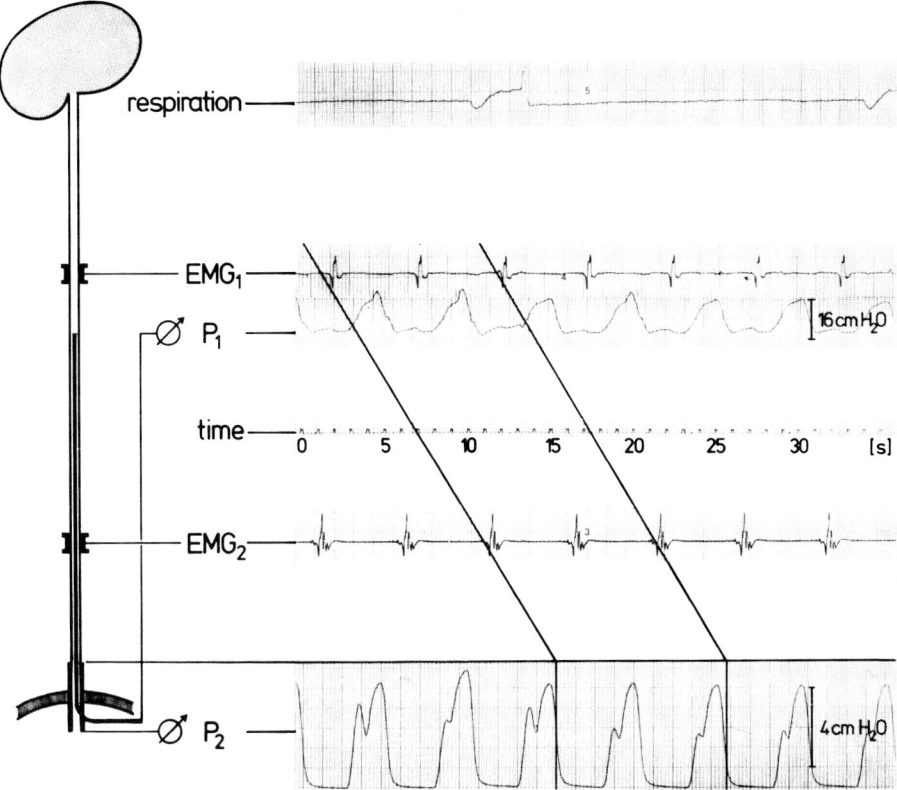

Fig. 5. Time-Distance Diagram combined with recordings of the electric muscle potentials (EMG) and the time-pressure course

Pressure Course Along the Ureter

To eliminate temporal changes of the local measured values during the investigation all the parameters of external influence (like diuresis, abdominal pressure, intravesical pressure, drugs etc.) must be kept constant. Even then comparative pressure measurements at various locations of the ureter show amazingly deviating results.

Therefore, we measured the pressure course along the ureter and compared it with the Time-Distance-Diagram. For that purpose a pressure measuring catheter which had been inserted into the renal pelvis via the bladder, was moved through the ureter in defined steps. After each change of the catheter's position a refractory period must be allowed before any other measurement until the parameters reach a stationary course.

Figure 7 shows the time-pressure course at various locations of the ureter. It appears that the amplitude of the maximal contraction pressure varies for every location of the ureter, just as variations in the interior pressure of the bolus and in its

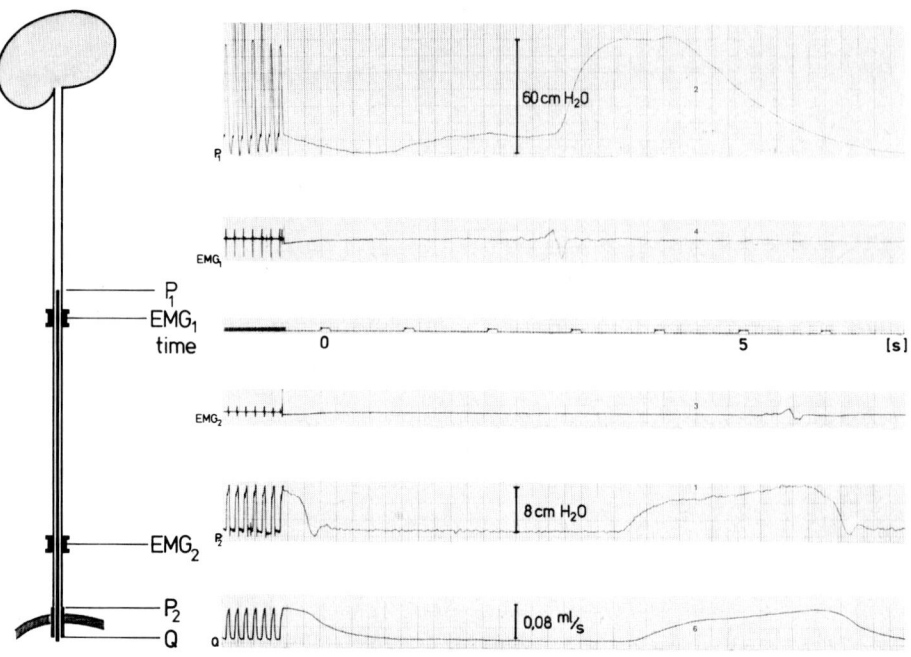

Fig. 6. Analysis of the respective recordings at different velocities of the plotter

graphical course were recorded. The arrows indicate the moments of breathing, which in most cases creates artefacts in the course of the pressure curve.

Plotting the maximum contraction pressure and the maximum interior pressure of the bolus as a function of the ureter's length, we find an almost similar course of the maxima (Fig. 8, also see the definition of the pressure maxima in Fig. 9). Only close to the renal pelvis where the muscular ring is developed and where the measuring parameters are superposed by the contractions of the renal pelvis, we find no distinct correspondence.

The ureter and the renal pelvis illustrated in Fig. 8 (on the right) were copied from an X-ray film which we received after the examined organ had been explanted and filled entirely with X-ray contrast medium at the end of the experiment. The physiological ureteral isthmi and dilatations (Fuchs 1933) correspond quite well with the maxima and minima of the pressure courses.

At constant pressure within the ureter the changes in diameter can be explained by different elastic properties of the ureteral wall during the passive state of the musculature. As Fig. 8 shows, the highest contraction pressures and bolus interior pressures are observed at the narrow parts of the ureter, while the lowest pressures are found in the segment with low wall tension. It seems that the structure of the wall which is different for all ureter segments (Tanagho 1971) is responsible for the variable contraction force of the musculature and thus for the contraction pressure course.

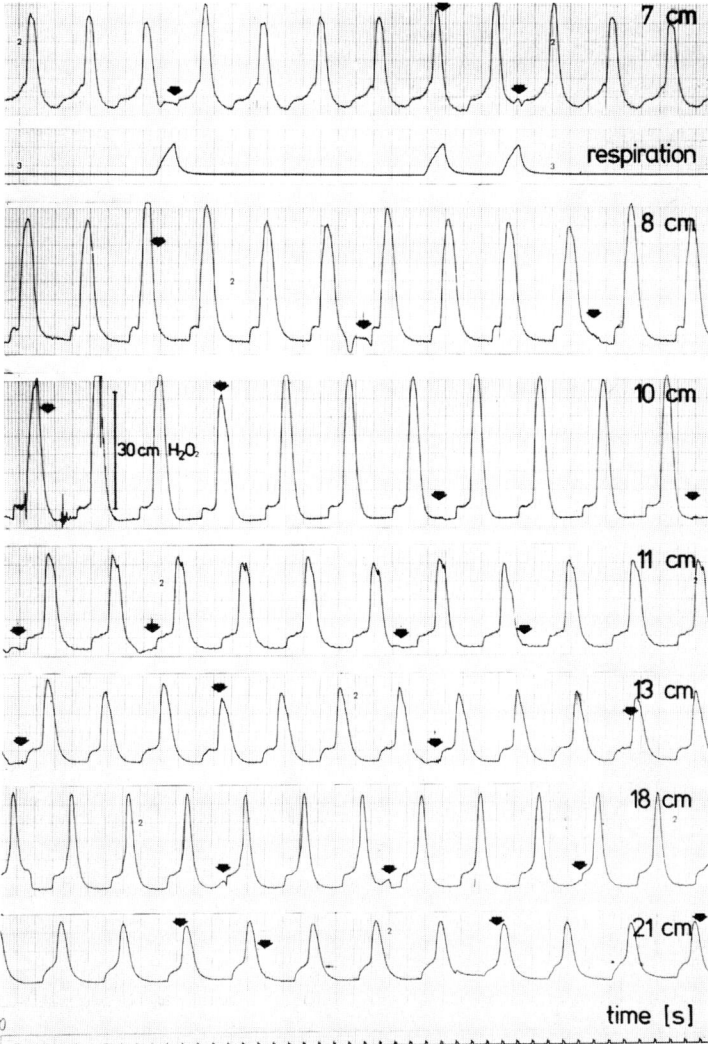

Fig. 7. Time-pressure course at different locations of the ureter. (The respective lengths in cm correspond to the respective distances from the pyeloureteral junction)

The calculated length of the contractile ring (Fig. 8, left) shows the same tendency along the ureter as the pressure course. Also, the 'steps' of the distal bolus end in the simultaneously erected Time-Distance Diagram (middle of Fig. 8) correspond to the pressure maxima. They are located directly in front of the ureter isthmi. These findings are confirmed by investigations of Kiil (1973), who simultaneously measured pressure and wall tension and found a good correlation between the two courses.

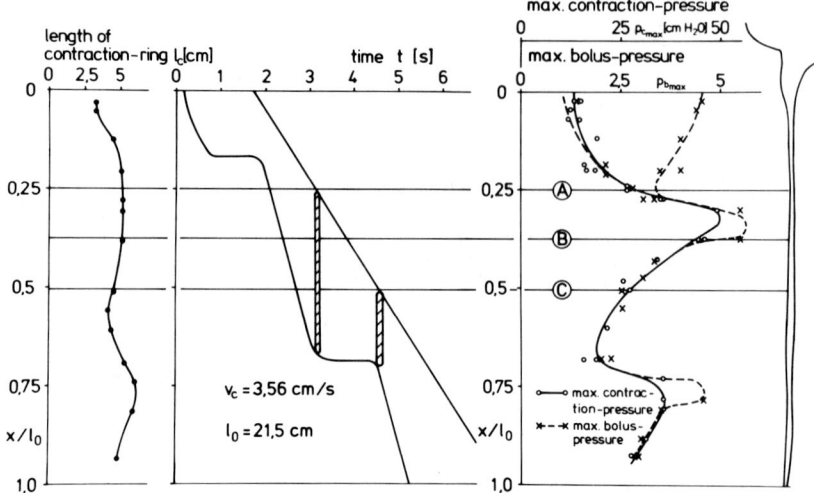

Fig. 8. The courses of the respective parameters along the ureter

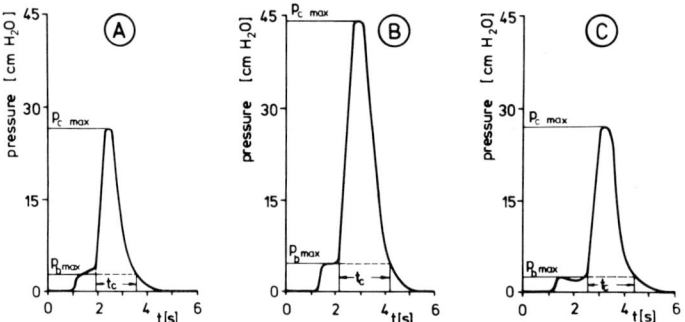

Fig. 9. Definition of the maximum bolus and contraction pressure

Influence of Diuresis and Urine Viscosity

For obtaining a Time-Distance Diagram an injection of a contrast medium with renal elimination is necessary. As the viscosity of these substances – the chosen contrast medium was three-iodized water-soluble Conray 70 – is about six times higher than urine, we have to consider different flow properties, which among other things depend on viscosity. Also, the contrast mediums cause an increase in diuresis due to their osmotic effect. This increased fluid volume can lead to altered flow-off conditions in the ureter.

For investigation of these influences we fixed a small funnel proximal to the ureter ostium after performing a sectio alta. By means of a tube system the voided urine is conducted into a receiver whose increase in weight within a given time is a measure of diuresis. At the same time samples can be taken for viscosity tests. As for this kind of tests a certain volume of urine is respectively needed, we had to collect urine over a longer period of time. The values given in Fig. 10 (below) are mean values for the respective interval of time.

According to Martin (1973) the increase in diuresis caused by the contrast medium is dependent on the injected dose, also the urine concentration of the contrast medium rises with increasing doses, and beside the dosage of the contrast medium the hydration condition of the organism is also decisive for the final urine concentration of the contrast medium.

In our example (Fig. 10) the initial diuresis was reduced to 0.1 ml/min by perfusion of ADH (500–700 µU/kg/h) as soon as the test started. The relative urine viscosity rises significantly (1.33). Further increase in diuresis up to middle and high values was obtained by infusion of 5% glucose solution and further doses of the contrast medium (see Fig. 10). After injection of contrast mediums with renal elimination a typical pattern of diuresis can be observed, as Fig. 11 illustrates by an example. About 30 to 60 s after the end of injection diuresis increases significantly, until after about 4 to 6 min a maximum has been reached. After exceeding this maximum diuresis the graph initially shows a steep slope and is then, after the 10th minute post injectionem decreasing less and less. After about 20 to 30 min the diuresis is approaching its initial value. Similar results were found by Constantinou et al. (1974).

Parallel to the diuretic loading of the urinary tract we find a physiologic distinct increase in the peristaltic frequency during the first 20 minutes post injectionem. Similar to diuresis, these values return to normal only after 30 min. However, over a longer period of time there are still whole number multiples of the initial base-line frequency to be found (interrupted lines in Fig. 11, below).

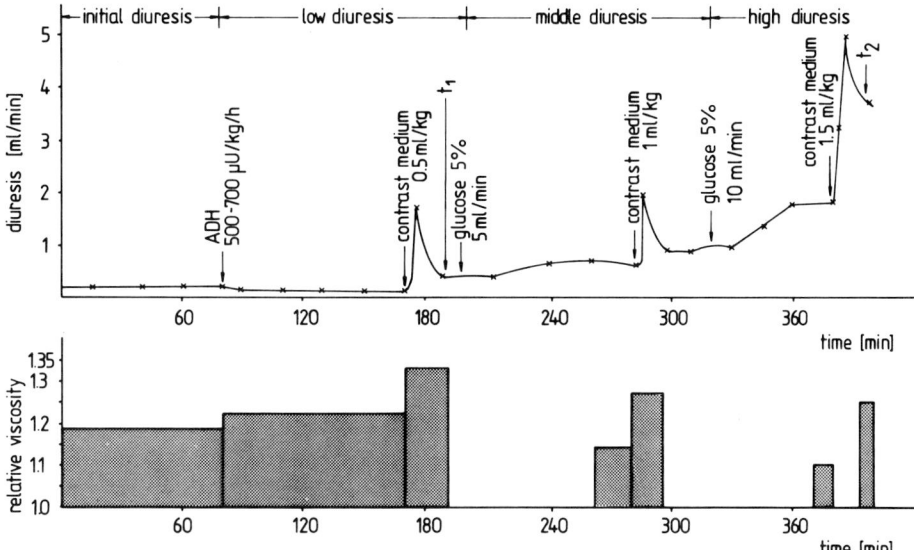

Fig. 10. Diuresis course and mean viscosity during an examination (according to Friedrich 1982). Fig. 13 shows the Time-Distance Diagrams for t_1 and t_2

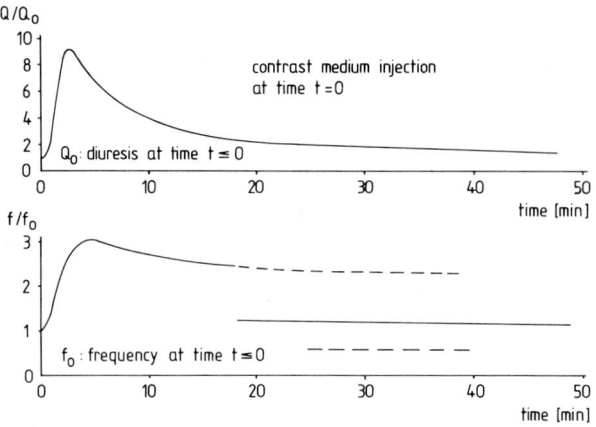

Fig. 11. Changes of diuresis and frequency after injection of the contrast medium

Plotting the maximum diuresis Q_{max} in relation to the initial diuresis, which means the diuresis increase, and the initial diuresis ante injectionem, we obtain the graph illustrated in Fig. 12a. In spite of the limited number of measured values, the typical hyperbolic graph can easily be recognized. When the initial diuresis is extremely low, the injection of small doses of contrast medium causes an immense increase in diuresis, while in spite of high doses of contrast medium only a slight increase can be recorded, when we started with a very high initial diuresis. The different dosages of contrast medium were chosen empirically, in order to supply a high contrast urine for the X-ray kinematographic evaluation.

In our experiments we found an increase in viscosity after the injection of the contrast medium for all the different steps of diuresis. Thereby the following two phenomena have to be differentiated:
1) As Fig. 12b demonstrates, the relative viscosity rises with increasing diuresis, which can be explained by the lower concentration of dissolved substances. This is valid for the normal urine as well as for the urine enriched with molecules of contrast medium.
2) The percental viscosity increase rises according to the dosage of the injected contrast medium (Table 1).

Though in our experiments we did not define the urine concentration of the contrast medium, it can be concluded, that the viscosity increase can only be attributed to the high viscous contrast medium molecules. In our experiments the physiologic range of the urine viscosity of the dog lay between 1.05 and 1.23, which means 17.1%. Proceeding from the highest physiological viscosity it was exceeded by a maximum of 8.9% in our investigations.

Table 1. Percental increase in viscosity after different doses of contrast medium at different initial diuresis rates

Initial diuresis (ml/min)	Contrast medium dose (ml/kg)	Increase of viscosity (%)	
		min.	max
0.1–0.2	0.5	8.9	9.9
0.3–0.8	1.0	11.1	12.2
1.4–2.7	1.5	12.5	13.6

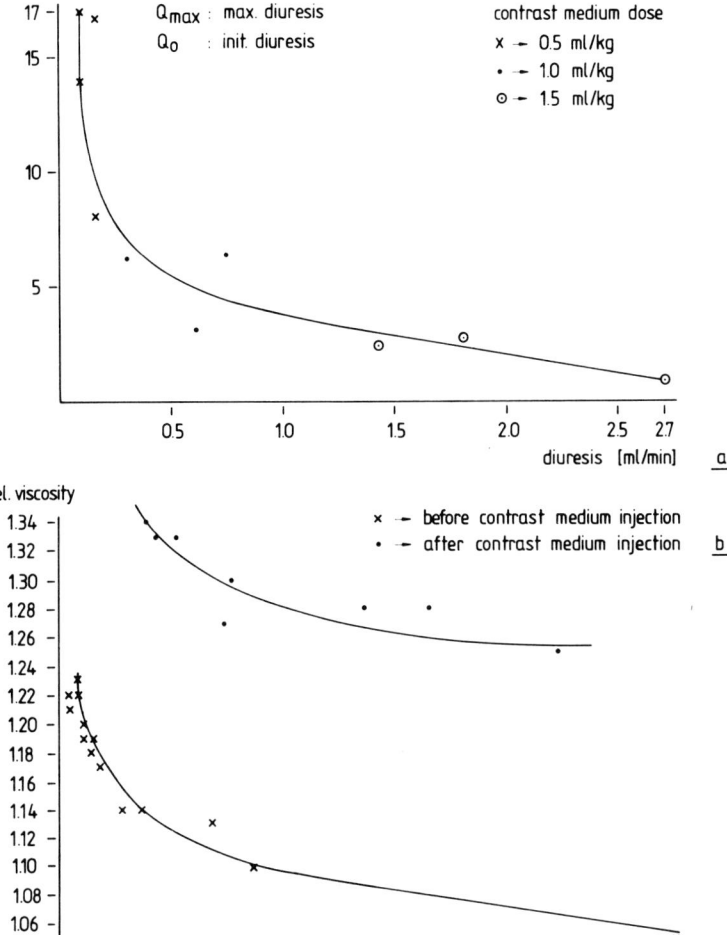

Fig. 12. a Increase in diuresis in relation to the injected contrast medium. **b** Change of the relative viscosity after contrast medium injection

Discussion of the Influence of the Contrast Medium

The viscosity deviations due to the highly viscous contrast medium usually lie within the physiological range and exceed it only in extreme cases. As viscosity is a linear parameter in the basic equation for flowing fluids, no significant influence of the contrast medium on the peristaltic flow is to be expected.

However, the distinct changes in diuresis and peristaltic frequency especially within the first 20 minutes post injectionem can simulate an unrealistic peristalsis. The most pronounced change in diuresis occurs when the hydration condition of the organism is very low. As, however, a sufficient contrast is a basic requirement for the X-ray examinations and as the organism should not be charged with too high dosages of the contrast medium, these changes need to be accepted. Exact investigations and an assessment of the urinary tract dynamics should not start before 20 min after the contrast medium injection.

Compensation Mechanisms of the Ureter

The physiological filtration rate of the kidney covers a wide range from oliguria to polyuria, whereby the diuresis rate reaches and even exceeds the factor 10. The ureter has to adjust to these variations in the fluid volume. With increasing diuresis the ureter has four possibilities of compensation: 1) increasing the bolus volume, 2) raising the peristaltic frequency, 3) enhancing the propagation velocity, 4) increasing the contraction force of the muscles.

The ureter's function is to intermittently propel the urine from the renal pelvis into the bladder. Due to the constant filtration the renal pelvis and the proximal ureter segment (conus ureteralis) are filled with urine and function as reservoirs (Kiil 1957). After a certain degree of filling a muscular contraction of the ureter occurs in the pyelo-ureteral junction and runs distad towards the bladder. Directly in front of the muscular contraction ring a muscle potential difference can be derived electromyographically. The muscular contraction moves with constant velocity towards the bladder and propels the bolus. In contrast to the results of van Mastrigt and Tanecchio (1984), who performed similar experiments in vitro, the propagation velocity of the contractile ring in vivo is constant until the bolus is ejected into the bladder.

Ad 1: Increase of the Bolus Volume

With increasing diuresis the proximal ureter segment can be filled with urine to a large extent. The entire ureter can also be filled with urine before a peristaltic wave starts. The comparison in Fig. 13a and b illustrates this phenomenon qualitatively. In this experiment diuresis was increased by a factor 10 from 0.39 ml/min to 3.9 ml/min. The lengths of the respective boli allow an estimation of the increase of the bolus volume. Weinberg (1977) also observed a correlation between bolus length and bolus volume and reports an increase of both parameters in accordance with diuresis.

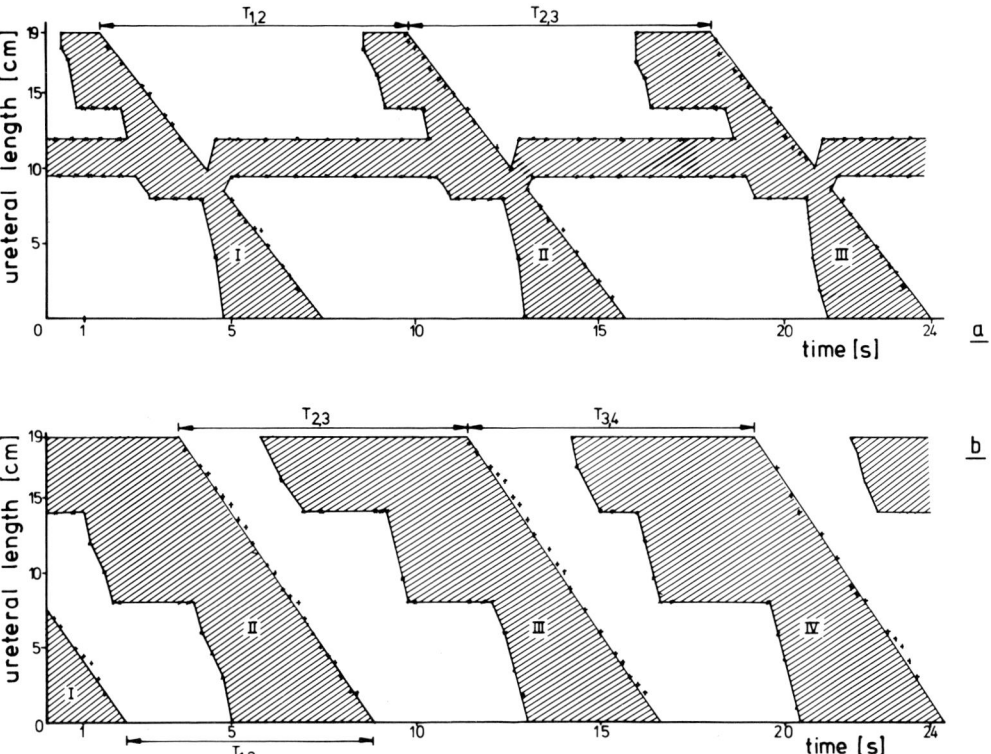

Fig. 13. Time-Distance Diagram of the urine transport at **a** low (0.39 ml/min) and **b** high (3.9 ml/min) diuresis rates (according to Friedrich 1982)

Ad 2: Increase of the Peristaltic Frequency

In literature we find considerable contradictions concerning the frequency reactions of the ureter to increasing diuresis. Rutishauser (1970) reports an increase in frequency up to a diuresis rate of 2.0 ml/min and a frequency decrease when diuresis exceeds this limit. Hannappel (1983) found a large variability of the normal peristaltic frequency and a dependence on species with changing diuresis. Olsen (1981) describes a continuous frequency increase up to a maximum diuresis, which I could confirm in all of my experiments on dogs and pigs. As an example for this, I want to refer to Fig. 13a and b, in which a frequency increase has also been measured in accordance with increasing diuresis, which can be recognized by the diminishing distance between the consecutively running peristaltic waves.

Ad 3: Enhancement of the Propagation Velocity

The active muscular contraction ring moves with a constant velocity towards the bladder. Thus, the gradient angles of these graphs in the Time-Distance Diagram (Fig. 13a, b) are a direct measure for the velocity. The steeper the graph is, the higher is the velocity. In the experiments described above a velocity increase from 2.7 cm/s at low diuresis rates to 3.7 cm/s at maximum diuresis was observed. Kiil (1978) even reports on changes from 1 to 7 cm/s.

This compensation phenomenon of the ureter can be explained as follows: After a fast emptying of the urine-filled ureter the time interval during which the proximal ureter can be re-filled, becomes longer.

Ad 4: Increased Contraction Force of the Musculature

A residual urine depot that is found in the ureter at low diuresis rates can disappear again after an increase in diuresis (Fig. 13 a, b). This means, that the active muscular contraction ring raises its contraction force in accordance with the increasing propelled volume and that it is functioning occlusively on the entire length of the ureter. In Tanagho's and Meyers' (1973) as well as Morales' et al. (1952) reports on their investigations they mention residual urine depots which were temporarily found in the ureter only under the condition of oliguria. Campbell (1966) and Schmidt (1978) also found residual urine depots in the human ureter in about 12% of the cases during their investigations.

Pathological Pressure Course

When during the pressure measurement in the ureter distinct differences in the described time-pressure courses occur, the transport mechanism must be disturbed, if exterior influences and technical artefacts can be excluded. The pressure course shows for example several maxima for each bolus (Fig. 14). The corresponding

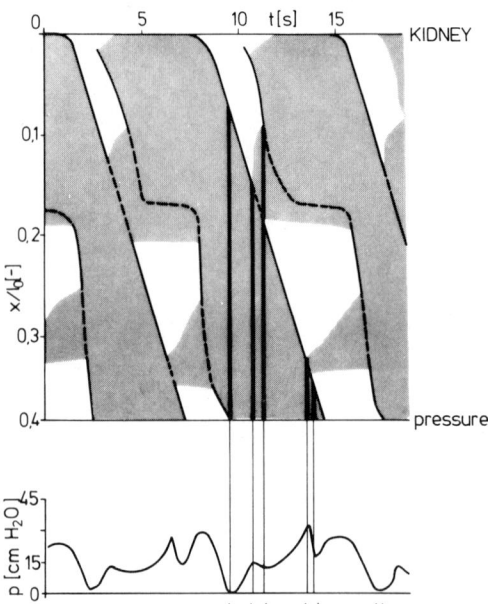

Fig. 14. Pressure course and Time-Distance Diagram during the formation of residual urine depots in the ureter

Time-Distance Diagram demonstrates the ureter segment between kidney and the catheter's tip. The shaded areas represent the urine-filled ureter, in the intervening ureter segments the contraction ring is closed, which means no contrast urine can be detected on the X-ray film.

At the moment of t_1 the bolus reaches the catheter's tip. Afterwards the continuous movement of the fluid column causes a continual pressure rise in the circular gap between catheter and ureter until the time t_2. The aperture of the contractile ring is detected by contrast urine, which is suddenly and with a high velocity propelled in retrograde direction and leaves behind a residual urine depot in part of the ureter. The repeated pressure increase at the moment of t_3 and the urine free segment make us assume that the musculature is again occluded until the time t_4. The repeated pressure drop till t_5 results from another aperture of the contraction ring followed by a residual urine depot. In the Time-Distance Diagram the graphs of the two bolus ends drawn as interrupted lines, could represent an undisturbed transport without any formation of residual urine.

The course of the pressure maxima along a ureter without any pathological alterations (Fig. 8) show, that the slightest contraction pressure occurs, as soon as a congestion of the bolus (step) is observed in the Time-Distance Diagram. Therefore, the phenomenon of residual urine in the ureter (Fig. 14) can be explained by an increase in the interior pressure, which cannot be overcome by the previously affected musculature (long test period, wide diameter of the catheter).

A similar behaviour of the ureter can be expected, when obstructions (e.g. stones) disturb the flow-off, when the organ is locally compressed or when changes in the pressure conditions occur in the lower urinary tract. Long-term alterations of these parameters lead to a congestion of urine within the entire organ.

We examined this phenomenon on an experimental animal (in collaboration with D. J. Griffiths, Rotterdam, The Netherlands, within the framework of the 2nd Joint Meeting of the International Continence Society and the Urodynamics Society in Aachen, 1983). After filling the bladder up to 40 cm H_2O, the initially occlusively functioning ureter was not able to propel urine into the bladder. The high bladder pressure opens up the contraction ring, thus allowing the ureter to be filled with urine.

Conclusions

These investigations show that with every punctional measuring technique a determined parameter can be measured. However, the reciprocity among the various parameters can not be analysed. All the techniques can give only local evidence, they can not describe the kinematics and dynamics of the entire ureter.
- For all locations of the ureter we find different pressure values, which in addition to that are subject to temporal fluctuations.
- The propelled urine volume varies from bolus to bolus and is therefore not very reliable.
- Electromyography demonstrates locally nothing but a peristaltic wave, it can not make statements about its efficiency (occlusive or non-occlusive).

– The velocity of the bolus, the length and diameter of the bolus vary permanently, only the muscular contractile ring moves from the kidney to the bladder with constant velocity.

We examine the influence of contrast mediums with renal elimination. We observe – especially within the first 20 to 30 minutes after the application of the contrast medium – a distinct increase in diuresis and peristaltic frequency. Because of these changes in the parameters, whose values can then exceed the physiological ones, no measurements should be carried out during this interval of time. The dependence of urine viscosity on diuresis and dosage of the contrast medium is discussed. As the values within the physiological range are exceeded by 8.9% in the most unfortunate cases only, we can not expect a significant disturbance of the peristaltic transport. The ureter compensates a volume loading at increased diuresis by raising bolus volume, peristaltic frequency, propagation velocity and contraction force.

The Time-Distance Diagram has a comparatively high value as evidence, as it allows an interpretation of the entire ureter, even under pathological conditions. Only when the entire ureter is dilated, this technique fails, as then an interpretation would be very difficult or would not be possible at all. It is perfectly sufficient for routine examinations, especially because it does not demand too much of the patient as a non-invasive method. The manual interpretation of the films and videotapes which at the moment is quite time consuming, could be replaced by the digital substraction method.

Summary

In order to investigate the peristaltic urine transport on animals various parameters (pressure course, electromyogram, propelled volume, flow, velocity) were recorded simultaneously and compared by their respective yield of information. The evaluation of synchronously shot X-ray films allows us to relate the measured signals to the respective position of the propelled boli within the transport system.

Using the X-ray kinematographic investigations, we developed the Time-Distance Diagram, a technique which allows a graphic demonstration of the function of the entire ureter. This non-invasive method proves to be of high information yield and to be superior to all punctual measuring procedures.

The application of the contrast medium for an excretion urogram causes an increase in urine viscosity and a distinct rise of diuresis. Our investigations show that these changes in viscosity have a neglectible influence on the peristaltic transport mechanism. However, the increase in diuresis, which even under physiological conditions is subject to enormous deviations, should be taken into account after the application of the contrast medium. Exact evaluations of the peristalsis should not start before 20 minutes post injectionem. In order to receive good contrast low hydration conditions of the individuums should be chosen for an excretion urogram, though they cause the highest diuresis increases.

The compensation mechanisms of the ureter at rising diuresis rates are discussed. We find an increase in bolus volume, frequency, propagation velocity and contraction force.

Acknowledgements. This work could develop by support of the Deutsche Forschungsgemeinschaft in the framework of the Sonderforschungsbereich 109. I want to use this opportunity to thank the Aerodynamic Institute of the RWTH Aachen and Dr. med. G. Durben (Dortmund) for their good cooperation.

References

Campbell JE (1966) A cinefluorographic analysis of normal pyelo-ureteral dynamics. Invest Radiol 1:198–209
Constantinou CE, Granato JJ Jr, Govan DE (1974) Effects of radiopaque contrast media on the characteristics of ureteral function. Urol Int (Basel) 29:401–413
Durben G, Gerlach R, Eichhorn F, Friedrich R, Schäfer W, Lutzeyer W (1980) The Time-Distance Diagram: A new method to analyse ureteral peristalsis by cineradiography. Invest Urol 18:207–208
Friedrich RK (1982) Einfluß kontrastmittelbedingter Steigerung von Diurese und Harnviskosität auf die Harnleiterperistaltik des Hundes. Thesis, RWTH Aachen
Fuchs F (1933) Theorie der Harnwegefunktion. Urol Chir 37:154–212
Gerlach R (1980) Harnleiterdynamik und Harnleiterersatz. In: Forschung und Lehre, Heft 11. Stippak, Aachen
Griffiths DJ, Notschaele C (1983) The mechanics of urine transport in the upper urinary tract: 1. The dynamics of the isolated bolus. Neurourol Urodyn 2:155–166
Hannappel J (1983) Motorik des Harntraktes, Physiologische Grundlagen und Pharmakologie. In: Forschung und Lehre, Heft 13. Stippak, Aachen
Kiil F (1957) The function of ureter and renal pelvis. Oslo University Press
Kiil F (1973) Urinary flow and ureteral peristalsis. In: Lutzeyer W, Melchior H (eds) Urodynamics. Springer, Berlin Heidelberg New York, pp 57–68
Kiil F (1978) Physiology of the renal pelvis and ureter. In: Campbell's Urology, vol 1. Saunders, Philadelphia, pp 55–86
Lutzeyer W (1963) Harnleiterdruckmessung (Eine zusätzliche diagnostische Methode zur Erfassung der Harnleiterfunktion). Urol Int 16:1–15
Martin K (1973) Der Einfluß nierengängiger Kontrastmittel auf die physikalischen Eigenschaften des Urins. Thesis, Mainz
Mastrigt R van, Tauecchio EA (1984) Bolus propagation in pig ureter in vitro. Urology 23:157–162
Morales PA, Crowder ChH, Fishmann AP, Maxwell MH (1952) The response of the ureter and pelvis to changing urine flows. J Urol (Baltimore) 67:484–491
Olsen PR (1981) The renal pelvis and ureteral peristalsis. Scand J Urol Nephrol 1:53–57
Rutishauser G (1970) Druck und Dynamik in den oberen Harnwegen. Fort Urol Nephr 2. Steinkopff, Darmstadt
Schmidt H (1978) Motilität der oberen Harnwege. Springer, Berlin Heidelberg New York
Tanagho EA (1971) Ureteral embryology, developmental anatomy and myology. In: Boyarsky S, Gottschalk CW, Tanagho EA, Zimskind PD (eds) Urodynamics. Academic Press, New York London, pp 3–27
Tanagho EA, Meyers FH (1971) Ureteral peristaltic activity. In: Boyarsky S, Gottschalk CW, Tanagho EA, Zimskind PD (eds) Urodynamics. Academic Press, New York London, pp 119–124
Weinberg SL (1977) Ureteral function. IV. The urometrogram at increased urine output. Invest Urol 12:307–311

Mechanics of the Upper Tract

D. Griffiths[1]

In this chapter I shall try to fit the results that Dr. Gerlach has described into a framework that is based partly on theory and partly on some simple experiments in vitro. I aim to give a short and provisional description of the mechanics of urine flow through the normal ureter. This work has been presented elsewhere (Griffiths and Notschaele 1983; Griffiths 1983), but has been modified in the light of experimental work carried out by Mortensen and Djurhuus (1983, and in this book).

As Dr. Gerlach has made clear, it is necessary to distinguish different flow regimes, which occur at different characteristic mean flow rates. Obviously at least three regimes are possible: isolated boluses (i.e. far apart, moving independently); boluses in contact (i.e. close together, not independent); open-tube flow (i.e. no boluses, continuous fluid column). In fact we shall see that this list is not comprehensive.

In the following I shall often refer to the bolus pressure. Since the bolus is launched from the pelvis, the pelvic pressure is approximately equal to the bolus pressure during the launching phase, assuming that there is no obstruction at the pelvi-ureteric junction. I shall assume further that viscous losses associated with flow through the open ureter (e.g. within the bolus) are relatively small. This is probably an oversimplification.

Isolated Boluses

An idealized diagram of a propagating bolus and a contraction ring is shown in Fig. 1. The contraction ring propagates at a myogenically determined speed of 3 or 4 cm/s. The leading edge of the bolus propagates into the resting ureter, which has been squeezed shut by the preceding contraction wave. Experiments show that the apposed walls tend to stick together, so that an overpressure is needed to separate them (the unsticking pressure). Thus the bolus pressure must at least be equal to the unsticking pressure for leading-edge propagation to be possible at all. If, however, the bolus pressure exceeds the unsticking pressure, the leading edge propagates very fast through the ureter. In practice this means that, if the bolus pressure is too low, the leading edge remains virtually stationary. Therefore the bolus shortens, its cross-section increases and correspondingly its pressure rises, until the leading edge begins to move. If the bolus pressure is too high, the leading edge moves much faster

---

1 Erasmus University Rotterdam, P.O. Box 1738, NL-3000 DR Rotterdam

Mechanics of the Upper Tract

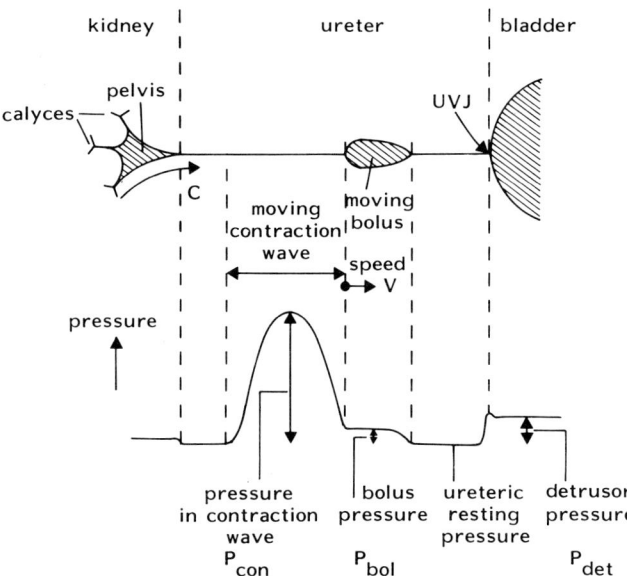

Fig. 1. Sketch showing morphological and pressure relationships in isolated-bolus flow. (From Griffiths and Notschaele 1983. Reprinted by permission of Alan R. Liss Inc., New York)

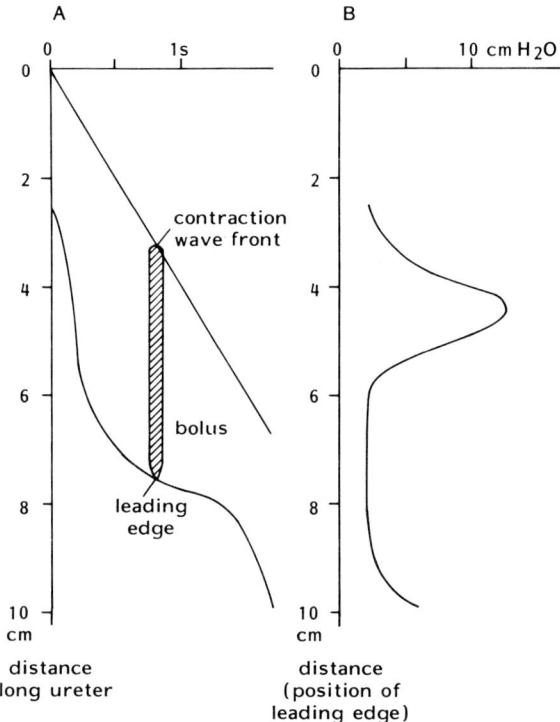

Fig. 2. A Time-distance diagram and **B** bolus pressure variation for the propagation of an isolated bolus through a non-uniform ureter, according to a theoretical model. (From Griffiths and Notschaele 1983. Reprinted by permission of Alan R. Liss Inc., New York)

than the contraction ring; thus the bolus lengthens, its pressure falls and the leading edge slows down. The leading edge thus tends to oscillate between a nearly complete stop and fast advance. Such oscillations in velocity are provoked by non-uniformities in the ureter (e.g. variations in unsticking pressure or in the cross-sectional area of the ureter) or by external non-uniformity (e.g. a crossing blood vessel). In Fig. 2 the results of a model calculation, assuming a non-uniform ureter, are shown. They should be compared with Gerlach's observations (1980, and in this book).

During this type of flow, which is characteristic of low mean rates of urine flow, the pelvic pressure and the pressure in the bolus remain quite close to the unsticking pressure (see Fig. 4). Measurements in the pig in vitro suggest that this pressure is about 7 cm H_2O on average (Bisballe et al. 1983).

Boluses in Contact

When the mean rate of urine flow increases, more fluid must be transported. The boluses tend to become longer and at the same time the frequency of peristalsis tends to rise, so that the distance between successive contraction rings diminishes. Thus the leading edge of each bolus contacts the contraction ring behind the preceding bolus. Under these conditions the leading edge is forced to travel approximately at the speed of the contraction ring (Gerlach 1980). The situation in the ureter is shown diagrammatically in Fig. 3.

Since now the leading edge is not propagating into a resting ureter, the bolus pressure is no longer related to the unsticking pressure. In fact it is determined by the elasticity (or rather, the viscoelasticity) of the ureter. Since both the length and the speed of the bolus are fixed, when the mean flow rate rises, the volume transported can only rise if the bolus cross-section (the lumen) is increased. Expanding the lumen of the ureter against its natural elasticity requires pressure. As the flow and the lumen increase the bolus pressure rises, first slowly and then more and more rapidly (Fig. 4). Measurements in pigs suggest that the pressure rise begins at mean flow rates of about 0.5 ml/min.

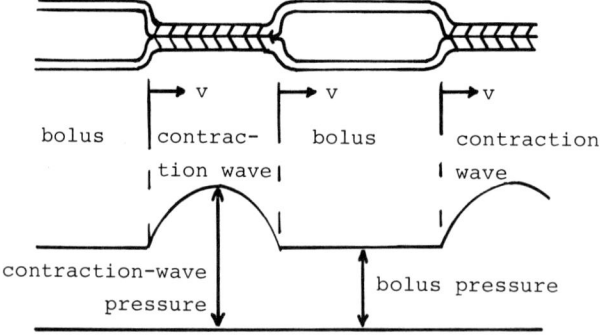

Fig. 3. Sketch showing morphological and pressure relationships in flow regime with boluses in contact

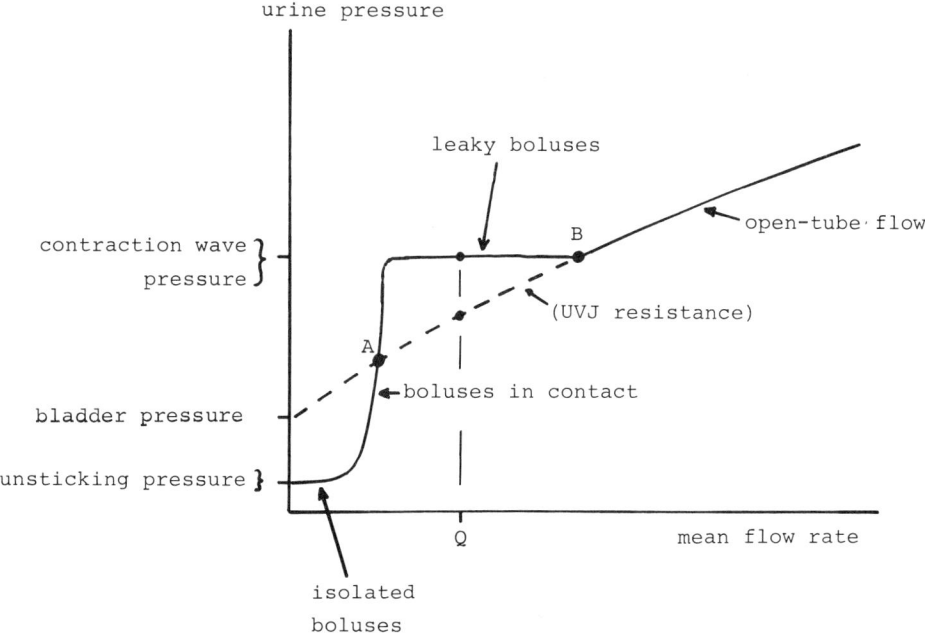

Fig. 4. Relation between mean urine pressure and mean flow rate, in the different flow regimes, according to theoretical prediction. Between points *A* and *B* the leaky-bolus regime (and the upper part of the boluses-in-contact regime) may in fact be unstable, being replaced by an oscillatory flow regime

Leaky-Bolus Regime

If the mean flow rate rises even further, it would appear at first sight that the bolus pressure, following the curve for boluses in contact, eventually should reach the maximum pressure in the contraction ring. The ring would then no longer be able to shut completely, and so fluid would leak through the ring from one bolus to the next. Under these conditions, the bolus pressure would be approximately equal to the maximum contraction-ring pressure (see Fig. 4) over a range of flow rates.

Open-Tube Flow

With increasing mean flow rates the leaky-bolus flow could be maintained only up to the point at which the pressure needed to force the flow through the uretero-vesical junction became equal to the maximum pressure in the contraction ring. If the flow rate were to exceed this value the contraction rings would be forced wide open by the overpressure due to the flow resistance of the uretero-vesical junction, so that open-tube flow would result, the contraction rings causing insignificant ureteral narrowing. Under these conditions the pressure in the ureter would be determined by the resistance of the uretero-vesical junction (see Fig. 4).

Stability of Leaky-Bolus Flow

In the leaky-bolus regime the pressure which is necessary to drive the flow (equal to the contraction-wave pressure) is higher than would be necessary for open-tube flow at the same flow rate (e.g. flow rate Q in Fig. 4). For reasons of stability we might therefore expect an open-tube flow to occur. However, steady open-tube flow is not possible because the contraction rings prevent it, demanding the much higher pressure needed for leaky boluses. An unsteady (oscillatory) type of open-tube flow may however be possible. Supposing that the flow rate oscillates between the points A and B in the figure in such a way that the average flow rate is equal to the given value Q, then the pressure must oscillate also, between the low and high values corresponding to points A and B, whereas the average pressure lies between these values. Since this average pressure is lower than that for leaky-bolus flow, such an oscillatory flow regime may be stable. In this case the leaky-bolus regime would not be observed.

Therefore, over a considerable range of flow rates (between the points A and B in Fig. 4) the pyelo-uretero-vesical system may function as a non-linear flow oscillator. The oscillator would almost certainly be entrained by the active pulsations of the pelvis and ureter. Pressure measurements should therefore show a large oscillation in the pressure accompanying each wave of active contraction, as is in fact observed (Mortensen and Djurhuus 1983). At certain stages of this process the ureteral walls are coapted by the contraction wave. The pressure at point A, however, is related to the bladder pressure. Thus the pelvic pressure is affected by changes in the bladder pressure, and to this extent the oscillatory flow regime has an open-tube character.

The exact conditions for the occurrence of such an oscillatory regime remain to be investigated. One important factor may be the number of contraction waves present in the ureter at any one time.

Concluding Remarks

Theoretically, in the normal ureter, there appear to be four or five possible flow regimes. In order of increasing mean flow rate they are:
1) isolated boluses (bolus pressure approximately equal to the unsticking pressure);
2) boluses in contact (bolus pressure varies with flow rate in a manner determined by the (visco)elasticity of the ureter);
3) either (A) leaky-bolus flow (bolus pressure approximately equal to that in the contraction wave), or (B) oscillatory flow (pressure oscillates between low and high values);

4) open-tube flow (urine pressure varies with flow rate, in a manner determined by the flow resistance of the uretero-vesical junction).

The predicted pressure/flow relation, corresponding to these regimes, is shown in Fig. 4. A similar relation has recently been demonstrated experimentally in the pig (Mortensen and Djurhuus 1983, and in this book).

In regimes 1, 2 and 3(A) the pressure/flow relation should be independent of the uretero-vesical junction and of the bladder pressure. Thus the peristalsis mechanically isolates the kidney from the effects of changing bladder pressure. In regimes 3(B) and 4, however, the flow has either a partial or a complete open-tube character, and changes in bladder pressure will certainly affect the pressure in the renal pelvis.

In practice, even in the normal ureter, non-uniformities may be very pronounced, as Gerlach has shown. Furthermore, pathology may be present. Thus the behaviour is likely to be even more complicated than that described here. In any event we can see that, in order to interpret clinical pressure/flow studies of the upper tract (e.g. Whitaker 1979), it is vital to know in what flow regime the measurements were made.

References

Bisballe S, Djurhuus JC, Mortensen J, Joergensen TM (1983) Pyeloureteral hydrodynamics − The pelviureteral junction resistance in the pig. Urol Int 38:55–57
Gerlach R (1980) Harnleiterdynamik und Harnleiterersatz. Thesis, RWTH Aachen. Forschung und Lehre, vol 11. Uhlenbruck, Cologne
Griffiths DJ (1983) The mechanics of urine transport in the upper urinary tract. 2. The discharge of the bolus into the bladder and dynamics at high rates of flow. Neurourol Urodyn 2:167–173
Griffiths DJ, Notschaele C (1983) The mechanics of urine transport in the upper urinary tract. 1. The dynamics of the isolated bolus. Neurourol Urodyn 2:155–166
Mortensen J, Djurhuus JC (1983) Pyeloureteral urodynamics − Renal pelvis pressure-flow relationship in pigs. Neurourol Urodyn 2:175–181
Whitaker RH (1979) The Whitaker test. Urol Clin North Am 6:529–539

The Propagation Velocity of Contractions of the Pig Ureter in Vitro

R. van Mastrigt[1]

Introduction

Under normal flow conditions, the ureter transports urine in isolated boluses (Boyarski and Weinberg 1973, Durben and Gerlach 1979). Each bolus of urine is propelled by a local, moving contraction of the ureteral wall (Rose et al. 1973; Weinberg 1974; Constantinou and Hrynczuk 1976; Weinberg and Labay 1977). The electrical signal (EMG) which accompanies the mechanical activity can be measured and modelled (Constantinou et al. 1974; Golenhofen and Hannappel 1973; van Duyl et al. 1978). In this study we used pig ureters to demonstrate the propagation of injected fluid boluses by electrical stimulation in vitro. The propagation velocity of the contraction ring was calculated from the electrical signals measured at various locations along the ureter. Ureters were stimulated at various points in order to induce contractions running antegradely as well as retrogradely. The influence of an obstruction on the propagation process was investigated by inflating the balloon of a Swan-Ganz catheter in the ureter.

Materials and Methods

Experiments were performed on twelve freshly dissected ureters from pigs which had been used for cardiovascular experiments. Various drugs had been administered to the pigs, including beta-blockers and Ca-antagonists, sometimes in very large doses, so that an influence on the smooth musculature of the ureter could not be excluded. The ureters were mounted horizontally in a groove in a block of plastic which was kept at 37 °C by circulating hot water through channels bored in it. The ureterovesical junction was tied over a Millar microtip pressure-measuring catheter. The size of the catheter was initially 8 FG, and later 4 FG. The groove was filled with a modified Krebs solution of the following composition in mMol/l: Na^+ 143; Ca^{2+} 1.9; K^+ 5.9; Mg^{2+} 1.18; Cl^- 126.5; SO_4^{2-} 1.18; $H_2PO_4^-$ 1.2; HCO_3^- 25.01; glucose 11. The fluid was constantly refreshed by a shower system of 9 injection needles which continuously dripped it onto the ureter. From the groove the fluid was circulated through an external heated container, where it was aerated with 95% O_2 and 5% CO_2, and pumped back to the shower. During stimulation of the ureter the

---

1 Department of Urology, Erasmus University Rotterdam, P.O. Box 1738, NL-3000 DR Rotterdam

shower was temporarily stopped. Four pairs of silver wires with a diameter of 0.1 mm were inserted into the ureter at regular intervals and were connected to four differential EMG amplifiers set at a bandwidth of 5 Hz–1 kHz and a full range of 200 µV. Boluses of the Krebs solution were injected into the ureter through a small tube inserted in the pyeloureteral junction, and the ureter was stimulated with a 10 V, 100 Hz rectangular wave for 0.5 s, using stainless steel field electrodes placed on either side of the ureter at this junction (unless explicitly stated otherwise). If the stimulation was successful, the injected bolus, or part of it, was transported down the ureter. The following signals were registered on a nine-channel ink jet recorder: time, stimulation duration, marker, the four EMG channels and the output from the pressure-measuring catheter at two different sensitivities. The two sensitivities were chosen so that both the (very low) pressure in the bolus, and the (sometimes high) pressure in the contraction ring could be measured. The marker button was pressed when the ureteral contraction ring was seen passing one of the EMG electrodes. In seven ureters the variations in the propagation velocity were studied as follows. For each ureter the first ten measurements were taken at regular intervals of five minutes, the next twenty measurements (if possible) were taken at two minute intervals and all the subsequent measurements were taken at one minute intervals. Alternate measurements were made with and without prior injection of fluid to form a bolus. The injected volume varied between 0.1 and 0.6 ml in steps of 0.1 ml. When there was no fluid injected, the measurement indicated whether the ureter had been emptied during the preceding measurement or not. The velocity of propagation between successive pairs of EMG electrodes was calculated by dividing the distance between the two electrode pairs by the time taken for the EMG signal to travel between them. The velocity of propagation between the stimulation electrodes and the first EMG electrode pair was estimated by dividing the distance between them by the time between the START of stimulation and the detection of the EMG signal at the first electrode pair. Since it is not certain at what instant during the 0.5 s of electrical stimulation the ureteral contraction started travelling, there is an uncertainty in the calculated value of this velocity, which therefore is always given as a minimum value. On the recorder chart the length of the bolus was determined as the distance from the first rise of pressure to the point of maximum pressure, and the contraction pressure was described by the height of this maximum pressure rise, see Fig. 1. In four more ureters antegrade and retrograde contraction waves were compared by stimulating the ureter alternately at the pyeloureteral and the ureterovesical junctions. In two of these ureters an obstruction was simulated by inflating the balloon of a 5 F Swan-Ganz catheter until it noticably dilated the ureter. In these two ureters this catheter replaced the pressure measuring catheter, and was positioned in such a way that the obstruction was between the 2nd and 3rd EMG measuring electrodes.

Results

In eleven of the twelve ureters fluid boluses were propagated successfully. In several cases we found that at the beginning of the experiment, the contractions produced by stimulation did not propagate to the end of the ureter, but after waiting for

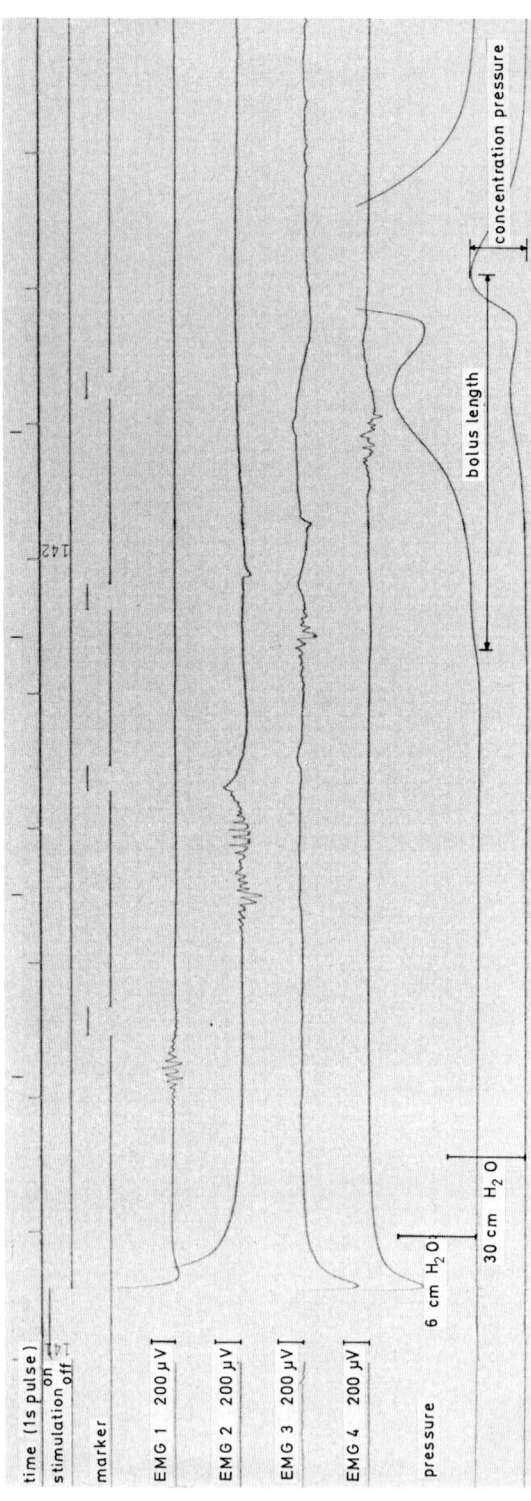

Fig. 1. Example of a recording of one measurement

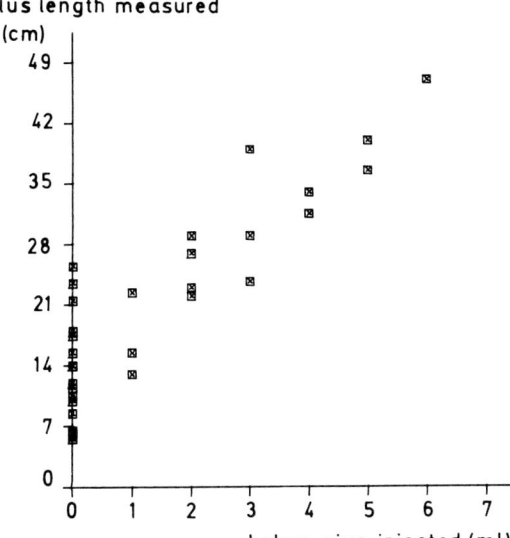

Fig. 2. Bolus length as a function of volume of injected fluid, for all measurements from one ureter. Bolus length is represented as cm measured on the paper chart and is not equal to the real length of the bolus

a considerable time (1 to 2 hrs) and injecting several large boluses, a proper propagation was finally established. On average about 30 measurements could be taken from one ureter, with a maximum of 39 measurements in one case. This number was strongly dependent on the time interval between stimulations; allowing an interval of 5 or 2 min a large number of measurements could be made, but using a one-minute interval the performance of the ureter deteriorated rapidly, soon resulting in contractions stopping before the end of the ureter. Figure 1 shows a typical result from one measurement. There is a systematic time lag, of about 0.2 s, between the EMG and the marker pulse, indicating that the electrical signal travels in front of the contraction ring. The pressure signal shows a typical sequence: a bolus with a rather low interior pressure, followed by a contraction ring with a considerably higher pressure.

Contractions Running Antegradely

We studied the influence of various parameters on the transport mechanism in seven ureters. Figure 2 shows a plot of the amount of fluid injected versus the measured bolus length for one of these ureters. Such a plot gives an impression of the efficiency of the transport mechanism. In this case there is a roughly linear relation between the variables, indicating that the injected fluid is indeed transported. The relation does not intersect the origin since to make the measurements easier bolus length was defined as the distance between the front end of the bolus and the maximum contraction pressure. It therefore includes part of the contraction ring. It can also be seen in Fig. 2 that, even when no fluid had been injected, quite long boluses were occasionally transported. Obviously in these cases the fluid injected previously

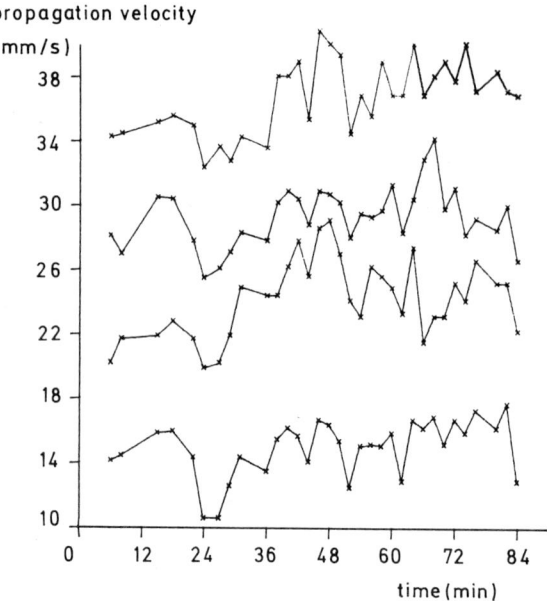

Fig. 3. Velocity of propagation of the ureteral contraction between stimulation electrodes and four pairs of EMG electrodes, as a function of time. Second, third and fourth tracings are shifted respectively 8, 16 and 18 mm/s upwards compared to the first tracing. Absolute values of the velocities for this ureter are given in Table 1, first row

had not been fully ejected. In fact the three highest of these measurements were made either very early or late in the experiment when the transport was not very efficient. In four of the seven ureters there was a linear relation like the one in Fig. 2. In the other three ureters no such relation was detectable. Figure 3 shows the four measured velocities as a function of time. Notice that the four velocities show a common trend as well as individual random variations. This indicates the influence of some variable which affects the propagation velocity in the entire ureter. These fluctuations are therefore also seen in the average value of the four velocities, as shown in Fig. 4, lower panel. In three ureters the average velocity tended to increase as time elapsed (as in Fig. 4), whereas in the other four ureters the average velocity decreased. There is also a systematic difference between the four velocities, as shown in Table 1. In six of the seven ureters the propagation velocity was higher in the distal section than in the third section. In the last four ureters the velocity was also higher in the most proximal section than in the second section. Although this does not seem to be the case in the first three ureters the fact that only a minimum value is given for the velocity in the proximal section should be taken into account. Thus we can conclude that in general the propagation velocity is higher in the proximal and distal parts of the ureter than in the middle. In four ureters one or more measurements were made at the beginning or the end of the experiment, in which the propagation of a contraction stopped about halfway along the ureter. In three of these ureters, the contraction ran significantly more slowly than normal just before

The Propagation Velocity of Contractions of the Pig Ureter in Vitro

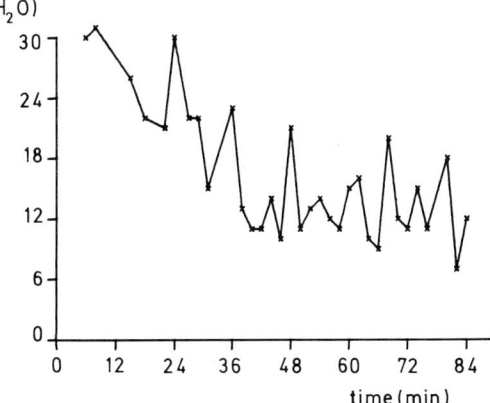

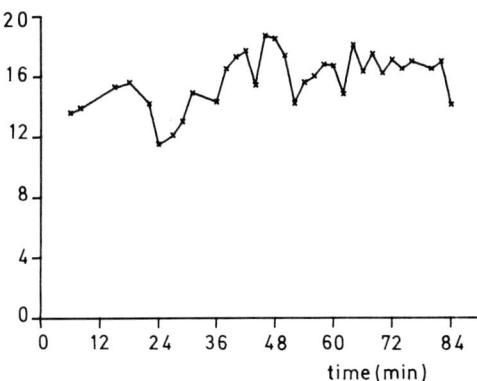

Fig. 4. Average propagation velocity, calculated from the data in Fig. 3, as a function of time (*lower panel*), and associated contraction pressure as a function of time (*upper panel*)

Table 1. Average propagation velocities of ureteral contraction between the stimulating electrodes and the four pairs of EMG electrodes, and overall average for the entire ureter. Data from seven ureters. Due to the uncertainty of the beginning of the contraction during electrical stimulation, the first velocity column shows a minimum value. Values in parentheses represent standard deviations

Number of measurements	Stim–1st el (mm/s)	1st–2nd el (mm/s)	2nd–3rd el (mm/s)	3rd–4th el (mm/s)	Average (mm/s)
n = 37	> 15.8 (4.7)	16.1 (2.3)	13.3 (1.8)	19.0 (3.0)	16.0 (2.3)
n = 19	> 16.7 (1.0)	20.6 (1.2)	17.4 (1.2)	17.4 (0.09)	18.0 (0.09)
n = 20	> 17.4 (2.6)	19.4 (2.1)	14.1 (0.8)	17.3 (0.09)	16.6 (2.4)
n = 12	> 25.4 (2.0)	22.7 (1.1)	26.0 (3.1)	34.1 (2.2)	25.4 (4.2)
n = 31	> 17.1 (3.6)	14.1 (2.4)	15.2 (1.3)	17.2 (1.1)	16.0 (1.8)
n = 39	> 18.6 (4.5)	16.2 (1.1)	21.1 (3.1)	21.5 (2.8)	19.3 (1.5)
n = 28	> 21.5 (6.1)	20.5 (2.7)	20.5 (3.0)	21.5 (3.2)	21.0 (3.0)

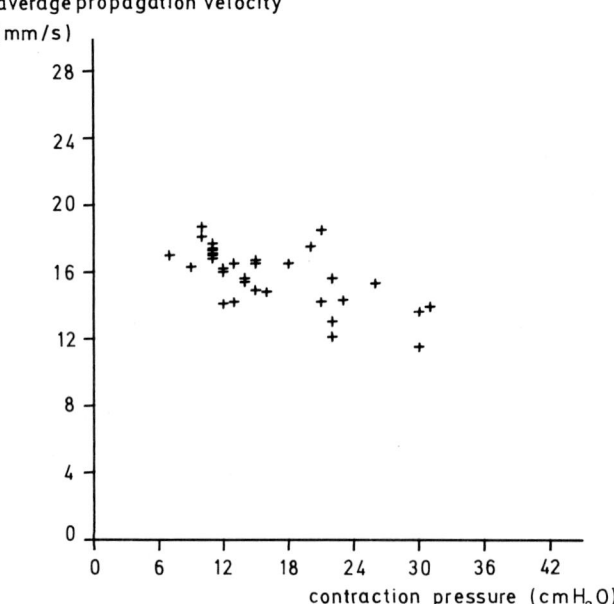

Fig. 5. Average propagation velocity plotted as a function of contraction pressure. Same data as Fig. 4. Spearman's rank correlation value for this data is –0.65, significant at the 1% level

stopping. An example is shown in Fig. 5, where the first two measurements of the propagation velocity between the second and third pairs of electrodes (third tracing) are significantly lower than the subsequent measurements, while the fourth electrode is not reached. In the fourth ureter this effect may have been masked by a measurement error. The upper panel of Fig. 4 shows the contraction pressure measured in one of the ureters as a function of time. It can be seen that not only the general trend is opposite to that of the average velocity in the same ureter (lower panel) but also that a number of small excursions from the general trend are oppositely directed in the two tracings. A scatter plot of the two variables (Fig. 6) demonstrates this inverse relationship. For these data Spearman's rank correlation coefficient is –0.65, significant at the 1% level. A similar inverse relationship was found in three of the seven ureters. In the other four ureters the contraction pressure was either so extremely low (three ureters) or so extremely high (one ureter) that it could not be reliably estimated. The possibility of a relation between the propagation velocity and the length of the bolus was investigated. Scatter plots of the two variables showed no correlation in any of the ureters.

Comparison of Antegrade and Retrograde Contraction Waves

Figure 7 shows the recording of a contraction running antegradely, Fig. 8 the recording of the following contraction running retrogradely in the same ureter. Table

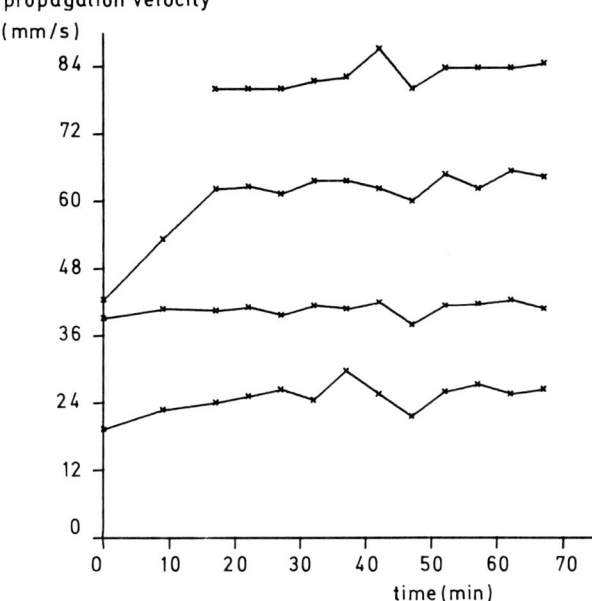

Fig. 6. Velocity of propagation of the ureteral contraction between stimulation electrodes and four pairs of EMG electrodes, as a function of time. In the first two measurements (made 0 and 10 min after the start of the experiment) the contraction stopped before reaching the end of the ureter. Second, third and fourth tracings are shifted respectively 18, 36 and 48 mm/s upwards compared to the first tracing. Absolute values of the velocities for this ureter are given in Table 1, fourth row (n = 12)

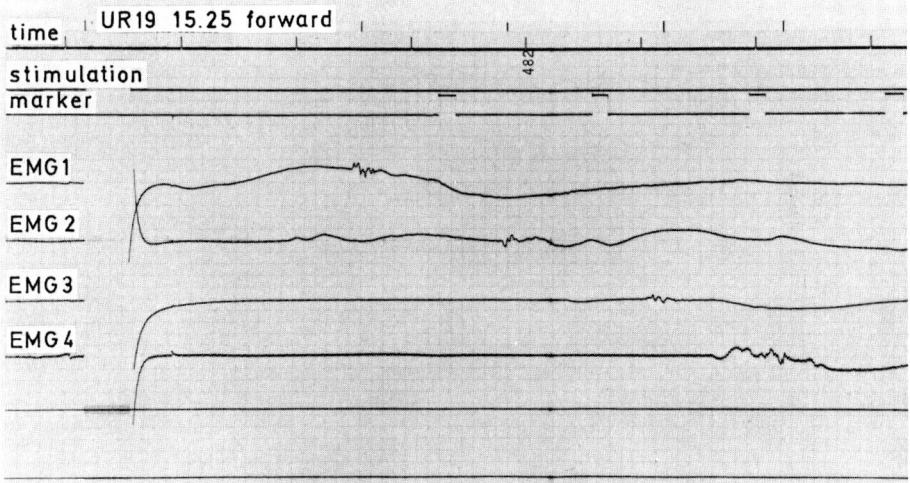

Fig. 7. Recording of antegrade contraction wave. Same scales as Fig. 1

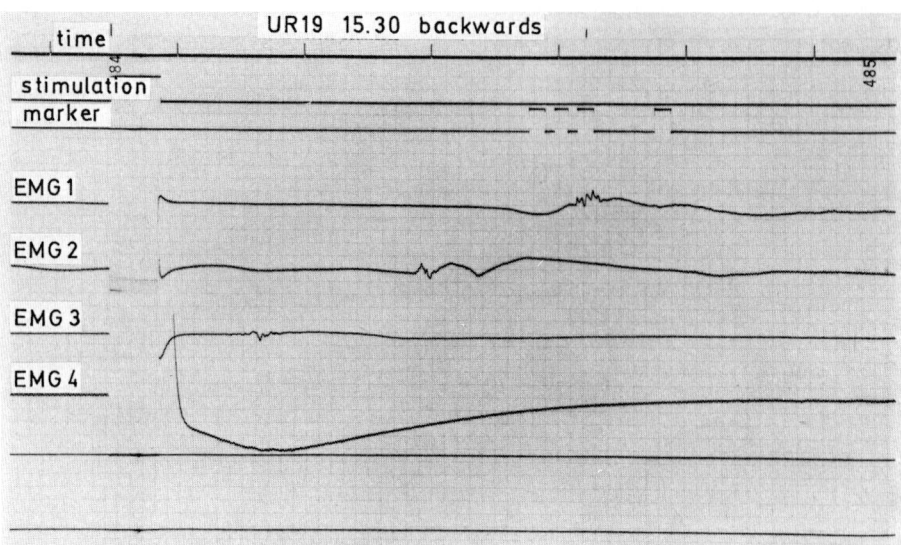

Fig. 8. Recording of retrograde contraction wave immediately following the contraction shown in Fig. 7

Table 2. Average propagation velocity of ureteral contraction between two EMG electrode pairs, for antegrade and retrograde contractions waves. Data from four ureters. Values in parentheses represent standard deviations

Direction	Number of measurements	1st–2nd el (mm/s)	2nd–3rd el (mm/s)
antegrade	n = 4	16.8 (1.0)	22.8 (3.0)
retrograde	n = 4/5	17.8 (1.8)	21.8 (1.6)
antegrade	n = 4	13.7 (0.5)	15.1 (0.3)
retrograde	n = 4	13.2 (0.1)	16.1 (0.6)
antegrade	n = 8/5	20.9 (1.8)	29.7 (0.7)
retrograde	n = 3	22.4 (1.9)	29.5 (0.5)
antegrade	n = 5	18.9 (0.4)	19.8 (1.3)
retrograde	n = 5	19.7 (0.7)	20.3 (0.1)

2 shows the propagation velocities of antegrade and retrograde contraction waves for four ureters. Although for one ureter (second row) a significant difference between the velocities exists (Student's t-test, 5%), there is no systematic difference in velocities. One ureter was stimulated several times at both ends simultaneously. It was observed that antegrade and retrograde contraction waves were mutually eliminated upon meeting.

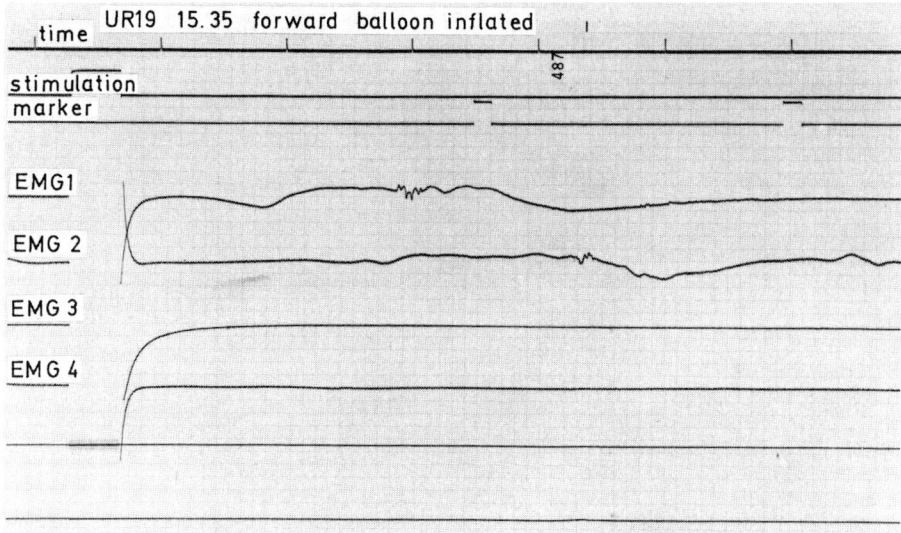

Fig. 9. Recording of antegrade contraction wave immediately following the contraction shown in Fig. 8. The balloon of a Swan-Ganz catheter was inflated between the 2nd and 3rd electrode. Propagation of the contraction stops at this point

Influence of Obstruction

Figure 9 shows a subsequent recording of the ureter illustrated in Figs. 7 and 8, but with the balloon of the Swan-Ganz catheter inflated between the 2nd and 3rd EMG electrodes. As can be seen, the contraction did not reach the 3rd electrode. Figure 10 shows the next recording, in which the balloon was again deflated, but the propagation of the contraction was not resumed. Figure 11 shows a subsequent retrograde contraction wave, which does not reach the 2nd electrode. In one ureter the propagation of a contraction past the point where the balloon had been inflated was never resumed. In the other ureter the propagation of the contractions was resumed after about one hour of waiting. This phenomenon was observed twice in this ureter.

Discussion and Conclusions

The electrical signals measured in our experiments reflect the depolarization of many cells near each pair of electrodes, so that the form of the signal cannot be accurately predicted or described. Nevertheless there seems to be some similarity among the signals obtained from the four electrode pairs as the contraction wave passes, indicating that the form of the electrical signal reflects at least partially some

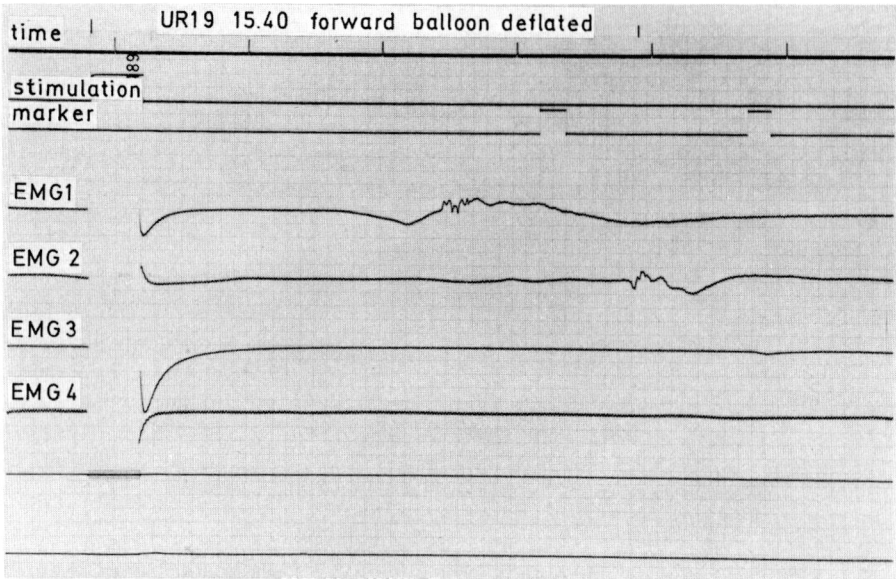

Fig. 10. Recording of antegrade contraction wave immediately following the contraction shown in Fig. 9. The balloon of the Swan-Ganz catheter was deflated. Propagation of the contraction still stops between the 2nd and 3rd electrode

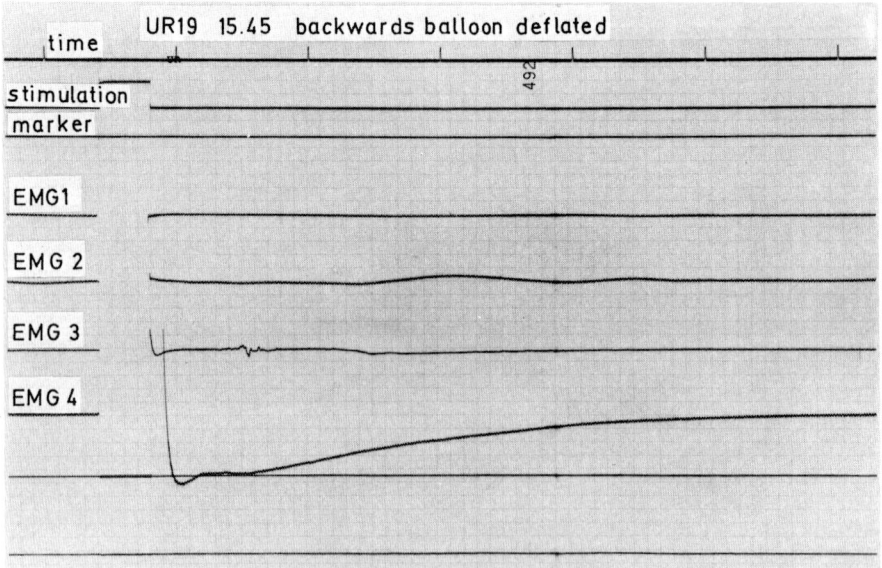

Fig. 11. Recording of retrograde contraction wave immediately following the contraction shown in Fig. 10. Propagation of the contraction still stops between the 2nd and 3rd electrode

constant characteristic of the contraction wave. The wave of pressure produced by the actual contraction travels behind the electrical signal. This time lag is probably due to the time necessary for activation of the muscle cells (van Mastrigt and Glerum 1984). When a bolus is propagated, its interior pressure is considerably lower than the pressure of the contraction wave. In the simplest model (Griffiths and Notschaele 1983) the pressure is uniform throughout the entire bolus. In our case a gradually increasing pressure has often been observed (compare Fig. 1), which is probably related to a similar variation in cross-sectional area of the bolus (Djurhuus et al. 1979). However, the pressure-measuring catheter obstructs the ureter and may affect the form of the signal in our experiments. The decrease in pressure which is often observed just before the contraction ring passes may be related to this obstructive effect.

The presence of a bolus is not a necessary condition for the propagation of a contraction wave. In half of our observations the empty ureter was stimulated and a contraction wave travelled its entire length. Furthermore, the fact that there is no relation between the velocity of propagation of the contraction wave and the size of the bolus that is propelled, suggests that the straining of the ureter due to the bolus does not facilitate (nor inhibit) the following contraction. On the other hand, the propagation velocity is clearly related both to the position in the ureter and to the contraction pressure, and also shows some (random?) fluctuations common to the entire ureter. The values which we found for this velocity in the pig are at the low end of the range reported for various other animals (Durben and Gerlach 1979; Weinberg and Labay 1977; Vereecken 1973). The velocity of propagation is highest near the beginning and end of the ureter and lower in the middle. This trend is parallel to that shown by the spontaneous intrinsic frequencies of ureter sections (Gruber 1928; Shiratori and Kinoshita 1961, cited by van Duyl et al. 1978), although in the modelling of the electrical activity (van Duyl et al. 1978) it was assumed that these latent intrinsic frequencies had no influence on the propagation velocity. Another interesting fact concerns the influence of metabolism on the velocity. The inverse relation which we found between the propagation velocity and the contraction pressure suggests that there is a trade-off between these two variables. A similar trade-off is represented by the well-known force-velocity relation for contracting muscle (van Mastrigt and van Duyl 1981). The present trade-off might be related to the force-velocity relation although the two velocities are of course quite different. Alternatively, it might be the result of a simpler mechanism, such as the following: When stimulated, muscle cells have a certain probability of entering the contractile state. In a fast-moving contraction wave, the stimulation time of a given cell is shorter, resulting in a smaller cumulative chance that it contracts. This means that fewer cells contract in a faster contraction wave, so that the contraction pressure is lower. In contrast to the increase in velocity as time elapses, the propagation velocity decreases before a contraction stops in the middle of the ureter. Arguments based on the Wenckebach phenomenon suggest that similar behaviour should be observed if contractions follow one another at (too) short time intervals (van Duyl and Groot 1982).

In four ureters the electrical stimulation was applied at various locations along the ureter. No directional preference was found in the propagation of a contraction ring. As we expected, contractions running in opposite directions were mutually eliminated upon meeting in contrast to contractions in the calyces which were reported to meet and progress undisturbed (Ohlson 1982). In our model a small dilatation of the ureter was sufficient to block the propagation of a contraction ring for a considerable time, even after removing the dilatation. In a physiological situation this could mean that an obstacle does not have to block the ureter in order to be obstructive; it only has to dilate the ureteral wall.

In summary, the propagation of the bolus in the ureter was investigated in vitro. It was found that considerable and understandable fluctuations exist in the propagation velocity, the latter depending among other variables, on position, time and metabolic circumstances. No directional preference was found for the propagation of contractions in the ureter, and this propagation could be blocked for a considerable time by a temporary slight dilatation of the ureteral wall.

References

Boyarsky S, Weinberg S (1973) Urodynamic concepts. In: Lutzeyer W, Melchior H (eds) Urodynamics. Springer, Berlin Heidelberg New York, p 1
Constantinou CE, Hrynczuk JR (1976) Urodynamics of the upper urinary tract. Inv Urol 14-3:233
Constantinou CE, Tsuchida S, Kavaney PB, Hayman WP, Govan DE (1974) Simulated vesicoureteral reflux. Urol Int 29:265
Djurhuus J, Constantinou CE, Andersen HR, Jorgensen F (1979) Bolus dynamics in ureter. Antwerp, 1st ISDU meeting
Durben G, Gerlach R (1979) The velocity of urine bolus under different conditions. Antwerp, 1st ISDU meeting
Duyl WA van, Groot RFH (1982) Evaluation of a model for the propagation of electrical activity along the ureter. Utrecht, 4th ISDU meeting
Duyl WA van, Brans JM, Coolsaet BLRA, Grashuis JL, Kingma YJ (1978) Provisional model for propagation of electrical activity in upper urinary tract. Urology XII-6:736
Golenhofen K, Hannappel J (1973) Spontaneous generation of excitation in pyeloureteral system and the effect of adrenergic substances. In: Lutzeyer W, Melchior H (eds) Urodynamics. Springer, Berlin Heidelberg New York, p 46
Griffiths DJ, Notschaele C (1983) The mechanics of urine transport in the upper urinary tract. 1. The dynamic of the isolated bolus. Neurourol Urodyn 2:155
Gruber CM (1928) The peristaltic and antiperistaltic movements in excised ureters as affected by drugs. J Urol 20:27
Mastrigt R van, Duyl WA van (1981) Mechanics of detrusor contraction. Determination of contractility. In: Coolsaet BLRA, Duyl WA van (eds) Principles of bladder function and urodynamics. Lameris Instrumenten, Utrecht, p 31
Mastrigt R van, Glerum JJ (submitted for publication) Electrical stimulation of smooth muscle strips from the urinary bladder of the pig
Ohlson L (1982) The principle of impulse conduction in the normal upper urinary tract. Utrecht, 4th IDU meeting
Rose JG, Gillenwater JY, Attinger F, Sim P, Wyker AT (1973) Ureteral wall tension. Inv Urol 10-6:480
Shiratori T, Kinoshita H (1961) Electromyographic studies on urinary tract. III. Influence of punching and cutting the ureters of dogs on their EMGs. Tokohu J Exp Med 73:159
Vereecken R (1973) Dynamical aspects of urine transport in the ureter. Thesis, Catholic University Leuven, Belgium
Weinberg SL (1974) Ureteral function. I. Simultaneous monitoring of ureteral peristalsis. Inv Urol 12-2:103
Weinberg SL, Labay P (1977) Ureteral function. IV. The urometrogram at increased urine output. Inv Urol 14-4:307

Assessment of Ureteric Dynamics by Simultaneous Electric Conductance Measurements at Two Sites

S. Plevnik[1], S. Rakovec[2], and P. Vrtačnik[1]

Pyelo-Ureteric Dynamics: Current Methods of Assessment

Pyeloureteric function can be assessed by various methods, which have been reviewed by Struthers (1976).

A rough estimate of the geometry of the upper urinary tract can be obtained using the classical intravenous pyelogram (urogram). Modern cineradiographic methods offer assessment of geometry versus time patterns of the propagation of the urine bolus. Time-distance diagrams of ureteral peristalsis can be obtained in such a way (Gerlach 1983).

Kiil (1953, 1957) introduced "urometry", which measures baseline pressures and phasic contraction pressure waves in the renal pelvis and ureter using the perfusion method via a ureteric catheter, introduced into the ureter at cystoscopy and connected to an external pressure transducer. Four to six French size catheters were used, and pressures recorded at a single site in the ureter or renal pelvis. They are believed not to produce artefacts which could occur due to catheter-induced ureteric obstruction.

Rakovec et al. (1982) described simultaneous measurement of the pressures in the upper urinary tract at two sites. They used a cystoscopically introduced two channel 7 F Millar microtip pressure transducer catheter having two pressure sensors placed on the catheter 5 cm apart. In addition to the baseline pressures, the amplitude of the phasic contractions and the rate of contractions at two sites in the ureter, the method described provided information on the velocity (Fig. 2) and orientation of the contraction pressure waves; patterns indicating retrograde orientation of the pressure waves are clearly recognized from the recordings (Fig. 3).

Intermittent injection of a radiopaque solution was added to manometry by Ross et al. (1972), thus combining pyeloureteric pressure measurement with routine urography.

All the methods described above are frequently used clinically for diagnosing obstruction. They were criticized by Whitaker (1973a) who stated that the intravenous urogram does not represent a reliable means for assessment of a small degree of obstruction, while retrograde ureterography, with or without pressure measurement, introduces artefacts and involves unknown factors such as the fluid load of the patient, the pressure behind the injection and the fullness of the bladder.

---

1 J. Stefan Institute, E. Kardelj University, Ljubljana, Yugoslavia
2 Urological Clinic, University Clinical Centre, Ljubljana, Yugoslavia

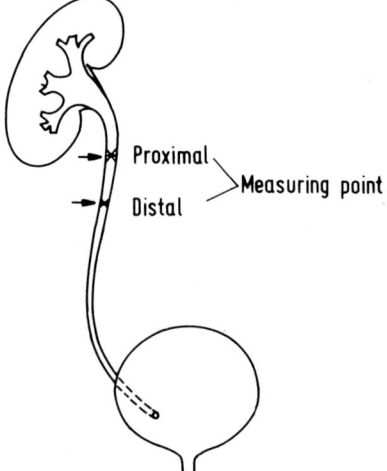

Fig. 1. Placement of the measuring sensors using pressure (Rakovec et al. 1982) or conductance measurement

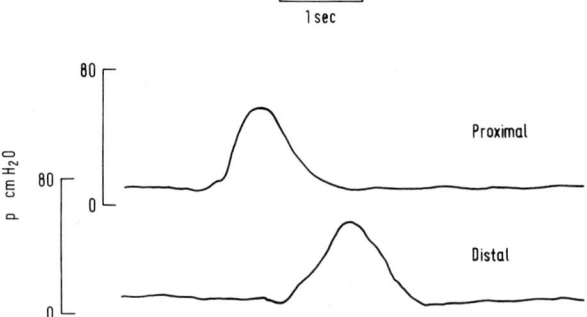

Fig. 2. Dual site pressure recording in the human ureter with placement of the pressure sensors as shown in Fig. 1. Kidney to bladder direction of the contraction waves is indicated from the recording with a velocity of 2.5 cm/s

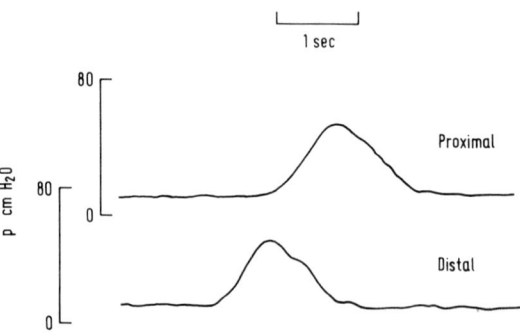

Fig. 3. Dual site pressure recording in the human ureter with placement of the pressure sensors as shown in Fig. 1. Antiperistalsis, i.e. bladder to kidney direction of the contraction waves, is indicated from the recording with a velocity of 5 cm/s

To overcome these problems, he introduced a new method (Whitaker 1973 a, b) by which the renal pelvis or ureter was perfused at known flow rates and simultaneously the back pressures to perfusion, as well as the pressures in the bladder were measured. Obstruction was diagnosed if the pressure drop between the renal pelvis or lower ureter and the bladder, at a flow rate of 10 ml/min, was greater than 10–12 cm H_2O.

More complex information on ureteral peristalsis was obtained by two different groups of investigators. Melchior and Simhan (1973) introduced a method of simultaneous measurement of pressure and flow rate at one site in the human ureter, which they called "uro-rheomanometry". The method uses pressure and flow measuring sensors placed on the tip of a 5F measuring probe. Djurhuus and Constantinou (1979) used the 4F flow velocity and cross sectional diameter probe developed by Rask-Andersen and Djurhuus (1976) for assessment of pyelo-ureteral function in the pig.

In our recent work a method for simultaneous measurement of electric conductance at two sites in the human ureter was developed and used to detect the presence, frequency, velocity, length and direction of the urine bolus and occlusiveness of the ureter between the two boli.

Electric Conductance Measuring Probe

A modified 4F ureteral catheter with two pairs of gold plated brass electrodes placed 5 cm apart was used for simultaneous electric conductance measurements (Fig. 4) at two sites in the human ureter. The presence of a urine bolus was detected by using the principle of the "electric fluid bridge test", described by Plevnik et al. (1983 a, b). The entry of the urine bolus in the ureter is detected from the change in electrical conductance between the two electrodes at each measuring site. The conductance of the inner ureteral wall is significantly lower than the conductance of urine. A constant sinusoidal voltage with an amplitude of 10 mV and a frequency of 50 kHz is applied to each pair of electrodes and the current which flows between each pair of electrodes is recorded.

Tracking the Urine Bolus

Measurements were performed on 26 patients without evidence of upper tract pathology, and in three patients with neurogenic bladders. The catheter was introduced into the ureter at cystoscopy and the electrodes placed in the upper third of the ureter (see Fig. 1). In 14 out of 26 controls stable patterns of ureteral peristalsis were obtained which lasted throughout the full length of the experiment (15 to 20 min) (Fig. 5). The frequency of peristalsis deduced from the recordings obtained in 14 controls are shown in Table 1.

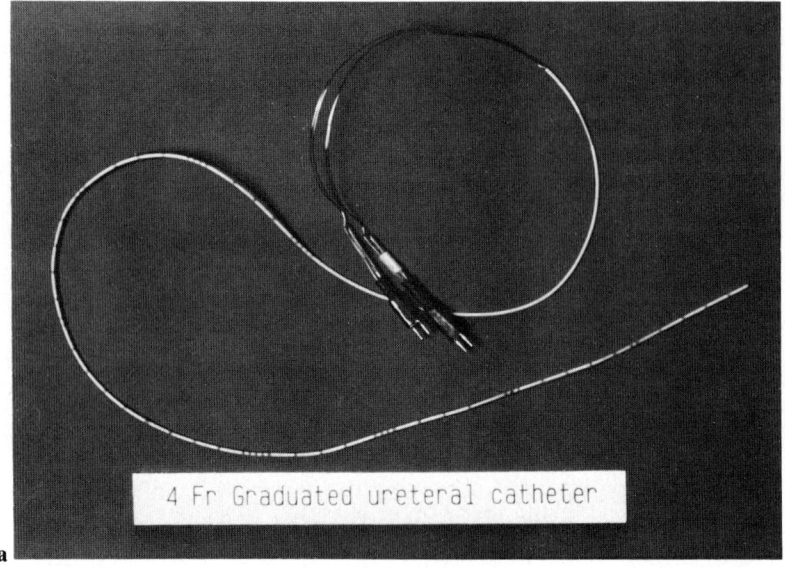
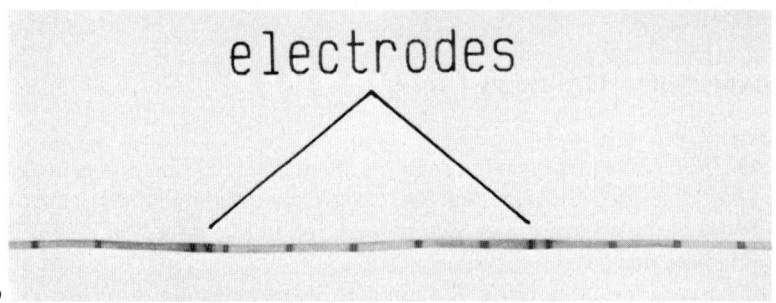

Fig. 4a,b. Probe for simultaneous electric conductance measurement at two sites in the human ureter

Velocity of the Bolus

The velocity and length of the urine bolus can be calculated from the recordings (Figs. 6, 7), but certain assumptions must be considered.

The theoretical scheme of passage of the urine bolus through points A and B, where the distance between the two points represents the distance between the two pairs of measuring electrodes (5 cm), is shown in Fig. 8.

Presuming that the front end of the bolus, D, travels along the length L from point A to point B at a uniform velocity, we can write:

$$v_{D(AB)} = \frac{L}{t_3 - t_1}.$$

Table 1

Material:	14 normal controls	
Frequency:	Mean:	3 bolus/min
	Range:	1.7–5 bolus/min
Velocity:	Mean:	2.75 cm/s
	Range:	2–5 cm/s
Length:	Mean:	6.15 cm
	Range:	2–10 cm

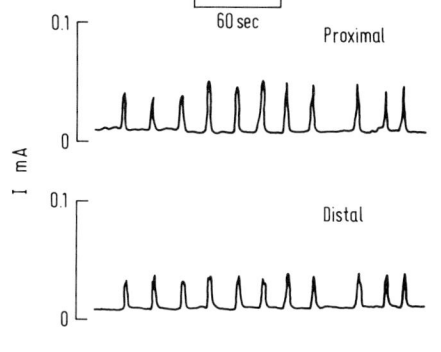

Fig. 5. Recording of peristalsis in control case M.D. frequency – 3.3 bolus/min

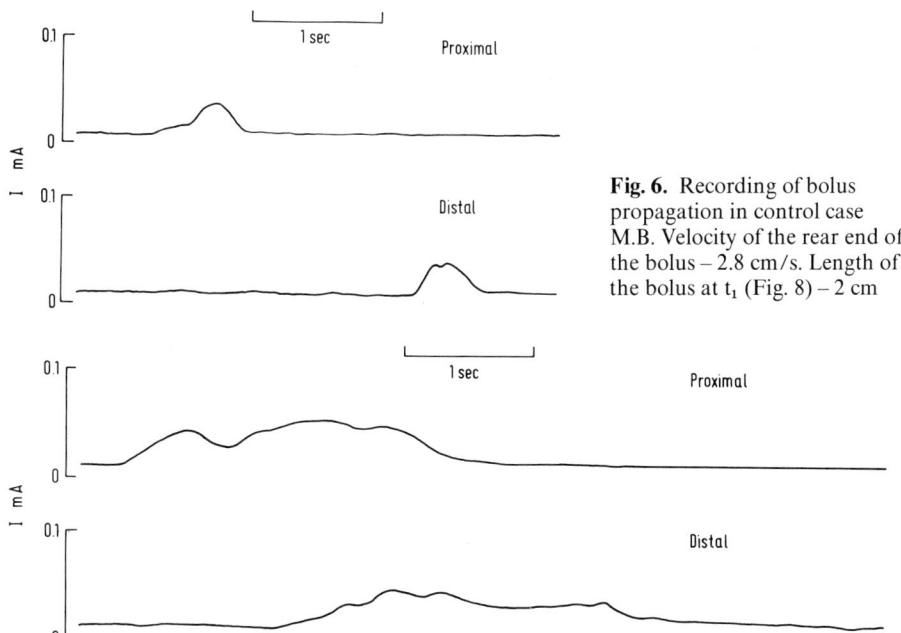

Fig. 6. Recording of bolus propagation in control case M.B. Velocity of the rear end of the bolus – 2.8 cm/s. Length of the bolus at t_1 (Fig. 8) – 2 cm

Fig. 7. Recording of bolus propagation in control case C.A. Velocity of the rear end of the bolus – 2.8 cm/s. Length of the bolus at t_1 (Fig. 8) – 7 cm. Note the significantly greater length of the urine bolus as compared to Fig. 6 for the same velocity of the bolus

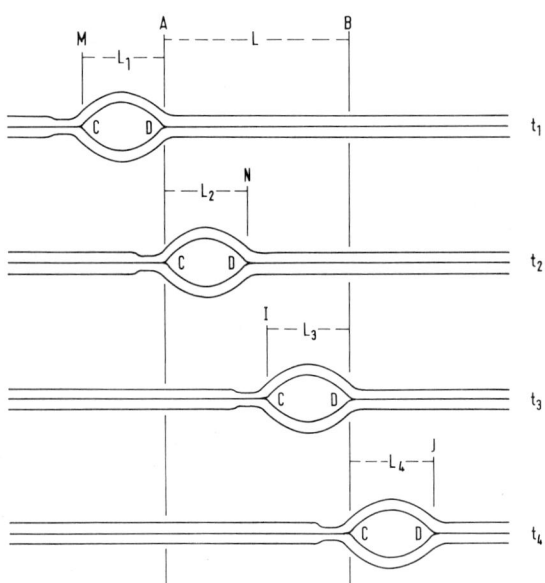

Fig. 8. Theoretical scheme of bolus propagation through the points A and B of the ureter at instants t_1, t_2, t_3, and t_4. L Length between points A and B

Considering similar assumption for the rear end of the bolus, we may write:

$$v_{C(AB)} = \frac{L}{t_4 - t_2}.$$

Thus the velocities of the front, $v_{D(AB)}$, and rear end of the bolus, $v_{C(AB)}$, at which they pass the ureteral part of length L, can be calculated.

Length of the Bolus

Lengths of the bolus at instants t_1, t_2, t_3, and t_4 (Fig. 8) can be calculated considering similar assumptions as before for the estimation of bolus velocity.

Assuming that rear end of the bolus, C, travels along the path MA (length of the bolus, L_1, at t_1) in time (t_2-t_1) at a uniform velocity $v_{C(MA)} = v_{C(AB)}$ the length of the bolus L_1 (at t_1) can be calculated from:

$$L_1 = v_{C(AB)}(t_2 - t_1).$$

Assuming that the rear of the bolus, C, travels along the path IB (length of the bolus L_3, at t_3) in time (t_4-t_3) at a uniform velocity $v_{C(IB)} = v_{C(AB)}$, the length of the bolus L_3 can be calculated from:

$$L_3 = v_{C(AB)}(t_4 - t_3).$$

Assuming that the front end of the bolus D travels along the path AN (length of the bolus, L_2, and t_2) in time (t_2-t_1) at uniform velocity, $v_{D(AN)} = v_{D(AB)}$, the length of the bolus L_2, can be calculated from:

$$L_2 = v_{D(AB)}(t_2-t_1).$$

Assuming that the front end of the bolus, D, travels along the path BJ (length of the bolus L_4, at t_4) in time (t_4-t_3) at uniform velocity, $v_{D(BJ)} = v_{D(AB)}$, the length of the bolus L_4 can be calculated from:

$$L_4 = v_{D(AB)}(t_4-t_3).$$

Velocities of the rear end of the boli and lengths of the boli (at t_1) deduced from stable recordings (14 controls) are shown in Table 1.

Direction of the Bolus

In all 14 controls from Table 1 peristalsis was directed from the kidney towards the bladder. This can be clearly recognized from the recordings (Figs. 5, 6, 7), since the change in conductance always occurred first at the proximal and later at the distal measuring point.

Occlusiveness of the Ureter Between Boli

In all 14 stable recordings of controls, the ureter was occlusive between the boli. In three patients with neurogenic bladder, peristalsis was not occlusive and was unsettled (Fig. 9).

Artefactual Measurements

In 12 out of 26 controls (46 percent) the catheter clearly caused obstruction which was seen as an unsettled and unocclusive pattern of peristalsis soon after the introduction of the catheter (Fig. 10).

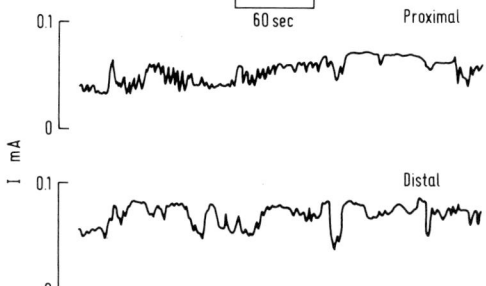

Fig. 9. Recording performed in patient F.G. with neurogenic bladder showing a nonocclusive and unsettled pattern of peristalsis

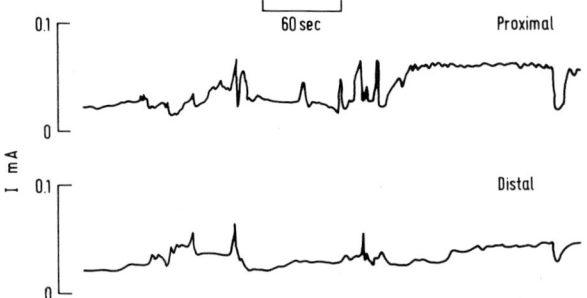

Fig. 10. Artefactual recording obtained in normal control G.I. Unsettled and nonocclusive pattern of peristalsis is seen soon after the introduction of the catheter

Conclusions

The main disadvantage of the method described is the presence of the catheter in the ureter which induced obstruction in 46 percent of the normal controls. If this could be avoided, the method could potentially provide an objective clinical index of upper tract pathology, such as for instance, ureteral obstruction.

It is interesting that such an artefact was observed, although a catheter was used of a size 4 F which, according to Kiil (1957), should not induce obstruction. This observation implies that conductance measurement as described is very sensitive in detecting obstruction, i.e. to the patency of the ureter which occurs as a consequence of obstruction, and which might not always be seen as a significant change in the base line pressure during manometric recordings.

Although it seems that the method as described at present causes too many artefacts to be of clinical use, it certainly has the potential to be used in physiological studies of the upper urinary tract. By appropriate modifications of the method, time-distance diagrams of ureteral peristalsis could be detected with greater accuracy compared with the results of cineradiography (Gerlach, 1983) in cases where the catheter causes no obstruction.

References

Djurhuus JC, Constantinou CE (1979) Assessment of pyeloureteral function using flow velocity and cross sectional diameter probe. Invest Urol 17:103–107
Gerlach R (1983) The time-distance-diagram of ureteral peristalsis. Abstracts of Workshop on Upper Urinary Tract Urodynamics, Aachen
Kiil F (1953) Pressure recordings in the upper urinary tract. Scand J Clin Lab Invest 5:383
Kiil F (1957) The function of the ureter and renal pelvis. Saunders, London
Melchior H, Simhan KK (1973) A new uro-rheomanometer. In: Lutzeyer W, Melchior H (eds) Urodynamics of the upper and lower urinary tract. Springer, Berlin Heidelberg New York, pp 30–34

Plevnik S, Vrtačnik P, Janež J (1983a) Detection of fluid entry into the urethra by electric impedance measurement: electric fluid bridge test. Clin Phys Physiol Meas 4:309–313

Plevnik S, Brown M, Sutherst JR, Vrtačnik P (1983b) Tracking of fluid in urethra by simultaneous electric impedance measurement at three sites. Urol Int 38:29–32

Rakovec S, Plevnik S, Vrtačnik P (1982) Urodynamic criteria for obstructions in the upper urinary tract. Abstracts of the 4th Congress of the European Association of Urology, Vienna

Rask-Anderson H, Djurhuus JC (1976) Development of a probe for endoureteral investigation of peristalsis by flow-velocity and cross section area measurement. Acta Urol Scand 472:59

Ross JA, Edmond P, Kirkland IS (1972) Behaviour of the human ureter in health and disease. Churchill Livingstone, Edinburgh

Struthers NW (1976) The physiology of the ureter. In: Williams DI, Chisholm GD (eds) Scientific foundation of urology. Heinemann Medical Books, London, pp 11–17

Whitaker RH (1973a) Methods of assessing obstruction in dilated ureters. Br J Urol 45:15

Whitaker RH (1973b) Diagnosis of obstruction in dilated ureters. Ann R Coll Surg Engl 53:153

Imaging of Peristaltic Urine Transport in the Ureter Using ^{123}Jodine Hippurate

K. U. Laval[1], K. Vyska[2], and F. Höck[2]

Clinical investigations of ureteral dynamic function are usually carried out by endoluminal techniques e.g. pressure (Boyarsky and Labay 1972; Lapides 1948; Lutzeyer 1963) and flow (Melchior and Simhan 1971) measurements, or by radiographic methods e.g. videodensitometry (Tscholl et al. 1974; Weinberg and Labay 1977) and cineradiography (Durben et al. 1980). Ureteral catheterism carries the risk of infection and also obstructs the urine transport whereas radiographic procedures have the well known disadvantages of reaction to radiopaque (Shehadi 1975), diuretic effects and radiation charge. The aim of our investigation was to find a concept of ureteral dynamic examination which avoids the disadvantages mentioned but nevertheless gives as reliable information on ureteral function as the techniques used so far.

Methods and Material

For our investigation we used ^{123}J-hippurate (Cyclotron of the E.I.R., Würenlingen/Swiss). The ^{123}Jodine used as the tracer was derived from the reaction: ^{127}J $(d, 6n)$ ^{123}Xe (β, EC) ^{123}J (Stöcklin 1977). The examination was carried out in supine position by means of a Gamma Camera (Nucl. Chicago LFOV) equipped with a high resolution parallel hole low energy collimator. The data were first computerized in list mode technique (Digital Equipment pdp 50). The data processing was usually done by printing series of matrices with a frequency of 1 matrix/s. On integral images of about 30 matrices we marked different regions of interest over the adrenal, mid and prevesical part of the ureter and also over the periureteral background tissue. The regions were designed as thin slices of the ureter extending about 2 to 3 cm in cranio-caudal direction. For these regions activity curves were calculated and plotted out at a frequency of 1 s beginning at the 10th second after a bolus like intravenous application and lasting till the 600th sec for normal individuals and until 30 min after the application for obstructed patients. Background activity was subtracted automatically.

Altogether 11 persons representing 20 reno-ureteral units have been investigated including 6 healthy volunteers and 5 patients. The patients suffered from uni- or bilateral ureteral obstruction caused by prevesical calculi or cancer invasion of the prevesical ureteral shead. The mean age of the group was 49.6 years.

---

1 Urodynamisches Laboratorium Düsseldorf, D-4000 Düsseldorf
2 Nuklearmedizinische Abteilung KFA Jülich, D-5170 Jülich

Before the examination no special preparation or diet was required except fluid intake abstinence for 2 hours before the examination, to achieve a physiological steady state of diuresis. For examining the diuretic effect on ureteral peristalsis we used furosemide 40 mg intravenously applied. We made sure that a constant peristaltic frequency and approximately steady bolus volume was registered before application. All the individuals recieved 2 mCi ^{123}J hippurate intravenously. The maximal radiation charge for the bladder as the critical organ was calculated at 100 mrem.

Results

After application of ^{123}J hippurate the ureter could be seen as a continuum of activity running from the kidney to the urinary bladder. The activity in the ureter was remarkably higher than in the background tissue and under normal non-obstructed conditions would be registered about 200 s after the bolus-like intravenous application. When the urine transport was obstructed the time between application of the activity and its appearance in the ureter was prolonged. In cases of decreased renal function the resolution of the ureter got worse and was prolonged according to the degree of renal failure.

The activity within the ureter was calculated over the marked regions of interest as described above. We could identify waves of activity. Both minima and maxima of the waves had a recurrent frequency of 25 to 30 s in all the examined individuals. Typically the maximum was immediately followed by the periodic minimum of activity.

The activity waves showed a directed propagation from the kidney to the bladder. The latency time between the adrenal and the mid-ureter region was about 1 s while between the mid-ureter and the prevesical region we found a latency time of about 4 s.

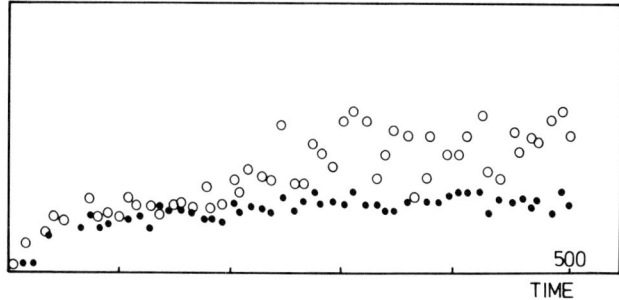

Fig. 1. Activity recording from the right mid-ureter region (○) and the periureteral tissue (●) between the 9th and the 500th second after application. Both curves show a rapid increase after bolus-like application of the isotope and stay at the same level for approximately 3 minutes. Thereafter rhythmic changes of activity are recorded from the region of the mid-ureter. The oscillations are superimposed on the background level

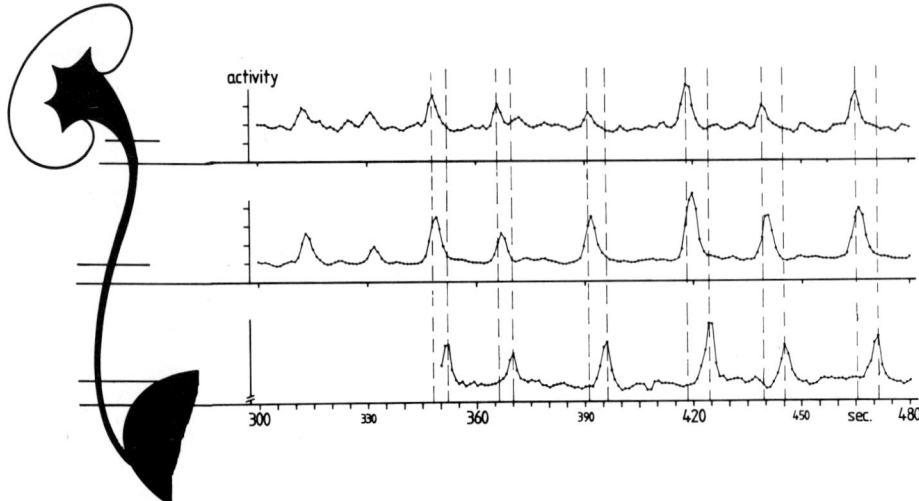

Fig. 2. Activity curves taken from the adrenal, mid-ureter and prevesical region of a normal, non-obstructed ureter. The analysis is carried out by activity calculation of one frame/s. Accumulations of activity are seen in all regions. The curve registered over the mid-ureter shows a most accurate separation of the single activity boli. In between the boli the activity remains at background level demonstrating an empty, closed ureter. The time distance between the maximum points is about 25 s. Over the adrenal ureter oscillations of activity between the maximum spikes are registered, suggesting a higher frequency of peristalsis

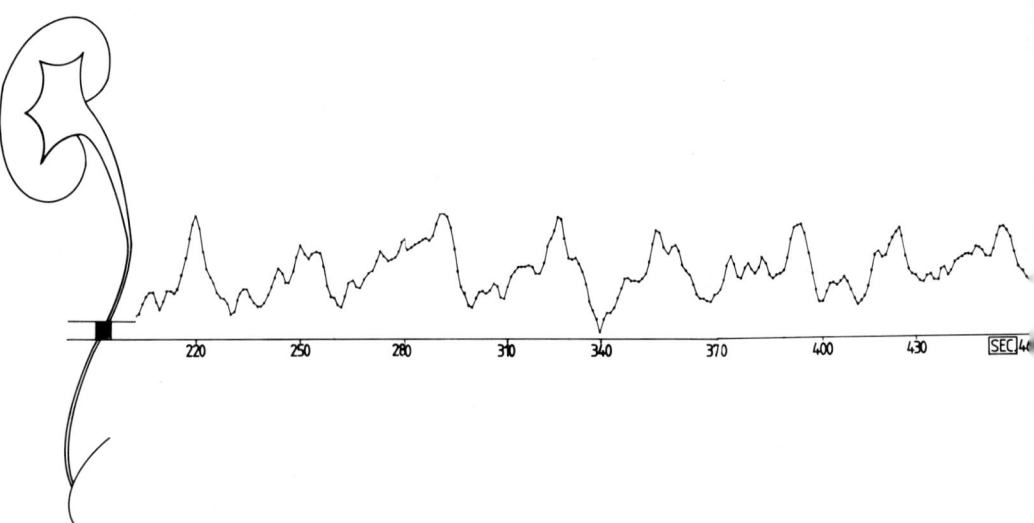

Fig. 3. Activity curve registered from a mid-ureter segment of a normal non-obstructed ureter. The analysis is carried out by activity calculation of one frame/s. About 3 min after application activity waves are recorded with a frequency of about 2/min. In this patient in contrast to Fig. 2 the shape of the curve shows a more continuous increase of activity up to the next maximum which is then followed by an abrupt decrease to the next minimum. Oscillations of a higher frequency are superimposed on the curve

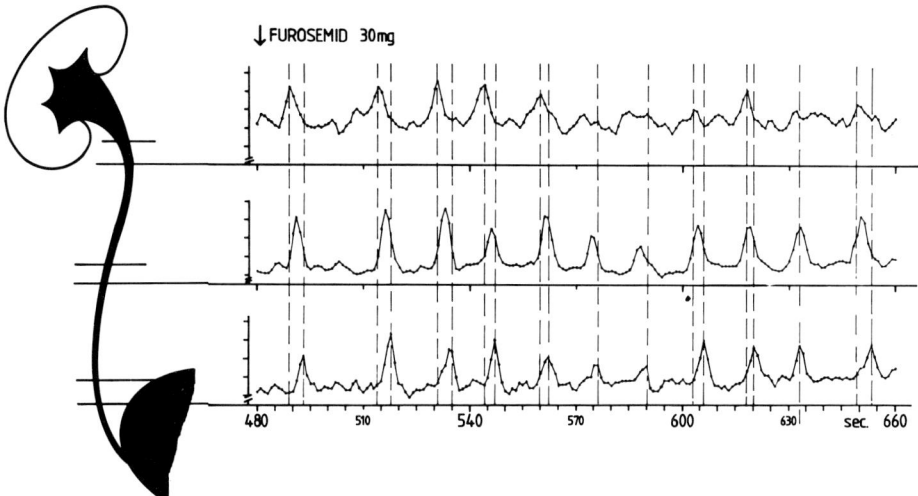

Fig. 4. Activity curve taken from the adrenal, mid-ureter and prevesical region of a normal ureter after furosemide-induced diuresis. The analysis is carried out by activity calculation of one frame/s. After application of furosemide an immediate increase of frequency of peristalsis is seen. In the mid-ureter region frequency is doubled. Between the boli background level is registered. Under diuresis progression time from the adrenal to the prevesical region seems to be shortened from 5 s to 3 s

The shape of the activity curves registered over the different regions showed typical variations in accordance with the region they were taken from. The activity waves derived from the adrenal region displayed oscillations within one single recurrence period of the wave. The oscillations showed a relatively low amplitude compared to the maxima of the activity wave. The time distance between the maximum point of the wave and the maximum point of the oscillation was about 10 to 14 s.

In most individuals the activity curves derived from the mid ureter region and with small reservations also from the prevesical ureter showed a short, limited bolus-like activity volume which passed the region in about 6 s. Between two boluses there was an almost equable niveau of activity at background level. However, in a few cases we found a different shape of the activity curve. In these individuals the maximum was also followed by a sharp decrease of activity to its periodic minimum corresponding to our findings in most of the individuals, but starting from the minimum point there was an approximately steady increase of activity till the following maximum. In these cases we also found oscillations of activity in the rising part of the curve very similar to the oscillations registered over the adrenal region. The frequency of the oscillations was also about 10 to 14 s.

The studies on the diuretic effects on ureteral peristalsis were performed, when an approximately steady bolus volume with a constant frequency was registered. 30 s after intravenous application of 40 mg of furosemide we found a rapid increase of the number of activity waves. The intervals between the maximum points of activity were about 15 s and the frequency almost doubled compared to the curves from the mid ureter as well as from the prevesical region before application.

In the adrenal ureter we found a further increase of persistaltic frequency. The intervals between the maximum points of the boluses were usually 8 s in this part of the ureter under the condition of forced diuresis. The activity spikes were flatter than in the more caudal parts of the ureter, and also only every second activity spike was propagated further downwards, when the frequency was 8 s in the adrenal ureter. Even the propagation speed of the activity wave was increased. The latency time needed to propagate the bolus maximum from the adrenal to the prevesical region was about 3 s.

Discussion

The purpose of examining the ureter transport function is to describe physiological phenomena and their pathological changes in order to find a way to cure the patient. By means of the common endoureteral as well as periureteral techniques pressure, flow and electromyographic phenomina of the physiological urine transport as well as their pathological changes can be registered sufficiently. However, the diagnostic procedures charge the patient considerably because endoluminal or even surgical manipulations are necessary in order to place the probe properly. Moreover, the endoluminal probe will obstruct the urine transport according to its diameter and the result of the examination will be only an approximate description of the actual process in the ureter.

The disadvantages of the common techniques have been the motive to look for non-invasive procedures. For an adequate alternative procedure we therefore require that the procedure
1) has no influence on the patho-physiological steady state situation of urine transport,
2) brings out the characteristic details of urine transport convertible to the results of invasive techniques so that well-known phenomena of ureter dynamics can also be formed in the information obtained by the non-invasive procedure.

We used ^{123}J-hippurate in the experiments because in our opinion the physical as well as pharmacokinetic properties of the radionuclide made it most fitted. The short half-life of the isotope limits the radiation dose to the patient and allows its application even in cases of restricted renal function, when the endocorporal circulation time is prolonged. The decomposition product Xenon will be expired by the lung. The renal pharmacokinetic properties of hippuric acid provides the highest possible concentration of the radionuclid in the urine by glomerular filtration as well as tubular secretion. Because of this a sufficient gradient of activity between the ureter and the background as well as the blood vessels will be achieved, though under physiological conditions the diameter of the ureter is small and also the organ is not continuously filled. Studies carried out by using ^{99}Tc-DTPA (Laval et al. 1979) showed us that the activity gradient achieved by a substance only filtrated glomerularly will be insufficient for examinations on physiological ureter dynamics.

The results obtained from our studies show a good correlation to the findings of many authors who used the classic invasive or even in vitro experimental techniques. By using ^{123}J-hippurate the ureter of normal healthy individuals which had not been previously hydrated, could be seen as a continuum of activity running from the kidney to the bladder. By using the technique of different regions of interest over the ureter we could register a periodic transport of activity from the kidney towards the bladder. These peristaltic activity waves showed a time distance between the maximum points of about 25 to 30 s, corresponding to the results of other investigators who used the endoluminal and electromyographic techniques on humans (Durben et al. 1980; Hannappel et al. 1982; Zödler et al. 1978). Forced diuresis induced an increase of peristaltic frequency. In general we found a multiplication of the frequency by the factor 2 to 4, corresponding to the results of other authors (Durben et al. 1980; Zödler et al. 1978). The shapes of the peristaltic boli were very similar for each individual, but they differed on a large scale among the individuals examined. However, in all individuals we constantly found the maximum activity directly followed by the next minimum. We would like to interpret this minimum of activity as the mark of the contractile ring which follows the urine bolus and has been identified as the propagating force of the ureter muscle (Durben et al. 1980; Zödler et al. 1978). A scale of variations in the ascending part of the curve could be seen between the minimum and the next maximum point. In most individuals the incision made by the contractile ring was followed by a period of activity at background level. During this period the ureter seemed to be empty and closed, whereas the urine which is continuously produced would be stored in the renal pelvis for a short while. Other individuals showed a more constant increase of activity beginning right after the minimum (Fig. 3). This type of curve indicated that an increasing amount of urine was almost reaching the mid-ureter region without being stored in the pelvis.

References

Boyarsky S, Labay PC (1972) Ureteral dynamics. Williams & Wilkins, Baltimore
Durben G, Gerlach R, Eichhorn F, Friedrich R, Schäfer W, Lutzeyer W (1980) The time-distance diagram. A new method to analyze ureteral peristalsis by cineradiography. Invest Urol 18:207
Hannappel J, Golenhofen K, Hohnsbei J, Lutzeyer W (1982) Pacemaker process of ureteral peristalsis in multicalyceal kidneys. Urol Int 37:240
Lapides J (1948) Physiology of the intact human ureter. J Urol 59:501
Laval KU, Höck F, Freundlieb Chr (1979) Visualisation of the ureter by radioisotopic methods. Urol Res 7:43
Lutzeyer W (1963) Harnleiterdruckmessungen. Urol Int 16:1
Melchior H, Simhan KK (1971) Zur Problematik der Uro-Rheomanometrie. Biomed Technik 16:99
Shehadi WH (1975) Adverse reactions to intravascularly administered contrast media. A comprehensive study based on a prospective study. Am J Roentg 124:145
Stöcklin G (1977) Bromine-77 and Jodine-123 radiopharmaceuticals. Int J App Radiat Isot 28:131
Tscholl R et al. (1974) Measurement of the velocity and rate of ureteral contractions with a video integrator in a model, in animals and in humans, preoperatively and with intact body surface. Invest Urol 12:224
Weinberg SL, Labay PC (1977) Ureteral function. The urometrogram at increased urine output. Invest Urol 14:307
Zödler T, Geisler R, Hannappel J, Schulman CC (1978) Frequenzverteilung der Harnleiterelektromyogramme bei verschiedenen Spezies. Urol Res 7:42

The Nuclear Medical Space Time Matrix Approach to Ureteral Motility

W. MÜLLER-SCHAUENBURG[1] and K. ANGER[2]

Introduction

Ureteral peristalsis can be studied traditionally by tracing
- electrical excitation,
- pressure,
- X-ray morphology, or
- the elimination of heat, generated from an intra-ureteral rheographic probe (Melchior 1971).

In the past the clinical use of these methods was restricted by an imbalance between the information we got and the price we had to pay: either by being invasive when assessing electrical excitation, effective heat conductivity, or intra-ureteral pressure, or by a rather high radiation burden in cineradiography.

In addition, all those approaches somehow interfere with the physiology of ureteral peristaltic transport: Electrical excitation can be recorded only in animal experiments or during operations, the manometric and uro-rheographic probes introduce at least a transient perturbation into the ureter, and the contrast medium in cineradiography promotes diuresis.

Finally, if we focus on clinical feasibility, only manometry, uro-rheography, and cineradiography have to be considered, the latter being superior in documenting the full space time pattern of ureteral motility. But unfortunately the advantage of high information content is not complemented by a convenient way of imaging the cineradiographic space time information at a compressed level: In the present conference Gerlach compiles time distance diagrams of ureteral motion, and Ohlson describes his kinetic urography of the renal pelvis and the ureter. Though in principle they are important, these approaches are cumbersome and not yet suitable for clinical routine.

The set of accesses to ureteral peristalsis mentioned above was complemented by Müller-Schauenburg in 1978 by the introduction of the nuclear medical space time matrix. This technique (Müller-Schauenburg et al. 1979; Byrom et al. 1982)
- is almost non-invasive (needing only an i.v. injection),
- does not interfere with ureter function (e.g. working at any level of diuresis),
- permits various steps of data compression (displaying e.g. 5 to 20 min of motility information in a single frame) and

---

[1] Nuklearmedizinische Abteilung des Medizinischen Strahleninstituts der Universität Tübingen, Röntgenweg 11, D-7400 Tübingen
[2] Abteilung Radiologie der Medizinischen Fakultät der RWTH Aachen, D-5100 Aachen

– is based upon routine radioisotope renography with 123-I-hippuran, 99m-Tc-DTPA, or 99m-Tc-MDP.

In the case of 99m-Tc-MDP the approach is a by-product of routine bone scans, permitting to study the physiology of normal ureters (cf. Kiil 1973), without any additional radiation exposure to the patient.

The Nuclear Medical Space Time Matrix

What is a Matrix?

A matrix is the standard tool to display computerized nuclear medical images of radioisotope distributions obtained from a Gamma Camera, e.g. on a TV screen. The square image is subdivided into 32×32, 64×64, 128×128, or 256×256 square elements, called cells or pixels. The image consists of the number of decay events or counts, which had been registered within the individual cells by the Gamma Camera. Such a computerized scintigraphic image is displayed on a TV screen by converting count numbers per cell into an intensity or colour scale.

In contrast to this computer approach of digitized scintigrams, nuclear medicine can directly image analogous scintigrams on X-ray film by putting one tiny dot per registered event on the film, without reference to a grid of e.g. 64×64 image cells.

While the computer approach forms the basis of further quantification (e.g. resulting in compressed images of ureteral peristalsis), the analogous scintigrams on X-ray film are an important complement in outlining the ureter and documenting slow changes in its radioisotope content. Analogous scintigrams are superior in spatial resolution compared to digitized computer images, because the former ones are not impaired by the subdivision into cells or pixels.

The Space Time Matrix

How can we compress information on ureteral motility into a matrix? The answer is that we have to put the time into the image. The ureter is more or less a one-dimensional organ. Nuclear medicine cannot resolve changes in diameter directly, only indirectly by monitoring the varying radioisotope content in the ureter, i.e. measuring the increase caused by an urine bolus and the decrease during the following contraction.

Where to put the spatial coordinate, and where to put the time? It is straightforward to take the time as abscissa (x-axis) and the spatial coordinate along the ureter as ordinate (y-axis). Gerlach's time distance diagrams and the M-mode of sonography do it in the same way. To obtain a proper spatial coordinate along the ureter, we have to rectify the organ.

The rectification is achieved by dividing the ureter into a series of regions of interest, mostly rectangular ones (Fig. 1). Regions of interest are a standard tool of nuclear medicine to proceed from a series of scintigrams to time activity curves ob-

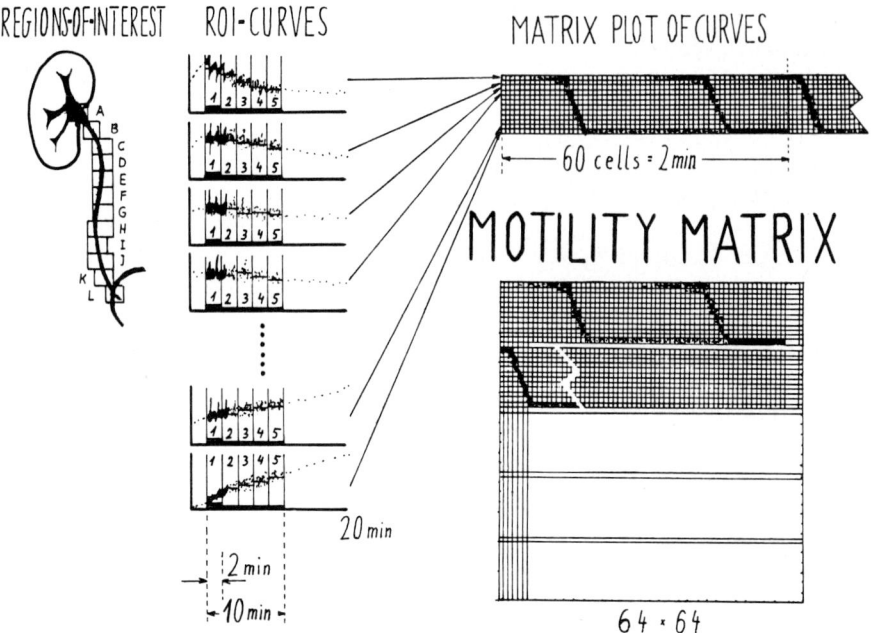

Fig. 1. The principle of the space time matrix (motility matrix). In the case illustrated, only 10 min within the first 20 minutes after injection had been acquired at a high frame rate of 1 frame per 2 s, showing the characteristic high scatter in each of the 12 region of interest curves. The 10 min are subdivided into 5 time segments, called 1, 2, 3, 4, 5, corresponding to 5 matrix segments in the motility matrix. Alternatively the full time interval of 20 min after injection can be imaged by using a frame rate of 2.5 s per frame, 8 time segments, and 7 regions of interest

tained from those regions. Each region creates one time activity curve. If we consider one special scintigram or frame, each region gives one count number added up from all cells in the region. A region works as a "super cell" or "super pixel", and a series of regions of interest covering the whole ureter compiles a set of count numbers, one count number per region, altogether forming a count profile along the curved ureter.

The basic step of the space time matrix is done by attributing the curved count profiles from the super pixels (regions of interest) to a normal straight count profile of a column of matrix cells, the number of cells in the column being equal to the number of regions of interest.

What has to be done by the software? Let us suppose that we use 7 regions of interest covering the ureter. These 7 regions compile 7 count numbers from frame one, and they may be inscribed (by a program) into the first column as profile number one, in the upper left corner of the 'motility matrix' or 'space time matrix', which we are just going to generate. The 7 count numbers from frame two are similarly inscribed into the 7 cells to the right of the first profile. Frame number three compiles profile number three which is inscribed into column number three. We thus fill one profile after the other into the upper 7 rows of our space time matrix.

What are those rows or lines of this new matrix? The top row or line of the matrix contains the counts obtained from region number one, the pelvic region. Row number two contains the counts from the subpelvic region, etc. until row number seven from a prevesical or a vesical region.

In summary, the basic step of generating a space time matrix is performed by inscribing count profiles from a series of regions of interest into columns of a matrix. The y-coordinate (or line number) in this "motility matrix" is the region number or the spatial coordinate along the ureter, the x-axis (or column number) is the frame number of the original scintigraphic series and corresponds to time.

For the sake of simplicity we do not fill all columns of the matrix. We stop at column 60. 60 columns (corresponding to 60 original frames) represent a time of 1, 2, or 2.5 min, depending on the frame rate of 1, 2, or 2.5 s per original frame.

How to proceed, when the top 7 by 60 cells of the 'motility matrix' are filled? It is nearly straightforward to leave one line of empty cells between, and to proceed below with the next segment of time, just as we write one line below the other in a text, always from left to right. If we keep to the example of 7 regions of interest, we may cope with 8 time segments, corresponding to 8×1 min, 8×2 min, or 8×2.5 min of motility information.

Basic Space Time Patterns

The basic pattern we are looking for is an oblique line, attributed to a travelling urine bolus and the following contraction wave. If the ureter is empty at rest, the line of increased radioisotope content of the travelling urine bolus is the dominating feature (Fig. 3). This is the normal case. For the hydroureter the line of decreased radioisotope content in the contraction wave is the trace of ureteral peristalsis (Figs. 5 and 2).

Background Subtraction

Both of the peristaltic patterns described above – the positive bolus lines and the negative contraction lines – are rather sharp in time compared to the interval between different peristaltic waves, if we consider one region along the ureter being attributed to a matrix line. In order to enhance the oblique line patterns a constant background subtraction has been applied to each matrix line individually by subtracting

– the average count value per matrix line or
– the minimum count value per line (minus one).

The first form gives a stronger enhancement of the positive bolus lines by setting all cells with count values below the average to zero. The second form (minimum subtraction) is especially suitable for contraction waves and preserves the full dynamics of the time course in the matrix line. What is the 'real' background, i.e. the activity time course of the tissue surrounding the ureter? For the mid-ureter it is a slowly decreasing function, but at least close to the bladder the functions look different.

Experiments with a slow varying background have been made, by subtracting from each ureteral region activity time course its own severely smoothed curve (reduced by a scaling factor to avoid areas of negative differences, which would be handled as unstructured areas of zero count pixels). This strategy is suitable if we consider the positive spindle lines. In order to also enable observation of slow phenomena like an increasing ureteral cone, we kept to the stepwise subtraction technique in the routine.

Further Contrast Enhancement by Display Manipulations

Statistical variations of the radioisotope decay numbers within the travelling peristaltic bolus are information which we want to discard in favour of the discrimination between the positive signal and the background noise. Overall we have three levels of interest:
- the very low level of a travelling contraction wave,
- the statistical pattern of the background, and
- the positive lines of a travelling urine bolus.

In order to get a somehow homogeneous intensity level displayed within the positive peristaltic lines, all cells above a count level chosen by the operator are displayed at maximum intensity. This level (the so-called upper threshold) is chosen to allow a maximal distinction between the three classes described above. This strategy supports the doctor's capability to recognize the pattern (Fig. 2).

Understanding Versus Generating Space Time Matrices

The space time matrix has been introduced by taking the count profiles along the ureter as elements.

Discussing the background subtraction, we considered the time course within individual ureter regions.

Both points of view, the radioactivity (count) profile at a chosen time, and the activity time course within a chosen ureteral region of interest, are equally important in understanding and interpreting the space time matrix.

The process of generating a space time matrix is dominated by the second point of view, referencing the region of interest curves. When the flagging of the ureter by

---

Fig. 2a–c. Motility of the left ureter of a 4 year old boy, showing a transition from retroperistalsis (segments 2 and 3) to a normal peristalsis (segments 4 and 5). Radioisotope dose: 18 MBq = 475 uCi 123-I-hippuran. **a** (*left part*) Enhancement of space time pattern, discarding information upon activity peaks. **b** (*left part*) By a different thresholding the retroperistaltic activity peaks in the renal pelvic matrix lines of segments 2 and 3 are retained. **c** 'Interpretation' of **b**. Adjunctive information: **a** (*right part*) A digital sum image (substitute for analogous imaging) shows the wide left ureter. **b, c** (*right part*) Curves from the left kidney with retroperistaltic activity peaks. The time interval of the motility matrix (scattering in the curves) is 0 to 10 min p.i. The first matrix segment is empty, corresponding to the phase before the radioisotope enters the ureter (rising phase of the kidney curve)

The Nuclear Medical Space Time Matrix Approach to Ureteral Motility 159

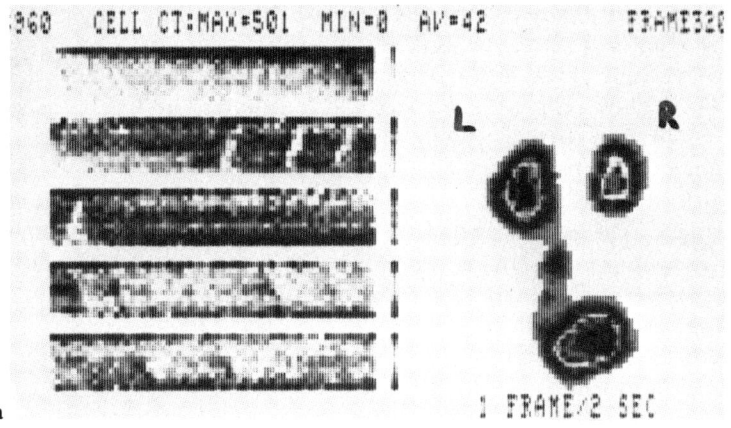

a

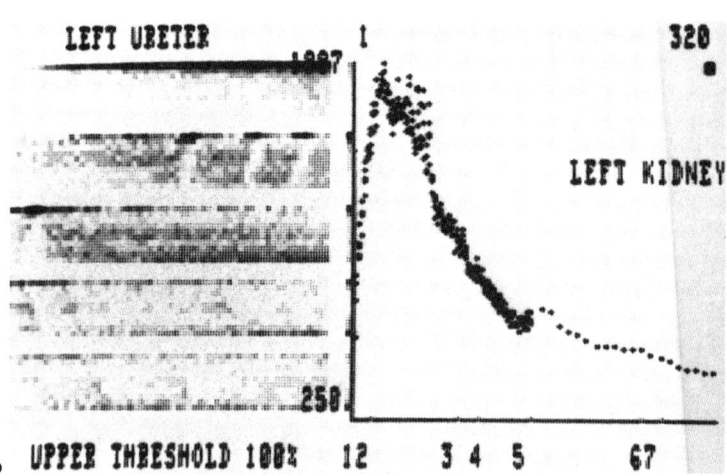

b

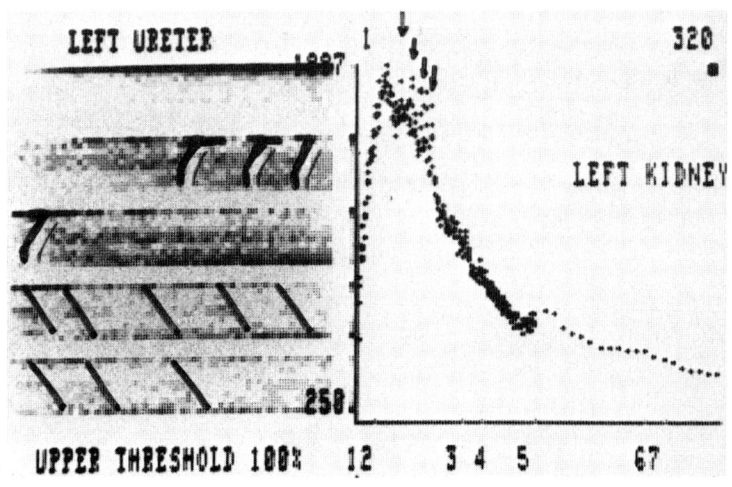

c

a series of regions of interest has been completed, standard data handling generates the corresponding region of interest curves. This process may be considered to be the central step in extracting the motility information from a series of e.g. 300 to 480 scintigrams. This data extraction process includes a data compression, since we discard count information from outside of the ureter and we reduce the spatial resolution along the ureter to the coarse set of regions of interest.

After the main step of data extraction and compression, a small special program enters the count values from the set of region of interest curves into the space time matrix. The final display manipulations are again within routine nuclear medical procedures.

Results

Space Time Matrix Information on Ureteral Function

The basic informations gained are
– the direction of the peristaltic wave,
  normally pointing downwards
  retroperistalsis being a pathological pattern,
– frequency,
  aperistalsis as the lower limit,
  stenosis peristalsis as high frequency limit,
– regularity, and
– an estimate of propagation speed.

Special patterns are
– intra-ureteral reflux,
– intermittent ureteral depots,
– long ureteral cones, and
– vesico-ureteral reflux.

Adjunctive Information on Ureteral Peristalsis by Different Ways of Data Compression Respectively Enhancement

The highly sensitive enhancement of space time patterns by the space time matrix enhances noise as well, and enhanced random patterns may be falsely interpreted as traces of motility. Alternative ways of data compression help to avoid such artifacts due to enhancement.

   Two types of information have proved to be useful:
– The kidney curve supplies information upon the *radioisotope input* into the ureter.
– The analogous series of e.g. 1 min per image delineates the ureter and documents the slow variation of the ureteral *radioisotope content.*

Both informations compile data about the chance to image ureteral motility in the different parts of the space time matrix.

The Nuclear Medical Space Time Matrix Approach to Ureteral Motility

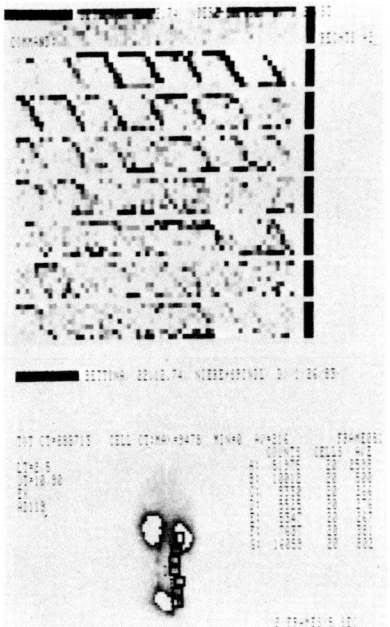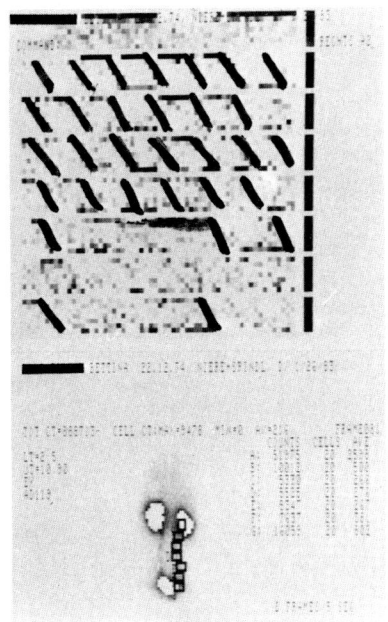

Fig. 3a, b. Normal and regular peristaltic pattern from an 8 year old girl with vesico-ureteral reflux on the contralateral side (cf. Fig. 4). Imaging interval 0 to 20 min after injection of 30 MBq = 800 uCi 123-I-hippuran. The bottom part shows the corresponding series of 7 regions of interest covering the right ureter. **b** 'Interpretation' of **a**

The point of view of data compression may guide us in comparing the types of information quoted above (Müller-Schauenburg 1982).

The space time matrix
- discards one spatial coordinate, and
- focuses upon time and the spatial coordinate along the ureter.

The kidney curve
- discards both spatial coordinates in favor of a single region of interest, and
- focuses upon counts and time.

The analogous series
- reduces the resolution in time and counts, and
- focuses upon the spatial coordinates.

Curves and analogous series are directly complementary and the space time matrix is an independent direction of focusing resp. data compression.

Nuclear medical imaging of function may be considered to be a spectrum of strategies of data compression and enhancement. Concerning ureteral motility the set described above is suitable to image repetitive patterns of peristaltic motion. The role of kidney curves and analogous series as adjunctive information to the space time matrix may be summarized as follows: The kidney curves
- support the documentation of retroperistaltic waves by showing the spikes of radioactivity in the renal pelvis (Fig. 2).

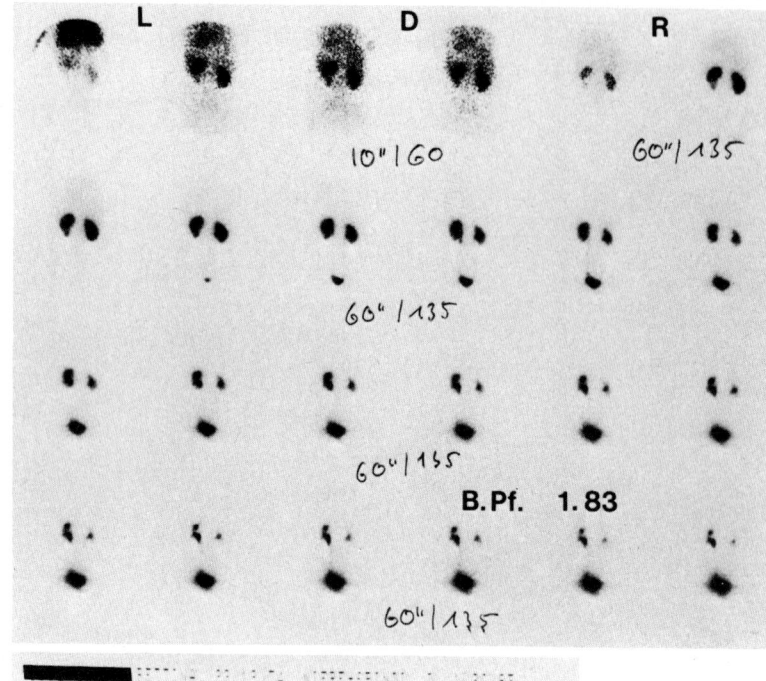

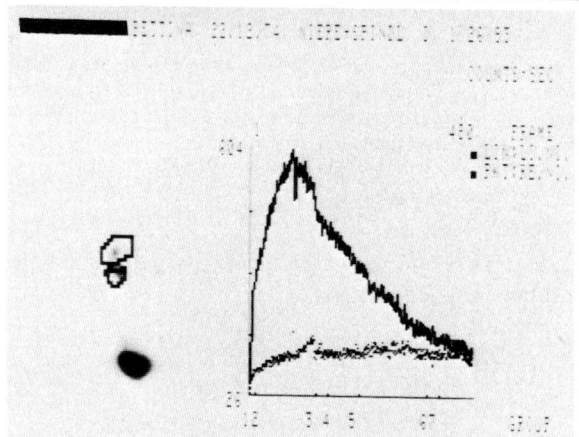

Fig. 4a–g. 8 year old boy with double ureter on the left side (same patient as in Fig. 3). **a** Analogous series, starting with 4 images, 10 s each, followed by images of 1 min duration. In the parenchymal phase (*top line, last image*) the two parts of the double kidney can be perceived distinctly. In the second line the upper left kidney fills its ureter and in the bottom line the second left ureter is filled by the lower left kidney (later the refluxive part). **b** Separate curves from the upper (normal functioning) and the lower (refluxive) parts of the doubled left kidney (artifact of motion close to the climax of the upper curve). **c** Analogous imaging of vesico-ureteral reflux during micturition, 10 s per image. **d** Radiographic assessment of reflux of the same ureter 4 years earlier, showing only a small ureteral reflux (with kind permission of Dr. K. Nolte, Paediatric Radiology, University of Tübingen). **e** ROI curves of the left kidney and the bladder, being the classical tool for documenting reflux. The severely scattering curve is already suspicious for retroperistalsis. **f** Space time matrix of the refluxive ureter, revealing retroperistalsis immediately after reflux. For the time preceding the reflux we lack any information on peristalsis. *Bottom part* 6 regions of interest covering the left double ureter. **g** 'Interpretation' of **f**

B.Pf. 26.1.83

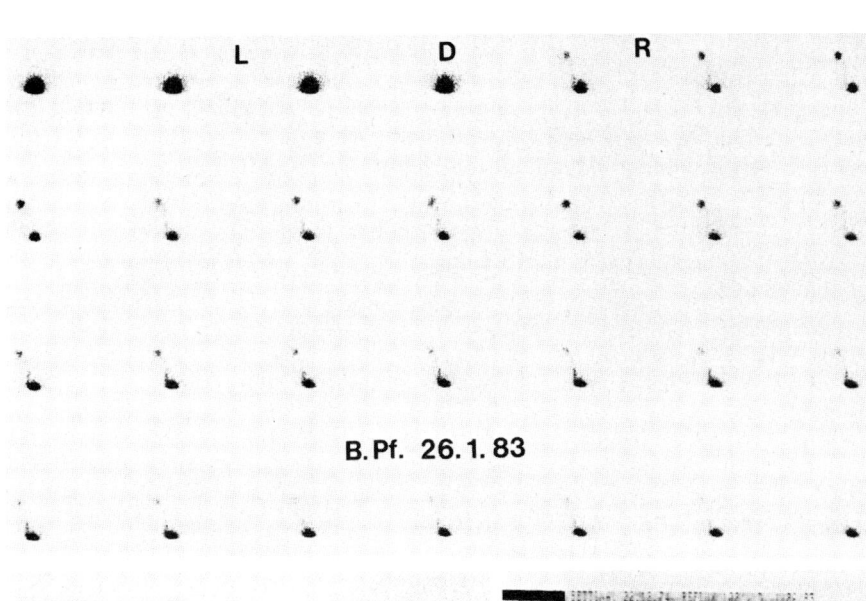

B.Pf. 28.11.78

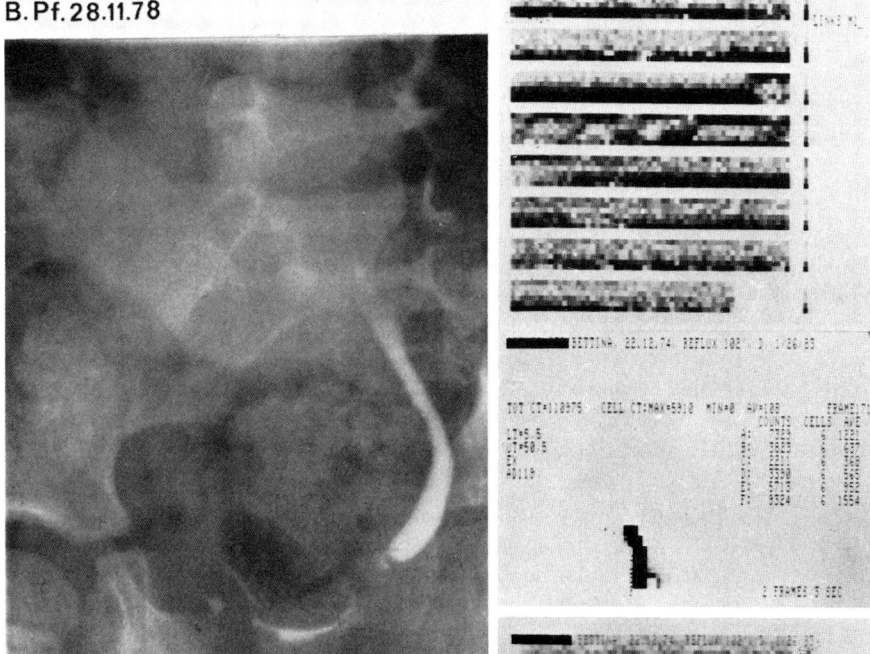

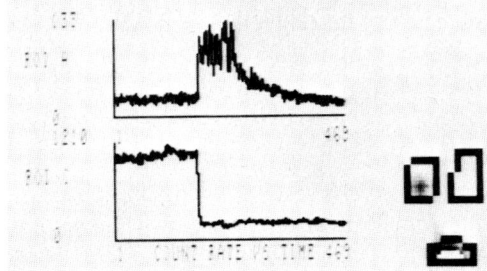

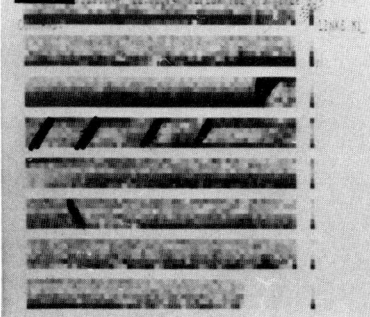

- In cases of double ureters renal pelvic curves may discriminate between the two ureters beyond the resolution of the space time matrix.
  pelvic curves document the radioisotope input into the different ureters (Fig. 4 b) as well as,
  the retrograde output in retroperistalsis or reflux.

The analogous images are helpful in imaging
- double ureters
- hydroureters,
- intra-ureteral depots
- ureteral irregularities in connection with intra-ureteral reflux, and
- ureteral cones.

Vesico-Ureteral Reflux and Retroperistalsis

Vesico-ureteral reflux and retroperistalsis are two different phenomena, but they may occur simultaneously.

The documentation of peristalsis during micturition requires a sufficient radioisotope content in the ureter during this phase. On the other side we try to have an empty upper urinary tract prior to the indirect test for vesico-ureteral reflux. Both requirements meet only in cases of sufficient reflux.

During the last month we had 4 such children with sufficient vesico-ureteral reflux. Two of them showed retroperistalsis in the refluxive phase (Fig. 4 f, g) and two of them did not. None of them showed retroperistalsis in supine position during the first 20 minutes after injection.

Several factors favour retroperistalsis during the test for reflux:
- the upright position during micturition (cf. Schmidt 1978)
- the elevated bladder pressure, impairing the emptying of the distal ureter into the bladder in the phase preceding micturition.

These factors have an influence even in the absence of reflux, thus stressing the importance of discriminating vesico-ureteral reflux, retroperistalsis associated with reflux, and retroperistalsis without such reflux.

The space time matrix has not turned out to be sensitive in documenting vesico-ureteral reflux itself. This reflux has a high speed and is not as repetitive as peristaltic or associated phenomena like intra-ureteral reflux. Therefore, the classical region of interest curve technique, analogous images, and certain difference images (Müller-Schauenburg et al. 1980) are better in documenting vesico-ureteral reflux, but the space time matrix reveals the interrelationship between retroperistalsis and reflux, and it makes the indirect nuclear medical test for reflux more specific.

Megaureter Motility

Megaureters (cf. Coolsaet et al. 1980) are an ideal object for applying the space time matrix (Fig. 5). It is well known that the prognosis of operating such ureters correlates with pre-operative motility (Melchior 1981).

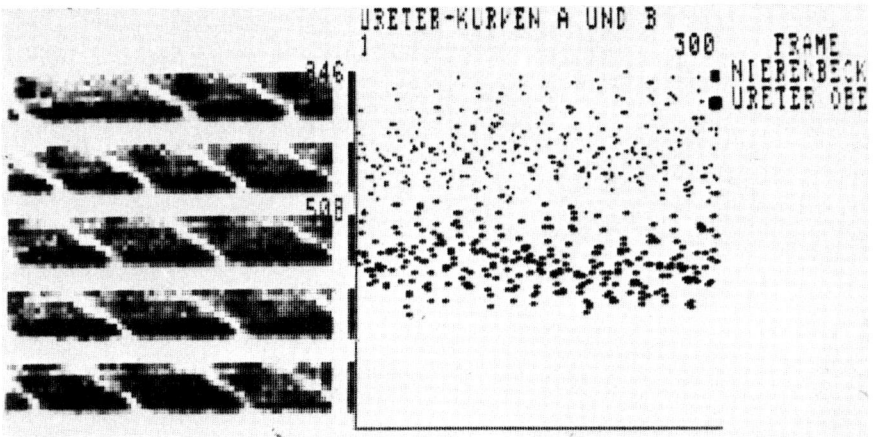

Fig. 5. Space time matrix of a megaureter, imaging 5 segments, one minute each, 35 to 40 min after injection of 70 MBq = 1.8 uCi 99m-Tc-DTPA. Two region of interest curves from the upper ureter part are displayed to the right. They demonstrate that peristaltic information may sometimes be drawn from classical ureter curves (cf. Laval, this volume), but this approach is less sensitive and less clear

The Problem of Aperistalsis

A crucial point of the imaging of peristalsis is to differentiate *the absence of peristalsis* from *the absence of information on peristalsis*.

For 123-I-hippuran, a quantitative parameter on radioisotope influx into the kidney and a qualitative judgement of the radioisotope transition from the kidney to the ureter, have proven useful in separating the majority of cases with absent information on peristalsis (Müller-Schauenburg 1983).

Aperistalsis is physiological at high diuresis (cf. Kiil 1973). Frusemide testing may thus induce
– a high frequency peristalsis due to relative stenosis,
– physiological aperistalsis, or
– a dilution of radioactivity below the level sufficient for space time imaging.

Discussion

The limitations of the space time matrix approach may be summarized as follows:
– The spatial resolution of the space time matrix is far below radiography. It is even lower than the resolution of the original scintigraphic images, and even inferior to the digital imaging, due to the region of interest technique.
– The limited resolution in space and time admits only a rough information on the speed of peristaltic propagation.

- Depending on the radioisotope dose and the radiopharmaceutical chosen, the time interval of safe imaging of peristalsis may be too short to reveal periodic patterns of peristaltic frequency as described by image intensified fluoroscopy (Hajós 1978).
- The method does not work in renal insufficiency, because of the lack of radioisotope concentration necessary to produce a signal above the tissue background underlying the ureter.
- In the absence of peristalsis (cf. Boyarsky et al. 1978), there is the danger of mistaking a statistical pattern for traces of motility. If there are clear peristaltic lines in the matrix, the comparison avoids such falsely positive judgements.

These limits are outweighed by a spectrum of advantages attributed to the space time matrix:
- It is non-invasive.
- It works even in hydropenia.
- Ureteral physiology (cf. Boyarsky and Labay 1981) can be studied in patients as a by-product of bonescans.
- Pathophysiology (cf. Weiss 1979) can be studied with bone tracers or as a by-product of routine renography with 123-I-hippuran or 99m-Tc-DTPA.
- The approach is simple compared to the extraction of space time information from cineradiography (Gerlach, this volume).

Summary

The principle of the nuclear medical space time matrix has been developed since 1978 as a routine tool for the imaging of ureteral motility. Limitations and advantages have been worked out. The sensitive technique is supplemented by standard adjunctive information from kidney curves, analogous images, and sometimes from difference images to increase specificity.

References

Boyarsky S, Labay P (1981) Principles of ureteral physiology. In: Bergman H (ed) The ureter, 2nd edn. Springer, New York Heidelberg Berlin, pp 71–104
Boyarsky S, Labay P, Teague N (1978) Aperistaltic ureter in upper urinary tract infection – cause or effect? Urology 12:134–138
Byrom E, Ryo UY, Pandya KK, Kim I, Pinsky S (1982) Computer visualisation of ureteral kinetics. J Nucl Med 23:P75
Coolsaet BLRA, Griffiths DJ, van Mastrigt R, Duyl WAV (1980) Urodynamic investigation of the wide ureter. J Urol 124:666–672
Hajòs E (1978) Telescreen and radiographic examination of urinary transport. Akadémiai Kiadó, Budapest, pp 39–61
Kiil F (1973) Urinary flow and ureteral peristalsis. In: Lutzeyer W, Melchior H (eds) Urodynamics. Springer, Berlin Heidelberg New York, pp 57–68
Melchior H (1971) Uro-Rheomanometrie (Simultane Uro-Rheographie und Elektromanometrie). In: Lutzeyer W, Melchior H (eds) Urodynamik. Thieme, Stuttgart, pp 125–129

Melchior H (1981) Urologische Funktionsdiagnostik. Thieme, Stuttgart New York, p 114
Müller-Schauenburg W (1982) General concepts of motion imaging and their application to ureteral, oesophageal, and gastric motility. In: Schmidt HAE, Rösler H (eds) Nuklearmedizin. Computer assisted functional analysis. Schattauer, Stuttgart New York, pp 114–117
Müller-Schauenburg W (1983) Ein Verfahren zur nuklearmedizinischen Darstellung der Ureterkinetik. Attempto, Tübingen
Müller-Schauenburg W, Anger K, Carl I, Feine U, Hippéli R (1979) Erste Erfahrungen mit einer neuen nuklearmedizinischen Darstellung der Ureteren (UKG). In: Schmidt HAE, Ortiz-Berrocal J (eds) Nuklearmedizin. Clinical value of the nuclear medicine methods. Schattauer, Stuttgart New York, pp 552–555
Müller-Schauenburg W, Anger K, Feine U, Hippéli R, Reifferscheid P, Wolf M (1980) Nuklearmedizinische Diagnostik des vesico-renalen Refluxes vom Säuglings- bis zum Erwachsenenalter. In: Schmidt HAE, Riccabona G (eds) Nuklearmedizin. Clinical significance of nuclear medicine. Schattauer, Stuttgart New York, pp 602–605
Schmidt H (1978) Motilität der oberen Harnwege. Springer, Berlin Heidelberg New York, pp 91 and 96
Weiss RM (1979) Clinical implications of ureteral physiology. J Urol 121:401–413

Dynamics of the Ureterovesical Junction

C. BLOK, G.E.P.M. VAN VENROOIJ, and B.L.R.A. COOLSAET[1]

Abstract. The ureterovesical pressure profile (UVPP) and the dynamics of the urterovesical junction (UVJ) were analysed with prevesical and intraluminal perfusion pressure measurements, and with an intraluminal micro-pressure sensor catheter.

The reliability of the measuring techniques was evaluated with different pressure measuring catheters under varying conditions.

Prevesical and intraluminal perfusion pressure measurements with F 8 or F 5 flexible catheters, at high perfusion rates, and intermittent or low withdrawal velocity of the catheter, produced the highest reproducibility.

The dynamical factors and anatomical structures, which possibly contribute to, or influence the pressure phenomena within the UVJ, were evaluated by the principle of addition and elimination.

Besides a baseline pressure, the UVPP showed fast and slow pressure waves.

The UVJ develops peristaltic activity by which it discharges fluid boli into the bladder. This UVJ peristalsis is responsible for the fast pressure waves in the UVPP.

The slow pressure waves represent the influence of detrusor activity upon urine transport through the UVJ, and reflect detrusor irritability.

Besides activity arteficially induced by an intraluminal catheter, the baseline pressure represents the resistance to continuous flow through the UVJ. It is determined by:
- The intravesical pressure in the bladder at bladder filling.
- The detrusor activity in the unexpanded bladder.
- The bladder wall stretch in the overdistended bladder.
- The bladder wall stress and intravesical pressure in the small volume, low capacity bladder.
  Similar pressure measurements in man seem to confirm these findings.

Clinical Introduction

Low compliant high pressure bladders and large volume, high compliant, low pressure bladders, with or without infravesical obstruction, may be associated with wide upper urinary tracts and deterioration of renal function (Bäcklund and Reuterskiöld 1969; Williams and Johnston 1982; Koff et al. 1979; Hald and Bradley 1982). Complications such as infection and stone formation aggravate the loss of renal function (Brat 1977).

Dilatation of these upper tracts is supposed to result from incompetence of the antireflux mechanism of the ureterovesical junction (UVJ) and outflow obstruction. This particular obstruction of the UVJ was postulated to be of functional origin as no obvious organic obstructive lesion was found in these cases (Bäcklund and Reu-

---

1 Department of Urology, State University Utrecht, Academic Hospital, Catharijnesingel 101, NL-3511 GV Utrecht

terskiöld 1969). However, morphologic changes of the ureteral sheaths have been described, which might contribute to this obstruction during filling of the bladder (Tokunaka and Koyanagi 1982). But also dynamics of the normal upper urinary tract and its dimension at IVU are influenced by bladder filling (Zimskind et al. 1969; Rose et al. 1971; Boyarski and Labay 1972). The results of pressure-flow studies of the upper urinary tract depend on bladder filling and intravesical pressure (Coolsaet et al. 1980).

Hence, further investigation of the UVJ dynamics is of clinical importance with regard to changes in its function related to infravesical obstruction, vesicoureteral reflux (VUR), detrusor dysfunctions and the interpretation of data obtained in urodynamic examination.

Until now, the urodynamics of the UVJ have been evaluated either by antegrade withdrawal, side-hole (Bruijnes 1978; Weiss and Biancani 1981; Leen et al. 1982), or open-end (Tanagho et al. 1968; Bäcklund and Reuterskiöld 1969; Hanna and Edwards 1972; Whitaker 1973) perfusion pressure measurements, and with combined manometric and electro-myographic studies (Tsuchida and Kimura 1967).

Statements about the dynamics of the UVJ are controversial and hypothetic. The development of peristaltic activity by the UVJ (Tsuchida and Kimura 1967; Mathisen 1964), and the presence of a pressure profile at the ureterovesical junction when the bladder is empty (Bruijnes 1978; Leen et al. 1982) have been advocated or denied. Near the UVJ a biphasic pressure profile has been described where the pressure increases or is attributed to the prevesical ureteral sphincter activity, and the passage of the measuring catheter through the ureteral orifice (Bruijnes 1978). Hypertrophy of the trigone could result in an increase of flow resistance through the UVJ, while trigonal insufficiency not only reduces this resistance but even may cause VUR (Tanagho et al. 1968).

The aims of our investigations were the evaluation of the hydrodynamic properties of the UVJ and the analysis of the ureterovesical pressure profile (UVPP).

Evaluation of Measuring Techniques

Initially ureterovesical pressure profilometry and prevesical ureteral perfusion pressure measurements were performed in order to select a reliable investigative method for the evaluation of UVJ dynamics.

Pigs were used for in vivo experiments because their upper urinary tracts highly resemble the upper urinary tract in man with respect to anatomy, except the ureteral orifice, which in the pig is situated more caudally at the bladder neck (Shehata 1977).

After the ureter was severed juxtavesically, different micro-pressure sensor catheters and perfusion pressure measurement catheters were withdrawn through the UVJ (see Fig. 1A). These pressure measurements were performed under varying conditions.

The F5 Millar, and the more flexible, as well as the highly flexible modified Philips-Honeywell micro-pressure sensor catheter were evaluated. According to our request the producer of the modified catheter levelled the cuplike micro-pressure

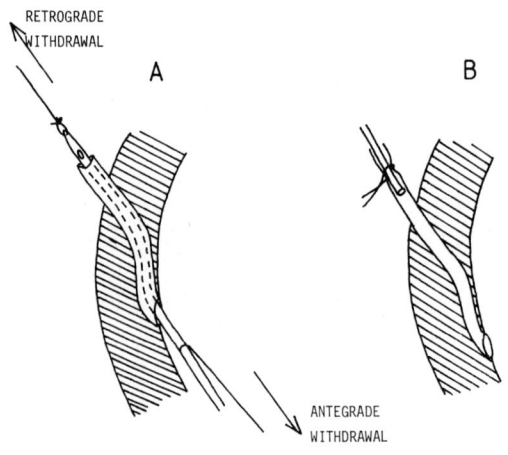

Fig. 1. **A** Antegrade or retrograde side-hole perfusion or micro-pressure sensor UVJ pressure profilometry. **B** Prevesical end-hole perfusion pressure measurement

sensor element with silicone. Intraluminal perfusion pressure measurements of the UVJ were performed with F5 and F8 flexible, polyethylene side-hole catheters with one side-hole which was located at 5 mm from the tip of the catheter. The inner diameters of the F5 and F8 perfusion catheters were respectively 0.8 and 1.3 mm. The side-hole had a surface area of 1 mm².

Similar catheters, but with an end-hole instead of a side-hole, were used for prevesical perfusion pressure measurement. For this purpose the catheter was introduced via a distal ureterotomy (see Fig. 1 B).

Highly reproducible UVPP's were only obtained at higher perfusion rates (> 1.0 ml/min), with intermittent or low withdrawal velocity (< 5 cm/min) of the measuring catheter (see Fig. 2). Reproducibility did not depend on whether the catheter was withdrawn in antegrade or retrograde direction.

Micro-pressure sensor UVPP's often showed artefacts (Coolsaet et al. 1982a), of which the most common were false negative and false positive pressure peaks. Artefacts were more pronounced when the less flexible catheters were used. At high withdrawal velocity flexible catheters behave like less flexible ones. The false negative pressure peaks were probably due to a suction effect of the ureteral wall upon the cuplike micro-pressure sensor element, when this slipped along the ureteral wall. Leveling the cup with silicone reduced, but did not eliminate these false negative pressure peaks. A significant false positive pressure peak was found when the rim of the ureteral orifice hooked into the cuplike micro-pressure sensor element, on its way through the orifice. Probably due to mechanical deformation of the UVJ, a less flexible catheter induced ureteral wall activity.

Prevesical perfusion pressure measurements of the UVJ invariably showed high reproducibility.

It was concluded that perfusion pressure measurements either prevesically or intraluminally of the UVJ, provided the most reliable results. Reliability was enhanced by using highly flexible catheters and by moving the catheter within the UVJ as little as possible.

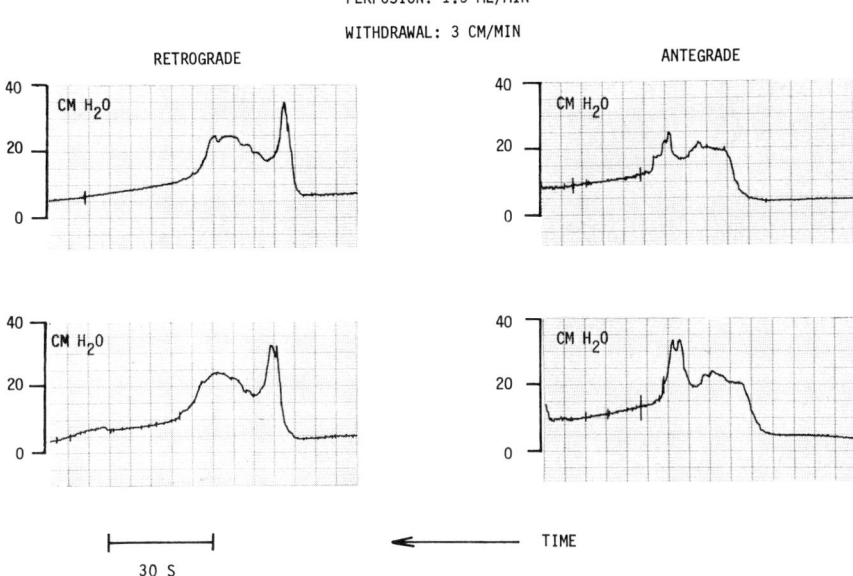

Fig. 2. Four successive ureterovesical pressure profiles (UVPPs)

Urodynamical and Anatomical Considerations

The UVPP showed a baseline pressure and fast and slow pressure waves (see Fig. 2), which also were detected with prevesical ureteral perfusion pressure measurement (see Fig. 3). This indicates that the pressure increases more likely originated from ureteral wall activity, rather than from a merely mechanical resistance to the passage of a catheter through the UVJ.

From the UVPP the following questions arise:
- What determines the baseline pressure and therefore the resistance to outflow of the upper urinary tract?
- What do these fast and slow pressure increases represent, and what is their clinical significance?

The UVJ contains the distal ureteral segment, which obliquely traverses the bladder wall and ultimately runs "submucosally" parallel to the bladder wall before it ends at the ureteral orifice.

Three ureteral segments can be differentiated at the UVJ, namely: the juxtavesical, intramural, and submucosal ureteral segment. These three segments are surrounded by the superficial and deep ureteral sheaths, both of which extend juxtavesically as well as in the trigone (Elbadawi et al. 1969; Elbadawi 1972). Only longitudinally arranged muscle bundles are found in the UVJ ureter segment.

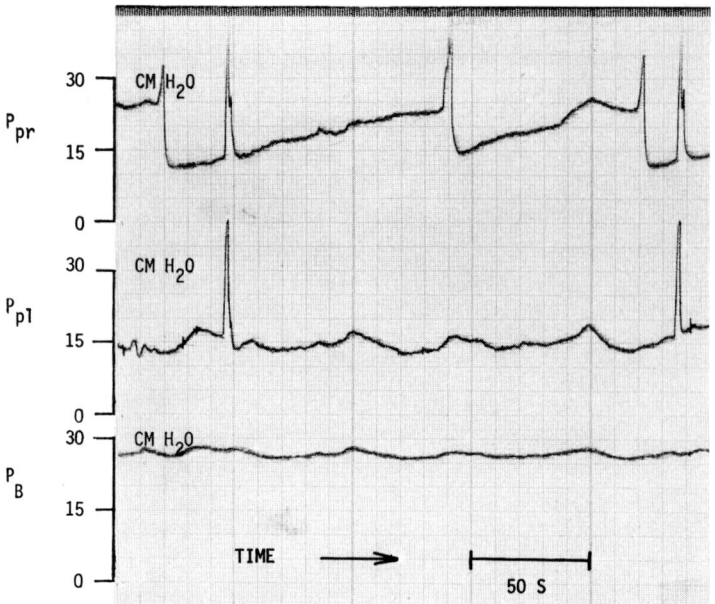

Fig. 3. Typical result of a prevesical ureteral end-hole perfusion pressure measurement. P_{pr} Perfusion pressure right ureter; P_{pl} perfusion pressure left ureter; P_B detrusor pressure. Note the decrease in basal pressure after a fast pressure wave above the level of 15 cm H_2O

From the anatomy of the UVJ it may be expected that intraluminal pressures within the UVJ could result from:
- The passive visco-elastic and active properties of the wall of the UVJ ureter segment with its ureteral sheaths.
- Forces in the bladder wall around the UVJ.
- Intravesical pressure which is transmitted upon the wall of the UVJ ureter segment.
- Prevesical ureteral pressure propagation into the UVJ and conduction of prevesical ureteral wall activity.

The role of each of these anatomical structures and dynamic factors in the pressure phenomena of the UVJ, was evaluated by the principle of elimination and addition during prevesical perfusion and by intraluminal micro-pressure sensor pressure measurements of the UVJ.

Materials and Methods

Materials

The following method was applied with minor variations in the majority of our experiments (see Fig. 4).

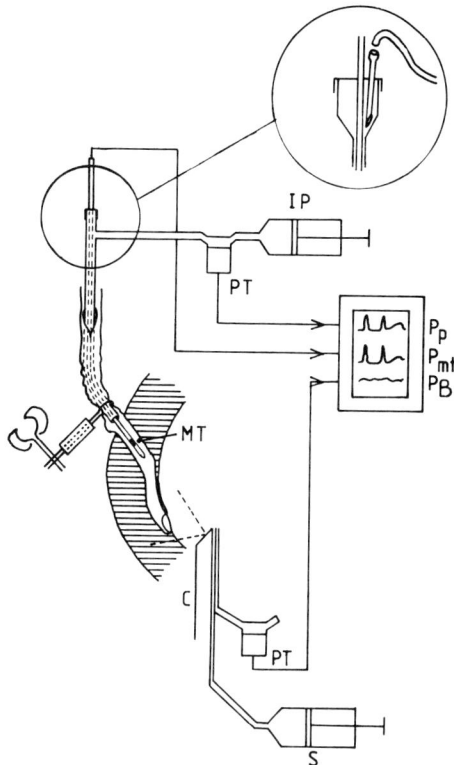

Fig. 4. Schematic view of the experimental set-up. *IP* Infusion pump; *PT* physiological pressure transducer; *S* syringe; *MT* micro-pressure transducer; *C* cystoscope; P_p perfusion pressure; P_{mt} micro-pressure transducer pressure; P_B detrusor pressure. The *inset* shows the combined introduction of the perfusion line and the micro-pressure sensor catheter into the system

60 female pigs with a weight of between 15 and 120 kg were used for in vivo experiments. These experiments were performed under general anaesthesia, with parenteral stresnil and hypnodil to which pavulon was added if necessary, and artificial respiration with O_2/N_2O mixtures.

The urinary tract was exposed via a midline abdominal incision. In vitro experiments were performed on bladder-ureter specimens which were either obtained from the slaughterhouse, or resected at the end of the in vivo experiments.

Prevesical ureteral perfusion pressure measurements were performed by using a flexible polyethylene F8 or F10 open-end catheter. This catheter was introduced into the ureter via a distal longitudinal ureterotomy. The inner diameters of the catheters were respectively 1.3 and 2.0 mm. The open end of the catheter was situated at 3 to 4 cm distance from the bladder, and the catheter was fixed with a ligature.

The ureteral segment which contains the catheter, was contused with a clamp before the catheter was introduced, in order to eliminate artificially induced ureteral wall activity (Blok et al. 1982).

Detrusor pressures were measured, and bladder filling volumes were adjusted, via two F8 end-side-hole catheters (AHS International) which were introduced into the bladder via the urethra. A distal urethral ligature prevented leakage.

A low compliant high pressure bladder was created by enveloping the bladder with fixonet, cranially to the level of the entrance of the neuro-vascular ligaments.

Perfusion pressures were measured with Hewlett-Packard physiological pressure transducers and registrated on a Polygraph or Hewlett-Packard recorder.

A Braun Unita I infusion pump was used for perfusion.

Two positive silver-platinum cup electrodes (diameter 11 mm), were implanted in the lateral bladder wall near the entrance of the neurovascular ligaments. A negative electrode was implanted into the trigone.

Methods

Prevesical perfusion pressure measurements were performed with the intact or bluntly contused juxtavesical ureters. These measurements were performed at different bladder volumes and detrusor pressures. Methylene blue coloured normal saline was used for perfusion. Perfusion rates varied between 0.08 and 8 ml/min.

Part of the prevesical perfusion studies were combined with intraluminal pressure measurements at different sites within the UVJ. For that purpose a flexible polyethylene F 10 catheter was introduced into the ureter in a similar way as the F 8 catheter. The proximal end of the F 10 catheter was closed with a rubber cap through which a G 14 infusion needle and the modified F 5 Philips-Honeywell micro-pressure sensor catheter were introduced into the system.

Unstable contractions of the detrusor quite often occurred in the low compliant bladders. However, the influence of detrusor activity was also evaluated with electrostimulation of the detrusor. Impulses of 10 to 15 V, at 10 to 20 pulses/s and a pulse duration of 10 to 20 ms resulted in clearly visible detrusor contractions.

In clinical practice, during cystoscopy one may observe urine spurts from the ureteral orifice in association with displacement of the orifice. The question arises whether this clinical observation correlates with a pressure phenomenon of the UVPP. In order to answer this question part of the perfusion pressure measurements were combined with cystoscopy.

For in vitro experiments the bladder was submerged in a buckett which was filled with water. The bladder trigone was kept at surface level. The bladder was dilatated for six hours by filling it with normal saline from a reservoir at 100 cm above the level of the bladder. Similar perfusion pressure measurements as in vivo were performed.

Results

Continuous observation of the ureteral orifice during the perfusion pressure measurements revealed that simultaneously with the fast pressure waves fluid spurts out of the ureteral orifice. During this action displacement of the open ureteral orifice with retraction of the submucosal ureter occurred.

The simultaneous occurrence of fast pressure waves and urine spurts from the ureteral orifice, suggests that these fast pressure increases represent a peristaltic mechanism which transports fluid boli. The fact, that the fast pressure waves also were associated with retraction of the submucosal ureter, indicates that they rep-

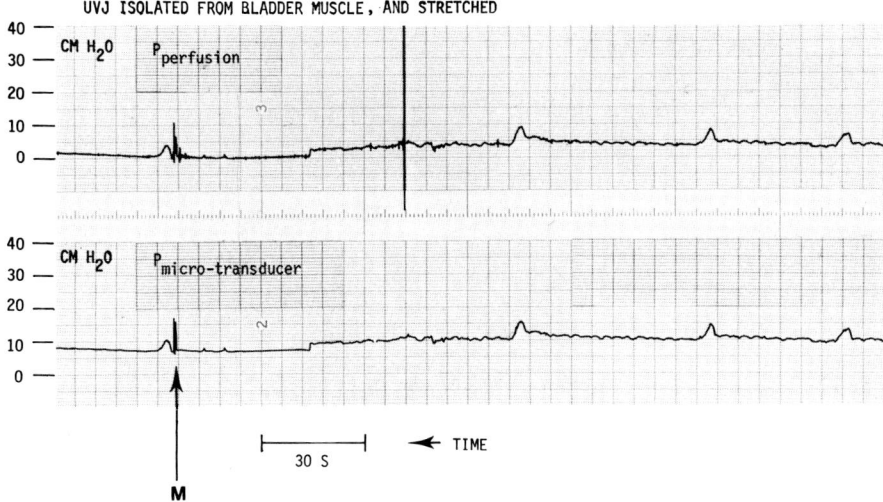

Fig. 5. Simultaneous pressure measurements on an isolated and stretched UVJ. *M* Mechanical detrusor stimulation

resent ureteral peristalsis. However, there should be at least some other mechanism that contributes to the fast pressure increases, as especially in the full bladder, retraction of the submucosal ureter slightly lags behind the fast pressure wave. This was further evaluated in a separate experiment.

Propagation of prevesical peristalsis was prevented by the ureteral ligature around the perfusion catheter, and the ureterotomy, through which the perfusion catheter was introduced, and which was left open.

Artificially induced activity of the juxtavesical ureteral wall was eliminated by blunt contusion of the juxtavesical ureter with a clamp. In our experiments it was clearly demonstrated that blunt contusion of the ureteral wall instantaneously and completely eliminates its activity for at least five hours, without interfering with the integrity of its wall (Blok et al. 1982).

The bladder wall was dissected from the ureteral sheaths in order to eliminate a possible contribution of detrusor activity to the fast pressure increases.

Finally retraction of the UVJ ureter segment, which only contains longitudinally arranged muscle bundles, was prevented by pulling on a stitch through the ureteral orifice.

Notwithstanding these procedures, fast pressure waves with simultaneous fluid spurts from the ureteral orifice could be detected at perfusion pressure measurement (see Fig. 5). At close observation of the UVJ under these conditions, it looks as if a sort of telescoping mechanism moves up and down within the UVJ, by which it produces a fluid spurt from the ureteral orifice.

According to these findings, it is most likely that the ureteral sheaths at the UVJ contribute to peristaltic urine transport through the UVJ, when this is stretched during bladder filling.

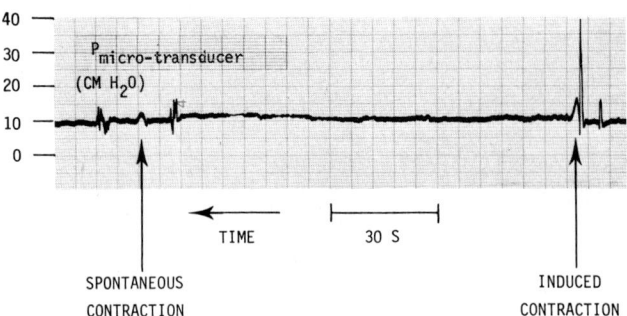

Fig. 6. Intraluminal micro-pressure sensor measurement in the completely isolated UVJ ureter segment

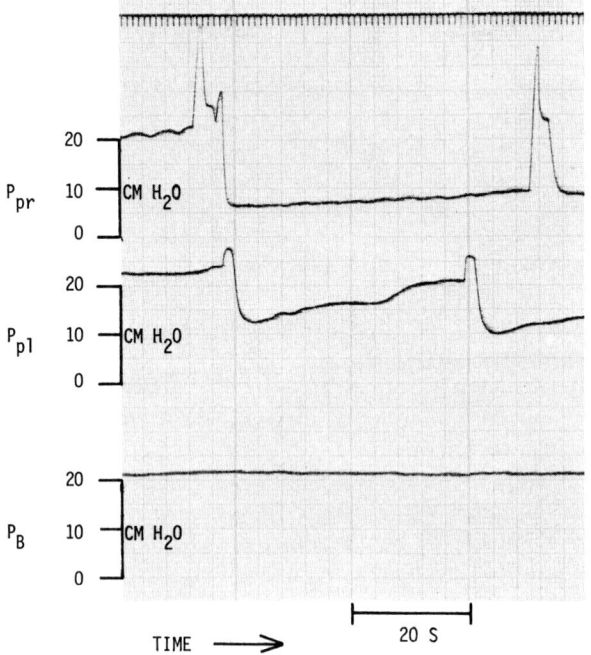

Fig. 7. Prevesical perfusion pressure measurements via the right intact (P_{pr}) and the left contused ureter (P_{pl}). P_B Detrusor pressure. Note monophasic fast pressure waves after juxtavesical contusion

Even after complete isolation of the UVJ spontaneous and mechanically induced pressure increases were measured with an intraluminal micro-pressure sensor catheter (see Fig. 6). Obviously the UVJ may autonomously develop peristaltic activity.

Especially at high intravesical pressures, a significant decrease of ureteral baseline pressure was observed after a fast pressure increase during which fluid spurted from the orifice (see Figs. 3 and 7). When such a fast pressure increase was shortly followed by another fast pressure increase, and when baseline pressure still was low,

Dynamics of the Ureterovesical Junction

hardly any fluid spurts from the orifice, and no further decrease in ureteral baseline pressure occurred (see Fig. 3). Obviously the decrease in baseline pressure is related to the amount of fluid which is evacuated from the UVJ at high intravesical pressures.

Thus, at high intravesical pressures, the decrease in ureteral baseline pressure at the UVJ, after a fast pressure wave, reflects the efficiency of UVJ peristaltic fluid transport.

When juxtavesical ureteral wall activity was not eliminated, biphasic or multiphasic fast pressure waves could be recorded, depending on the length of the prevesically perfused ureteral segment. After such a biphasic or multiphasic fast pressure wave the decrease in ureteral baseline pressure was greater, compared to the pressure decrease after a monophasic fast pressure increase (see Fig. 7).

From these findings, it may be concluded, that during UVJ peristalsis the juxtavesical ureter develops sphincter activity, which by preventing ureteral reflux, improves the efficiency of UVJ peristaltic fluid transport.

It is very likely that the ureteral sheaths contribute to this sphincter activity juxtavesically.

Slow pressure waves were neither accompanied by any displacement of the ureteral orifice, nor were they ever followed by a decrease in ureteral baseline pressure. Also during the slow pressure increases no fluid spurted from the ureteral orifice, but at higher perfusion rates, fluctuations in flow from the ureteral orifice were observed. Slow pressure waves were also recorded at intraluminal pressure measurement with a micro- pressure sensor catheter within the UVJ, when this was not perfused. These findings suggest, that the slow pressure waves represent an active mechanism which is not related to UVJ peristalsis, but which does interfere with flow through the UVJ. As the slow pressure waves disappeared from the UVPP (see Fig. 8) after the bladder wall was dissected from the ureteral sheaths, it was supposed that they originated from detrusor activity. This was established in a separate experiment.

A midureter segment of 5 cm was isolated and bluntly contused in order to eliminate the activity of its wall. Subsequently, it was obliquely passed through the bladder wall (see Fig. 9). Similar perfusion pressure measurements on this implanted ureter segment produced slow pressure waves which were comparable to those found at UVJ perfusion pressure measurement. No fast pressure increases could be detected.

During perfusion pressure measurement of the UVJ an increase of frequency and amplitude of the slow pressure waves could be observed when the perfusion rate was increased (see Fig. 8). Similar relationships were found at perfusion pressure measurement of the contused and transplanted mid-ureter segment (see Fig. 10). The results of these perfusion pressure measurements did not depend on whether the transplanted ureter segment was perfused in antegrade or retrograde direction.

From these findings it was concluded that the slow pressure waves of the UVPP represent the influence of detrusor activity on continuous flow through the UVJ.
The next question which had to be answered was: what is the influence of detrusor activity upon the flow through the UVJ?

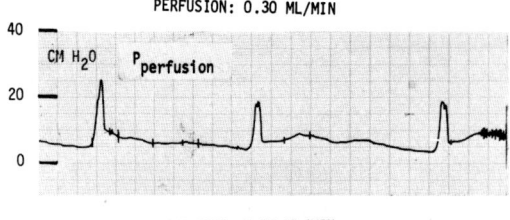
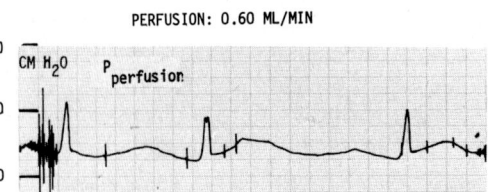
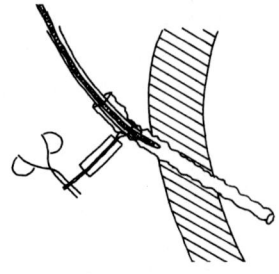

Fig. 9. Perfusion pressure measurement through an inactivated ureter segment, which is obliquely passed through the bladder wall

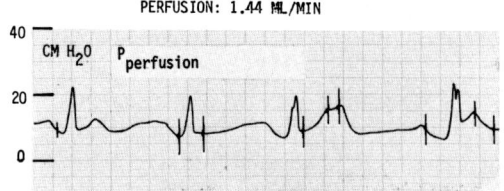
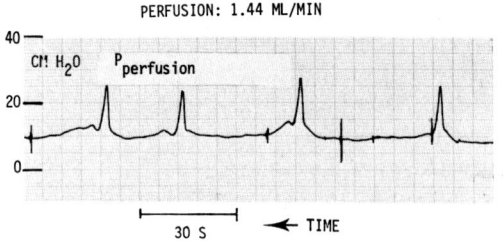

◄ **Fig. 8.** Prevesical UVJ perfusion pressure measurement results at increasing perfusion rates. The bottom registration represents perfusion pressure measurement results of a partly dissected UVJ

A momentary decrease in flow through the UVJ, with even distension of the prevesical ureter segment, could sometimes be observed at electrically induced detrusor contractions when the bladder was nearly empty.

Obviously, detrusor activity causes an increase in resistance to flow through the UVJ, and thus an increase of occlusion pressure of the UVJ, which is reflected by the slow pressure waves of the UVPP.

The next question which had to be answered was: how do detrusor tone and activity influence UVJ occlusion pressure and thus resistance to flow through the UVJ?

This inevitably leads us to the question: what determines the basal ureteral pressure at the UVJ and therefore baseline pressure at the UVPP?

At juxtavesical end-hole perfusion pressure measurements of the UVJ, the baseline pressure of the UVPP represents the resistance to continuous flow through the UVJ. The influence of the juxtavesical ureter upon this resistance to flow was eliminated by blunt contusion, and subsequent positioning of the end-hole of the perfusion catheter opposite to the entrance of the ureter into the bladder wall. Changes in

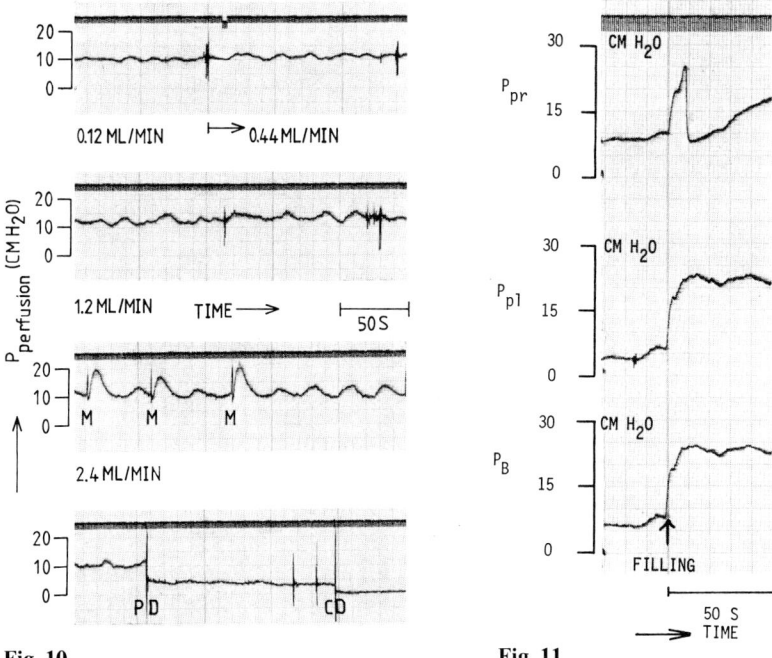

Fig. 10. Prevesical perfusion pressure registration of the transplanted ureter segment at increasing perfusion rates and after partly dissection (*PD*) and complete dissection (*CD*)

Fig. 11. Prevesical perfusion UVJ pressure measurement via the right (P_{pr}) and left ureter (P_{pl}). Note parallel increases of P_{pl} and P_B (detrusor pressure), unless bladder filling induces UVJ peristalsis (P_{pr})

UVJ perfusion pressure paralleled the changes in intravesical pressure at fast and slow filling or emptying of the bladder, unless UVJ peristalsis occurred, which by emptying the UVJ, lowered its basal pressure (see Fig. 11) (Coolsaet et al. 1982b).

The same pressure relationship was observed at intermittent manual compression of the bladder (Coolsaet et al. 1982b).

The stress of the bladder wall changed during filling and emptying of the bladder, but it does not change during manual compression of the bladder. However, both a change in bladder volume as well as manual compression of the bladder do alter intravesical pressure. These findings suggest, that the resistance to flow through the UVJ during bladder filling, and thus UVPP baseline pressure, depends on intravesical pressure (Coolsaet et al. 1982).

This was further evaluated in a separate experiment, in which the contribution of bladder wall stress to UVJ flow resistance was kept constant, while intravesical pressure decreased during bladder emptying. For this purpose a stiff plastic ring (diameter 45 mm) was sutured to the bladder wall around the UVJ region, when the bladder was full. During subsequent emptying of the bladder the decrease in UVJ perfusion pressure paralleled the decrease in intravesical pressure (Coolsaet et al. 1982).

The relationship between bladder wall stress (σ) and intravesical pressure can be approximated from bladder volume (V_B), intravesical pressure (P_B) and bladder tissue volume (V_t) with the following formula:

$$\sigma = \frac{3 P_B V_B}{2 V_t}.$$

From the relationship between bladder wall stress, perfusion pressure and intravesical pressure at different bladder volumes (Coolsaet et al. 1982b) it was concluded, that during bladder filling the resistance to flow depends on intravesical pressure, which in its turn, is influenced among other factors by detrusor activity. The conclusion itself provides its own restriction, namely: the bladder should indeed build up intravesical pressure at bladder filling.

This restriction is illustrated by the following experiment: Similar UVJ perfusion pressure measurements as in vivo, were performed in vitro on bladders, which were submerged in a bucket filled with water, and which were dilated for 6 hours at filling pressures of 100 cm H_2O. During the measurement the trigone was held at surface level within the bucket. Near the trigone intravesical pressures remained about zero during bladder filling up to 2 liters, which resulted in UVJ perfusion pressures between 8 and 10 cm H_2O, depending on the perfusion rate.

Obviously in the overdistended, high compliant, low pressure bladder, the stretch of the bladder wall contributes to the resistance to flow through the UVJ.

The influence of stress and stretch could be demonstrated in vivo on a thick-walled bladder. For that purpose stitches, which serve as reins, were placed through the bladder wall at the entrance of the ureteral hiatus, near the ureteral orifice, and laterally and medially of the UVJ. By pulling on these stitches longitudinally, laterally and multidirectionally bladder wall stress and stretch could be induced, all of which resulted in an increase of basal ureteral pressure (see Fig. 12). During stress and stretch of the bladder wall, UVJ peristalsis with intermittent decreases of baseline perfusion pressures, continued.

The small volume, low compliant bladder is also an exception to the conclusion, that in an expanded bladder the resistance to flow through the UVJ depends on intravesical pressure. This was demonstrated by the following experiment. In the bladder of a piglet resected 24 hours earlier the capacity was reduced by placing a clamp on the bladder above the level of the UVJ. At perfusion pressure measurement via the ureteral stump it was found that UVJ perfusion pressure increased more as the intravesical pressure at bladder filling and conversely decreased more at bladder emptying (see Fig. 13). This pressure relationship was more pronounced at increasing perfusion rates. The pressure change velocity depended on the rate of bladder filling.

Increases in intravesical pressure, which resulted from unstable and electrically or mechanically induced detrusor contractions, were also paralleled by the associated increases in UVJ perfusion pressures (Coolsaet et al. 1982b). Again, this only applies to a bladder which is filled so far, that it is expanded, and therefore builds up

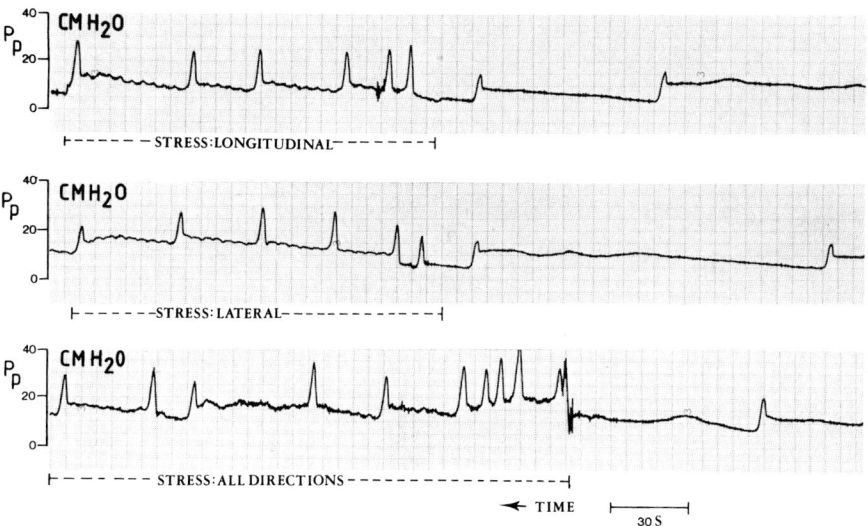

Fig. 12. Perfusion pressure measurement results (P_p) during bladder wall stretching in different directions

pressure during detrusor activity. In an empty or partly filled, unexpanded bladder, comparable electrically induced detrusor contractions resulted in increases of UVJ perfusion pressure, which were out of proportion with respect to the associated increases when the bladder was expanded (see Fig. 14).

At non-perfusion, intraluminal UVJ pressure measurements with a micro-pressure sensor catheter revealed that in the expanded bladder intraluminal pressure is highest in the submucosal ureter where transmission of intravesical pressure is maximal. In the unexpanded bladder it is highest in the intramural ureter where this is surrounded and compressed by detrusor muscle (see Fig. 15).

From these findings it is concluded that the resistance to continuous flow through the UVJ, and therefore baseline pressure of the UVPP is determined by: intravesical pressure in the expanded bladder; detrusor activity in the unexpanded bladder; bladder wall stretch in the overdistended bladder; bladder wall stress and intravesical pressure in the small volume, low compliant bladder (see Fig. 16).

Continuous or so-called open tube flow does not occur as long as the perfusion rate does not exceed the peristaltic fluid transport capacity of the UVJ.

The question arises, whether the resistance to peristaltic fluid bolus transport through the UVJ, similar to the open tube flow, is influenced by stress and stretch of the bladder wall, intravesical pressure, and detrusor activity.

Peristaltic UVJ fluid transport with intermittent decreases of basal pressure, not only continued, but may even be provoked, during increases of bladder wall stress and stretch (see Fig. 12), as well as by increases of intravesical pressure.

Reductions of baseline pressure up to 30 cm H_2O following the fast pressure waves were observed during UVJ perfusion pressure measurement at high intravesical pressures. This indicates that UVJ peristalsis discharges fluid boli into a high

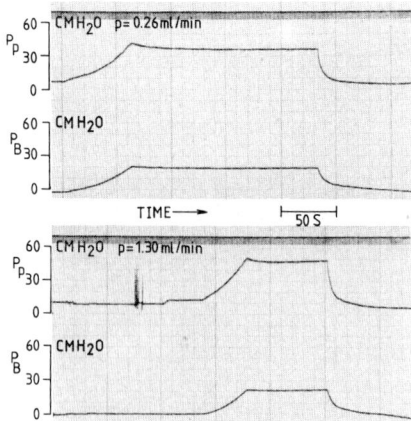

Fig. 13. Prevesical UVJ perfusion pressure measurement results in the low compliant, small volume bladder. Note the increase in discongruention between the increases in P_B (detrusor pressure) and P_p (perfusion pressure) at increasing perfusion rates

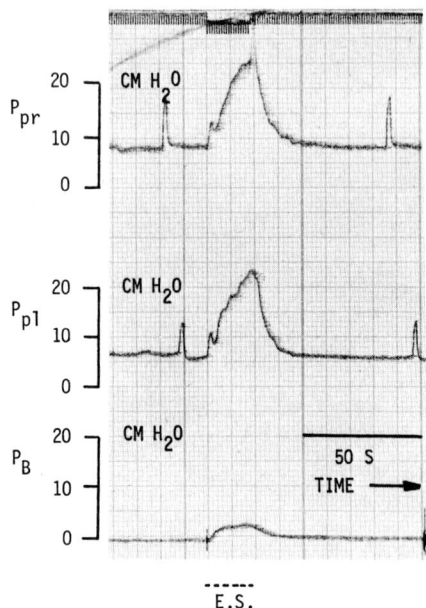

Fig. 14. The relation between detrusor pressure (P_B) and prevesical perfusion pressures (P_{pr} and P_{pl}) in the unexpanded bladder during electrostimulation (*E.S.*)

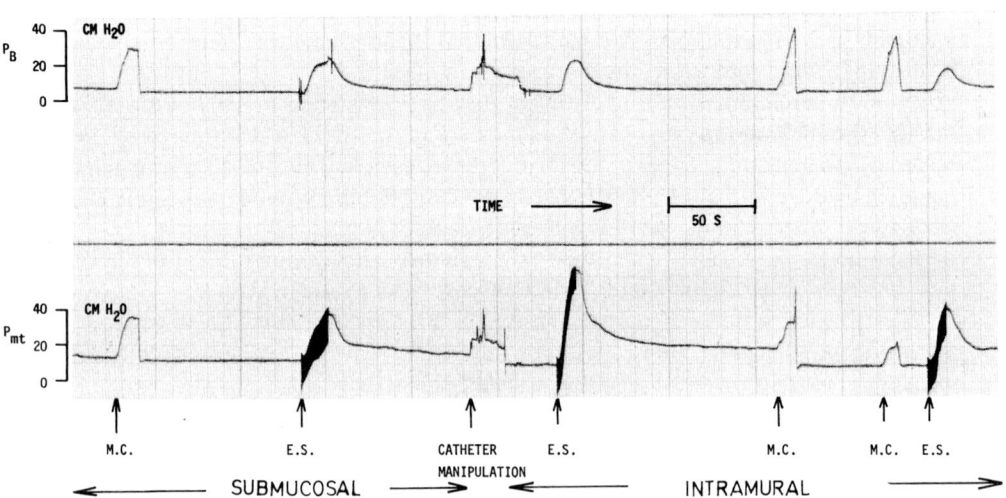

Fig. 15. UVJ pressure measurement results with a micro-pressure sensor catheter (P_{mt}) at two locations within the UVJ at an expanded bladder. P_B Detrusor pressure; *E.S.* electrostimulation; *M.C.* mechanical compression

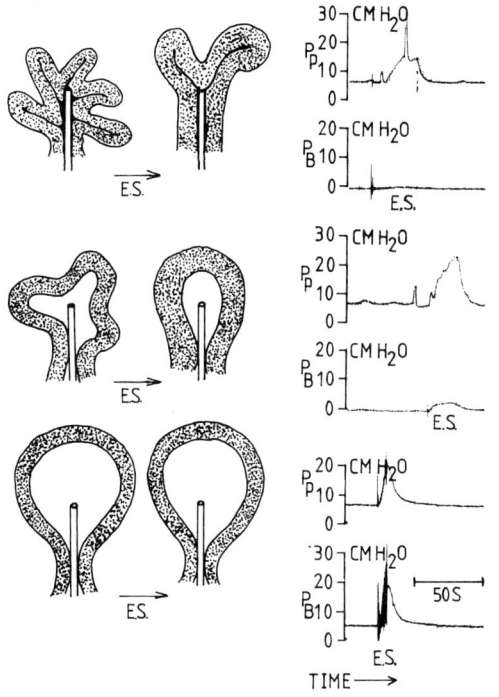

Fig. 16. Prevesical UVJ perfusion pressure measurement results (P_p) at an empty, partly filled and expanded bladder during electrostimulation (*E.S.*). P_B Detrusor pressure

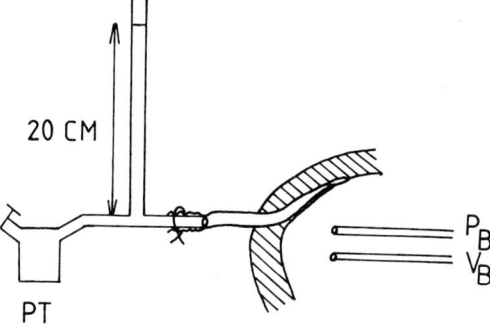

Fig. 17. Schematic view of UVJ pressure measurement with a prevesical fluid load. *PT* Pressure transducer; P_B detrusor pressure; V_B bladder volume

pressure bladder, and thus empties the UVJ with subsequent low pressure loading of the UVJ. This has been established in a separate experiment.

For this purpose the prevesical perfusion line was disconnected from the infusion pump and connected with a vertically positioned F 10 catheter, which was loaded with a column of 20 cm H_2O (see Fig. 17). Prevesical ureteral basal pressure, which now represents UVJ loading pressure, decreased from 20 to 13 cm H_2O after the first fast pressure increase. Notwithstanding the intravesical pressure of 20 cm H_2O further loading of the UVJ occurred at a pressure of 13 cm H_2O, as this was reduced to 10 cm H_2O after a second fast pressure increase (see Fig. 18).

These results clearly illustrate that UVJ peristaltic fluid transport may occur at high intravesical pressures, without increasing prevesical ureteral baseline pressure.

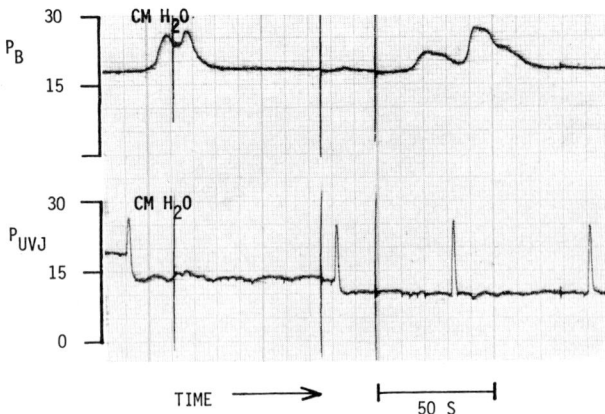

Fig. 18. Result of the UVJ pressure measurement (P_{UVJ}) with a prevesical fluid load. P_B Detrusor pressure

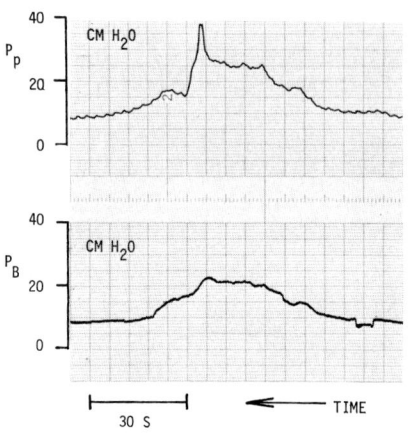

Fig. 19. Prevesical UVJ perfusion pressure measurement result (P_p) during unstable detrusor contraction (P_B). Note induced UVJ peristalsis which results in a decrease in basal pressure

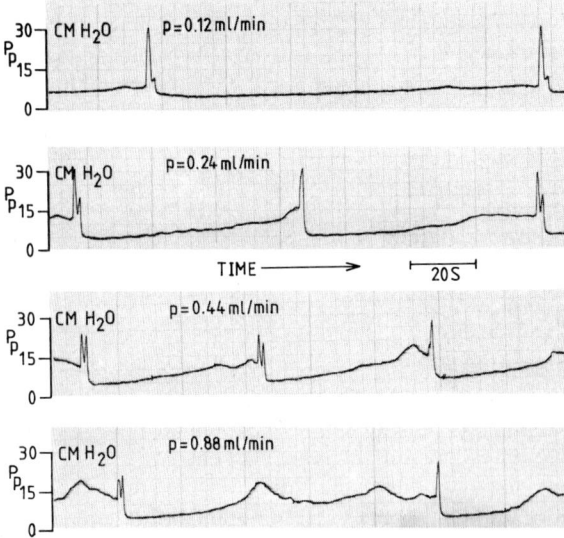

Fig. 20. Prevesical UVJ perfusion pressure measurement results (P_p) at increasing perfusion rates

In the expanded bladder a fast pressure increase, which seems provoked by, and is superimposed on a detrusor contraction, is usually followed by a decrease in UVJ perfusion pressure (see Fig. 19). In an unexpanded bladder, such a fast pressure increase never resulted in a reduction of UVJ baseline pressure. Obviously detrusor activity in the unexpanded bladder impairs loading of the UVJ.

Slow pressure increases occurred, once the UVJ baseline perfusion pressure reached a certain level, at which it stabilized, due to these slow pressure increases. This was more pronounced at higher perfusion rates, especially in the low compliant, high pressure bladder, when even visible unstable detrusor contractions were observed (see Fig. 20). The rate of bladder filling seems to influence these phenomena in a way that higher filling rates exert a provoking effect.

Obviously at a high perfusion rate, the cross sectional area of the open tube flow, and therefore the distension of the ureteral hiatus, interferes with the properties of the detrusor tissue around this hiatus. Such interference may then trigger unstable detrusor contractions.

Conclusions

The ureterovesical pressure profile (UVPP) showed:
- A baseline pressure which represents the resistance to continuous urinary flow through the UVJ at high diuresis. This baseline pressure is determined by detrusor activity in the unexpanded bladder and by intravesical pressure during bladder filling, once the bladder is expanded,
  In the large volume, low pressure bladder, resistance to flow through the UVJ is determined by the stretch of the bladder wall.
  In the small volume, low compliant bladder, UVJ flow resistance primarily is determined by the bladder wall stress.
- Fast pressure waves which represent peristaltic activity of the UVJ. This peristalsis promotes active urine bolus transport through the UVJ at low diuretic conditions. The difference between baseline pressures before and after such a fast pressure wave represents the efficiency of UVJ peristaltic urine transport at high intravesical pressures.
- Slow pressure waves which represent the influence of detrusor activity upon resistance to flow through the UVJ and which also reflect detrusor irritability.

UVJ Pressure Measurement in Man

In a few patients, with terminal renal insufficiency but otherwise normal upper urinary tracts, an F8 or F10 perfusion catheter was introduced into the ureter during nephrectomy, and was positioned with its end-hole prevesically. Similar UVJ perfusion pressure measurements as in the experiments with animals were performed. Fast pressure waves with associated fluid spurts from the ureteral orifice and retraction of the submucosal ureter were observed here as well. Also, at bladder filling, the increase in UVJ perfusion pressure paralleled the increase in intravesical pressure (Coolsaet et al. 1982b).

Discussion

In contrast to Tsuchida's statement (Tsuchida and Kimura 1967), our data clearly demonstrated that the UVJ develops peristaltic activity by which it evacuates fluid boli into the bladder. Moreover, the UVJ pressure registration curve of Tsuchida certainly does show activity in the intramural ureter, and not a silent baseline pressure profile.

Any measuring catheter within the UVJ may influence its motility. Similarly prevesical ureteral perfusion catheters influence ureteral wall activity, and also measure prevesical peristalsis. We eliminated these possible artefacts by blunt contusion of the prevesical ureteral wall at prevesical UVJ perfusion pressure measurement.

Ureteral manipulation, body temperature, dryness of the retroperitoneum, and temperature of the perfusate and of the bladder filling fluid, all influence ureteral wall activity and may inhibit UVJ peristalsis. Also these factors could well be responsible for the controversies in the results of UVJ pressure measurements by different investigators.

A peristaltic contraction of the UVJ may propel a fluid bolus into a high pressure bladder, with almost the same contraction force as in case of a nearly empty UVJ, when hardly any fluid transport occurs (see Fig. 3).

Obviously, UVJ peristalsis propels fluid boli but also reduces outflow resistance of the UVJ during the peristaltic contraction. This dual goal seems to be brought about by the ureteral sheaths and the UVJ ureter segment, which retract and probably, like cylinders, telescope into each other. As a consequence, the UVJ ureter segment shortens and is pulled back over the fluid bolus like a sleeve, which then is discharged into the bladder. During this action the submucosal ureter retracts intramurally (see Fig. 21).

When the bladder is filled so far, that it is expanded, the resistance to outflow of the upper urinary tract through the UVJ, is determined by:
- An end-hole outflow resistance at the ureteral orifice, which is determined by intravesical pressure.
- A resistance due to occlusion of the UVJ ureter segment by transmission of intravesical pressure upon the wall of the UVJ ureter segment, which is highest at the submucosal ureter.
- At high flows the cross sectional area of the flow may interfere with the distensibility of the UVJ ureter segment.

Momentary flow during fluid bolus transport should not be underestimated. Discharge of a bolus of 0.3 ml within 2 s into the bladder during UVJ peristalsis, is a common finding in the pig. During such fluid bolus transport the flow through the UVJ then equals a flow of 9 ml/min.

From what is mentioned above it may be clear that when the submucosal ureter is retracted intramurally during UVJ peristalsis, this will result in a significant re-

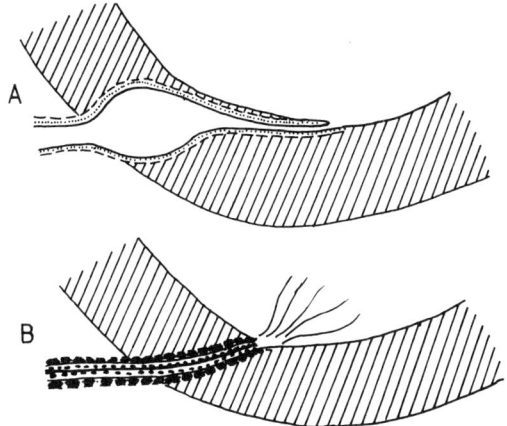

Fig. 21 A, B. Model of the probable mechanism of UVJ emptying

duction of resistance to a flow of about 9 ml/min (see Fig. 21). This reduction of flow resistance in its turn facilitates peristaltic emptying of the UVJ.

At a high flow, UVJ peristaltic fluid transport turns into a continuous open tube flow through the UVJ, with intermittent superpositon of peristaltic fluid transport. Resistance to this high open tube flow is significantly higher compared to the resistance to peristaltic fluid transport, as no reduction in flow resistance occurs.

As high intravesical pressures comprise continuous flow through the UVJ, but leave UVJ peristaltic fluid transport comparatively unaffected, it may be concluded that patients with high pressure bladders will benefit from equal distribution of their fluid intake, as this promotes the low diuretic peristaltic fluid transport by the UVJ and protects their upper urinary tracts and renal function.

In an unexpanded bladder, the resistance to continuous flow through the UVJ is determined by the compression of the intramural ureter by the surrounding bladder tissue. Consequently, detrusor activity impedes flow through the UVJ in such a bladder. However, in an unexpanded bladder, fluid bolus transport through the UVJ is also affected by detrusor activity. This happens because compression of the intramural ureter by detrusor muscle impedes loading of the UVJ, in contrast to high intravesical pressures, which increase outflow resistance of the UVJ. The impairment of the UVJ bolus loading is inversely related to the filling volume of the bladder.

The clinical implication of these findings is, that the upper urinary tract and renal function are even more in danger in patients with low compliant high pressure bladders, due to hyperactivity of the detrusor muscle with unstable contractions. Regular emptying of the bladders of such patients does not protect them against further detoriation of their upper urinary tracts and renal function. Therefore, the addition of anticholinergic medication to bladder catheterization in selected patients, as advised by McGuire (McGuire et al. 1983), should be strongly endorsed.

When such patients have wide upper urinary tracts, the only way of maintaining urine transport may be the erect position, as this enhances the hydrostatic loading of the UVJ, and therefore peristaltic urine transport by the UVJ. This is confirmed by the clinical observation of George (George et al. 1982), who found the erect position being of life-saving significance in patients with infravesical obstruction and wide upper urinary tracts.

Impaired fluid transport through the UVJ in cases of hypertrophy of the trigone (Tanagho et al. 1968), most probably results from reduced retractility of the submucosal ureter. As a consequence, UVJ peristalsis is less effective, as well as the resistance to flow through the UVJ is higher.

Similarly, in the overdistended bladder a reduced retractility of the submucosal ureter may be responsible for less effective urine transport through the UVJ.

Secondary reactive hypertrophy of the muscular components of the ureteral sheaths probably results from an increase in outflow resistance of the UVJ. Such hypertrophy of the ureteral sheaths in its turn may affect the distensibility of the UVJ ureter segment, and cause a further increase in UVJ flow resistance, especially in the full bladder. This seems to be confirmed by the findings of Tokunaka and Koyanagi (Tokunaka and Koyanagi 1982).

In an overdistended bladder the resistance to flow through the UVJ is primarily determined by the stretch of the bladder wall.

On the contrary during filling of a low capacity, small volume bladder, the resistance to flow through the UVJ primarily is determined by the stress of the bladder wall. Such small volume bladders, especially in the presence of detrusor hyperactivity, constitute a great threat for the upper urinary tracts and renal function. In patients with such bladders, an augmentation cystoplasty seems highly recommendable, especially when an artificial sphincter is implanted, because even an extra low artificial sphincter (P_{cuff} 50 to 60 cm H_2O) will create a high pressure bladder (P_B about 40 cm H_2O, as bladder leakage pressure shows a deficit of about 25% with respect to cuff pressure (Blok et al. 1983).

A remarkable finding was, that especially at higher UVJ perfusion rates, visible unstable detrusor contractions occurred in the high pressure bladders. This suggests, that the cross-sectional area of a high diuretic open tube flow, with distension of the ureteral hiatus and consequent elongation of the detrusor bundles around it, probably trigger unstable contractions in a patient with detrusor instability. The exact causative nature of this mechanism remained obscure.

Examination of UVJ-Dynamics in Clinical Practice

Pressure measurement of the UVJ during cystoscopy seems to be the obvious examination method in functional evaluation of the UVJ in clinical practice. Such a measurement should be performed under antidiuretic conditions, as these will reduce the influence of prevesical peristalsis on the measured results. In order to evaluate fluid transport properties of the UVJ, perfusion pressure measurement is preferred to pressure measurement with a micro-pressure sensor catheter.

High rate perfusion through special flexible crenel or rose catheters (see Fig. 22) seems advisable, as this will envelop the measuring end of the catheter in a fluid bolus. Consequently, the pressure effects of the catheter upon the ureteral wall at

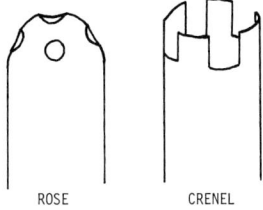

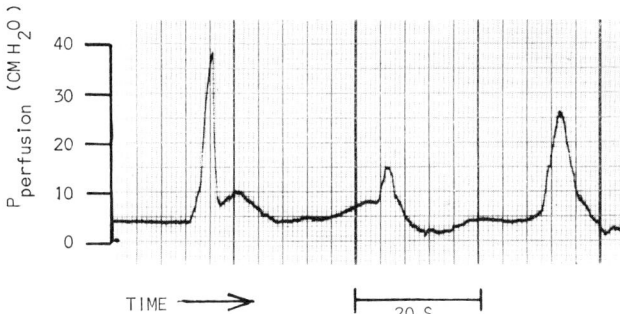

Fig. 22. Tip of recommended catheters for UVJ perfusion pressure measurements in man

Fig. 23. Typical result of intraluminal UVJ perfusion pressure measurement with a crenel catheter in a patient

the measuring site will be reduced. For the same reason the catheter should be withdrawn either intermittently, or at low withdrawal velocity.

High rate perfusion pressure measurement through a crenel catheter, which intermittently was withdrawn through the UVJ at cystoscopy in a patient, produced comparitive pressure profiles as in the experiments on animals (see Fig. 23).

High withdrawal velocity of any pressure measuring catheter through the UVJ should be rejected because:
- The greater the withdrawal velocity the more a flexible catheter will behave like a stiff one, and the more it will influence ureteral wall activity.
- With high withdrawal velocity, slow pressure waves and therefore the mutual influence between detrusor activity and flow dynamics of the UVJ may be missed.

Quality of fluid transport by the UVJ should be judged on the UVPP by:
- The baseline pressure, which represents resistance to continuous flow (high diuresis) through the UVJ.
- The decrease in baseline pressure after a fast pressure wave, which reflects the efficiency of UVJ peristalsis at high intravesical pressures. For this purpose, on a full bladder, the Credé manoevre should be exerted during the measurement.
- The slow pressure waves, which represent the influence of detrusor activity on resistance to flow through the UVJ, and which also reflect detrusor irritability.

Both, the examination technique and its clinical value need further evaluation.

References

Bäcklund L, Reuterskiöld AG (1969) The abnormal ureter in children. Scand J Urol Nephrol 3:219–228
Blok C, Venrooij GEPM van, Coolsaet BLRA (1982) Active urine transport through the ureterovesical junction. Abstract fourth meeting ISDU, Utrecht, The Netherlands, August 29 – September 1
Blok C, Riel MPJM van, Venrooij GEPM van, Coolsaet BLRA (1982) Artificial sphincter pressure versus bladder leaking pressure. Proceedings 2nd Joint Meeting ICS and UDS, Aachen, Federal Republic of Germany, August 3 – September 31 pp 96–98
Boyarski S, Labay P (1972) Ureteral dynamics. Williams & Wilkins, Baltimore London
Brat CG (1977) Renal function in patients with hydronephrosis. Br J Urol 49:249–255
Bruijnes E (1978) The ureteral pressure profile. Urol Int 33:381–392
Coolsaet BLRA, Griffiths DJ, Mastrigt R van, Duyl WA van (1980) Urodynamic investigation of the wide ureter. J Urol 124:666–672
Coolsaet BLRA, Venrooij GEPM van, Blok C (1982a) The ureterovesical pressure profile. Abstracts 77th Annual Meeting of the AUA, Kansas City, May 16–20, 1982, p 180
Coolsaet BLRA, Venrooij GEPM van, Blok C (1982b) Detrusor pressure versus wall stress in relation to ureterovesical resistance. Neurourol Urodyn 1:105–112
Elbadawi A (1972) Anatomy and function of the ureteral sheaths. J Urol 102:224–229
Elbadawi A, Amaku EO, Frank IN (1969) Anatomy of the submucosal segment of the ureter. Read at the annual meeting of the Northeastern section of the AUA, Quebec City, Quebec, September 1969
George NJR, O'Reilly PH, Barnard RJ (1982) Extra-renal factors which may influence drainage down the wide ureter. Abstract fourth meeting ISDU, Utrecht, The Netherlands, August 29 – September 1
Hald T, Bradley WE (1982) The urinary bladder. Williams & Wilkins, Baltimore London
Hanna MK, Edwards L (1972) Pressure perfusion studies of the abnormal ureterovesical junction. Br J Urol 44:331–335
Koff SA, Lapides J, Piazza DH (1979) The uninhibited bladder in children: a cause for urinary obstruction, infection and reflux. In: Hodson J, Kincaid-Smith P (eds) Reflux nephropathy. Masson, Paris New York Barcelona Milan, pp 161–170
Leen GL, Fegetter JGW, Stobbart D (1982) The ureterovesical pressure profile: fact or fiction. Abstract fourth meeting ISDU, Utrecht, The Netherlands, August 29 – September 1
Mathisen W (1964) Vesicoureteral reflux and its surgical correction. Surg Gynecol Obstet 118:965–971
McGuire EJ, Woodside JR, Borden ThA (1983) Upper urinary tract detoriation in patients with myelodysplasia and detrusor hypertonia: a follow-up study. J Urol 129:823–826
Rose DL, Constantinou CE, Sands JP, Govan DE (1971) Dynamics of the upper urinary tract: effects of changes in bladder pressure on ureteral peristalsis. J Urol 106:209–213
Shehata R (1977) A comparative study of the urinary bladder and the intramural portion of the ureter. Acta Anat 98:380–395
Tanagho EA, Meyers FH, Smith DR (1968) The trigone: anatomical and physiological considerations in relation to the ureterovesical junction. J Urol 100:623–632
Tokunaka S, Koyanagi T (1982) Morphologic study of primary nonreflux megaureters with particular emphasis on the role of ureteral sheath and ureteral dysplasia. J Urol 128:399–402
Tsuchida S, Kimura Y (1967) Vesicoureteral reflux. Tohoku J Exp Med 91:1–12
Weiss RM, Biancani P (1981) Characteristics of normal and refluxing ureterovesical junctions. Abstract third meeting ISDU, Aarhus, Denmark, August 31 – September 1
Whitaker RH (1973) Methods of assessing obstruction in dilated ureters. Br J Urol 45:15–22
Williams DI, Johnston JH (1982) Pediatric urology. Butterworth Scientific, London
Zimskind PD, Davis DM, Decaestecker JE (1969) Effects of bladder filling on ureteral dynamics. J Urol 102:693–696

**Upper and Lower Tract
Urodynamics – Reviewing
the Aachen 1971 Meeting**

Innervation and Histologic Characteristics of the Urinary External Sphincter

E. A. Tanagho[1]

Twelve years ago we met here and my assignment at that meeting was to discuss the physiology of micturition. We concentrated on the activity of the detrusor and on the sphincteric mechanism, placing much stress on its two divisions – the smooth component and the striated component. Our thinking about the function of the smooth component has not changed much since then. However, we learned a great deal more about the striated urinary sphincter. This is why the title of this presentation is "The Urinary External Spincter Revisited."

External Sphincter Length. In many books, illustrations and diagrams depicting the anatomy of the external sphincter, it is shown as a very short segment not exceeding ½ to ¾ of a centimeter. In reality, the external sphincter of the normal male seen in a sagittal section of a fixed pelvis is clearly much longer (Fig. 1). The extent of urinary sphincter extending from the apex of the prostate to the beginning of the bulbous urethra and the spongy tissue of the penis is approximately 1 to 1¼ inches (or 2½ to 3 cm) long; in the particular adult male specimen shown here it is about of the same length as the prostatic urethra – an anatomical fact we cannot really appreciate by endoscopic examination and/or visualize on radiological evaluations and studies. However, recent examination by nuclear magnetic resonance (NMR) of a sagittal section in a normal male confirms our anatomical description (Fig. 2).

The urinary external sphincter, wrapped around the membranous urethra, has its own intrinsic smooth muscular elements, constituting about half the thickness of the membranous urethral wall. The striated element wrapped around it is also an intrinsic element of the musculature of the membranous urethra. However, it is generally separate from it and can be dissected alone. On cross section of the membranous urethra we can see the abundance of the smooth component surrounding its entire circumference (Fig. 3). We also can see about the same thickness of striated muscle fibers, predominantly of circular orientation, surrounding the smooth muscular component (Fig. 3). It is worth noting that this striated musculature does not form an absolute complete ring; it is actually open in the midline posteriorly, probably where it gains attachment to the median raphe. That is why we say it is omega-shaped. However, from a functional point of view, it is a circular muscle wrapped around the membranous segment of the male urethra and the middle segment of the female urethra.

Innervation. The innervation of the external sphincter still remains a controversial subject. One would assume that such an anatomical fact would be a well agreed

---

[1] Department of Urology, U-518, University of California, San Francisco, CA 94143, USA

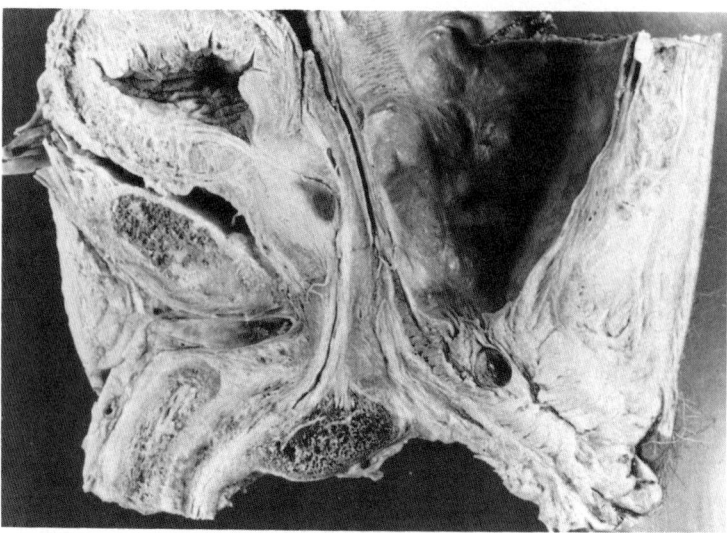

Fig. 1. Sagittal section of a fixed adult male pelvis, cut exactly in the midline to show the anatomical relationship of the pubic bone to the bladder, bladder neck, and prostatic segment as well as the membranous urethra and the penile urethra when it enters the spongy tissue of the penis. Also note the prominent anal sphincter as well as the rectum. Most significant is the length of the urethral segment traversing the pelvic floor before entering the spongy tissue of the penis. The distance between the apex of the prostate and the bulbous part of the urethra constitutes the membranous urethra, which is roughly the same length as the prostatic urethra – a fact confirmed by NMR studies (see Fig. 2)

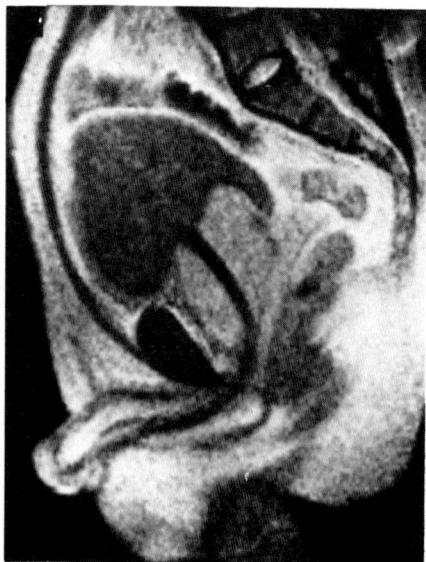

Fig. 2. NMR demonstration of a sagittal cut in an adult male with benign prostatic hypertrophy. Note the size of the prostate as well as the prostatomembranous urethra before it enters the spongy tissue of the penis. It is worth noting that the membranous urethra is clogged and its length is almost equal to that of the prostatic urethra

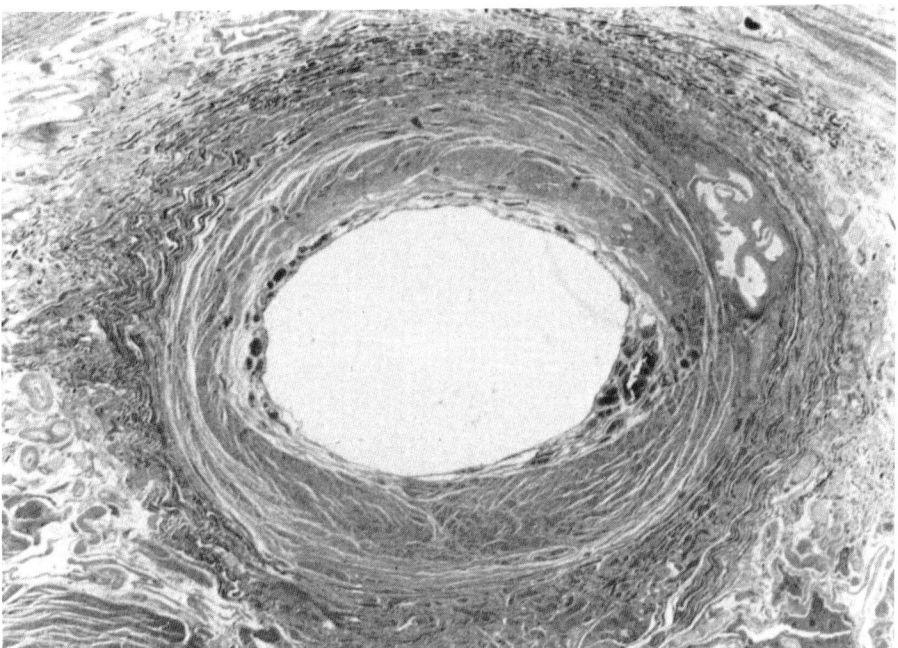

Fig. 3. Histologic section of the membranous urethra of a normal adult male shows the distribution of the smooth intrinsic musculature in the urethral wall, with circular fiber orientation; it is surrounded by an equally thick intrinsic coat of striated muscle fibers, essentially omega-shaped, with a defect in the midline posteriorly where it inserts in the perineal body. Note that the external sphincter constitutes an integral part of the musculature of the urethral wall at the level of the membranous urethra

upon issue, yet there are many divergent opinions about the origin and pathway of the nerve supply to the external sphincter. Most researchers maintain that it is mainly from the pudendal nerve. However, others believe that the external sphincter is supplied by the sympathetic autonomic nervous system, while others again maintain that this innervation is carried along the pelvic parasympathetic; it might be somatic in origin, but it is travelling along this nerve.

To identify the exact nerve pathway of the fibers innervating the urinary external sphincter, we utilized the technique of retrograde axonal transport of horseradish peroxidase (HRP) enzyme, in a technique combining histochemistry and autoradiography. A series of dogs received a direct injection of the HRP enzyme into the muscle fibers of the external sphincter, as well as in several other groups of muscles in the pelvic floor and bulbous spongiosus and ischiocavernosus muscles. On the contralateral side, HRP was injected directly into the cut end of the pudendal nerve to determine the location of the pudendal nucleus in the spinal cord and to compare it to the destination of the HRP injected in the various groups of striated muscle fibers. Direct injection of the pudendal nerve defined and localized the neuron cells supplying this nerve in the spinal cord, predominantly in S_1 and S_2 (Fig. 4). These cells were very similar to those described in the cell group in the human known as

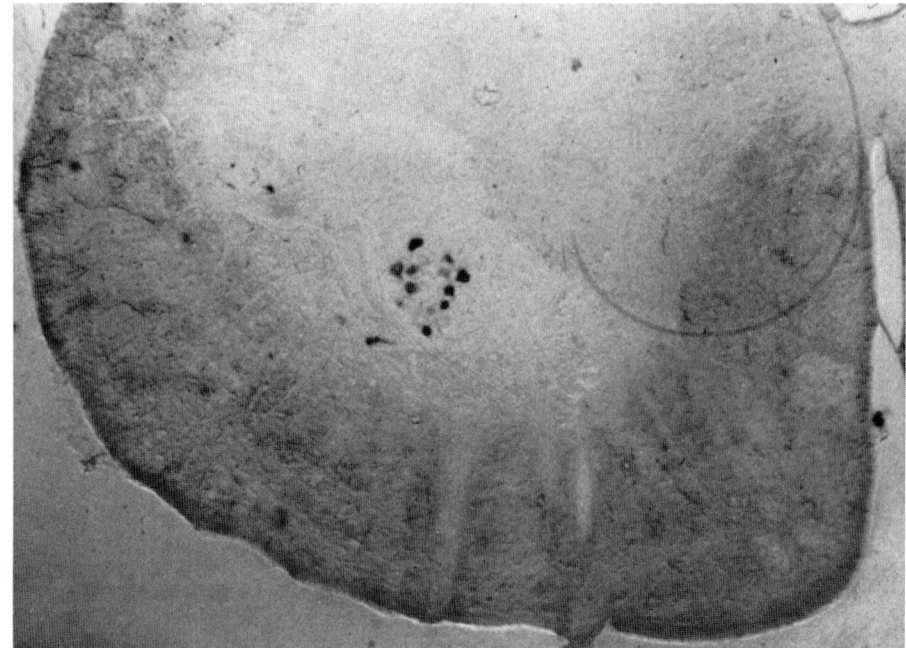

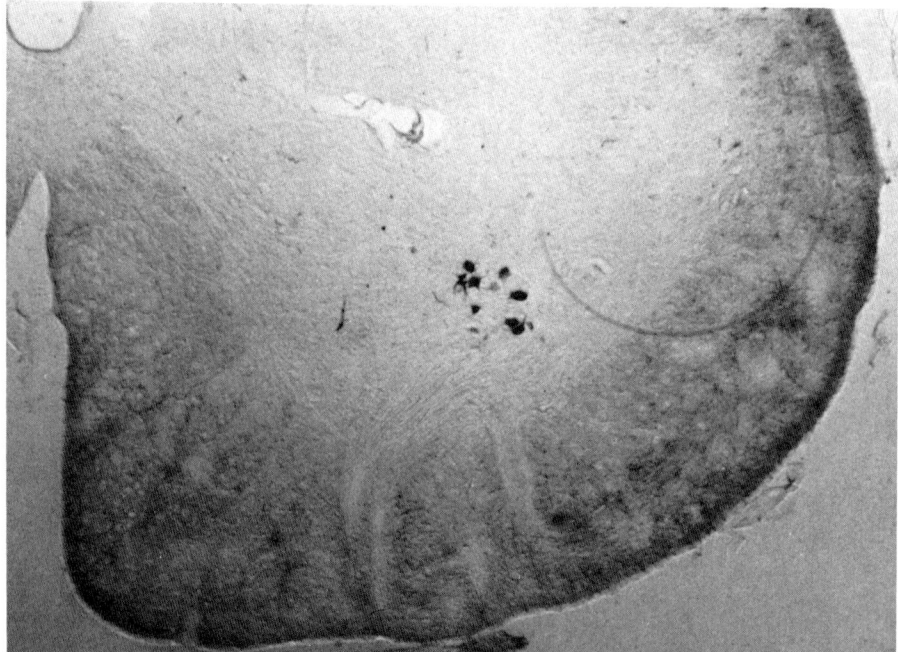

Fig. 4. a Cross-section of spinal cord at the S_1 level shows nuclei stained after direct injection of the cut end of the pudendal nerve. **b** Cross-section of spinal cord on the contralateral side of the above shows nuclei stained after injection into the striated external sphincter segment

nucleus of Onuf. Tracing of HRP from the injection site in the external sphincter showed that the location of the neuron cells was identical and a mirror image of Onuf's nucleus obtained by direct injection of the pudendal nerve. These data are definitive evidence that it is the pudendal nerve that carries the nerve fibers, the motor neuron fibers innervating the urinary external sphincter.

It was also impressive to see the confluence of the innervation origin of the urinary sphincter and of that of the bulbocavernosus and sphincter ani muscles; this tends to disprove the theory that the striated urethral sphincter is different in development and structure from the muscles of the pelvic floor and that it has no connection with them. On the contrary, our findings of single double-labelled neurons when injections in the striated urethral sphincter were combined with those in the anal sphincter or levator ani muscle suggest an even closer connection of these muscle groups than assumed previously. This neuroanatomic basis explains the functional synergism of different muscle groups and the comparable EMG readings from the urethral sphincter, anal sphincter, and bulbocavernosus muscle usually obtained during clinical evaluations. The new anatomical fact confirms the identification of the pudendal nerve as the primary motor supply to the external sphincter. Clinically, it presents a hopeful direction in the possibility of maintaining its sphincteric activity and controlling urinary incontinence through electrical stimulation.

Histochemical Studies. The characteristics of the smooth and striated components are of major interest. One can easily isolate, by conventional microscopic examination and with normal staining, the smooth component from the striated component – the latter's evident striations are clearly seen in the attached figure. However, unlike any other striated muscle, the striated sphincter is very specialized. The question is whether it is truly a voluntary sphincter, that is, a purely striated muscle like any other striated muscle, *or* a totally different structure, somewhere between the smooth involuntary musculature and the pure striated musculature. During the last few years we learned much about the structure of the striated urinary external sphincter, the results of which I would like to present to you.

In our studies of the functional patterns of the striated sphincter it became clear that the action of striated muscles is directly related to their twitch characteristics. It is well known that the twitch characteristics of striated fibers correlate with the specific activity of myosin-adenosine-triphosphatase (ATP'ase). Taking advantage of this staining, ATP'ase was used to study the details of the striated musculature element. Our animal histological studies, which were later extended to the human urethra, showed the presence of fast twitch striated muscle fibers as well as of slow twitch striated muscle fibers (Figs. 5, 6). The fast twitch fibers, which stain very darkly, are strongly ATP'ase in alkaline pH, while the reverse is true in the acid pH. By using the same segments with both alkaline and acid ATP, it is easy to show the different properties of each element of the striated muscle. In the figure shown, we can readily see the dark stained fast twitch fibers in ATP'ase in alkaline medium. In the second figure we can see the same section stained on the left hand side in an alkaline medium and on the right hand side in an acid medium; what was dark on one side became light on the other. Using these histological characteristics, we started to do muscle counting to identify the proportion of each fast and slow twitch fibers. It was apparent that the slow twitch fibers represent about 35 per cent of the

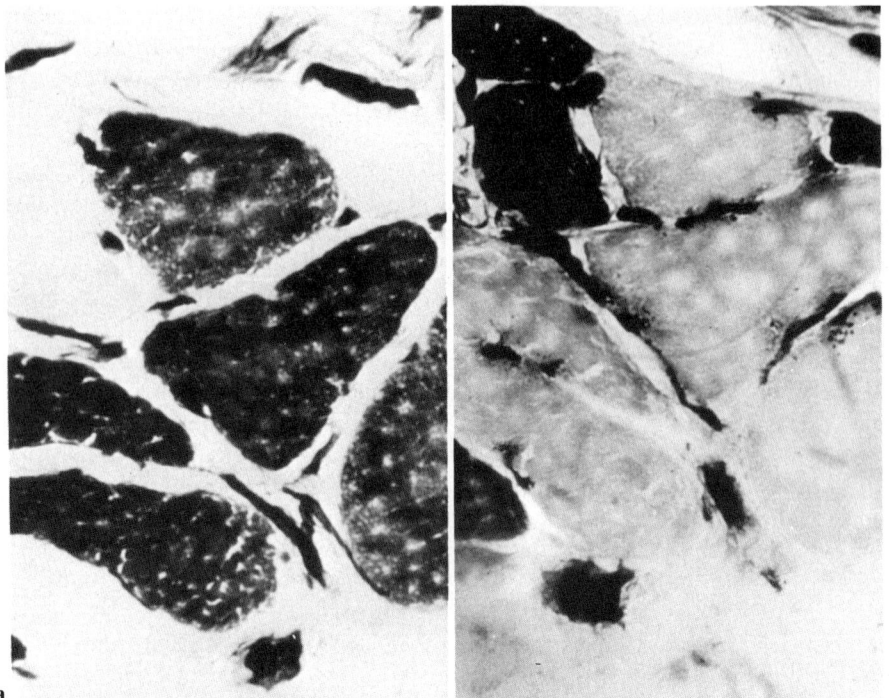

Fig. 5. Normal human male urethra with **a** alkaline and **b** acid adenosine triphosphate staining. Dark (fast-twitch) fibers in the left segment (alkaline medium) appear lighter with the acid stain on the right; the reverse is true for slow-twitch fibers

total striated muscle mass of the external urinary sphincter, and the fast twitch fibers about 65 per cent.

Another intriguing aspect of the external urinary sphincter that attracted our attention was resistance to fatigue. Our studies showed that this resistance to fatigue is directly related to the intensity of the oxidative enzyme staining of the muscle fibers. Using this histological advantage, we reexamined our sections of the human urinary external sphincter. As we became more familiar with the histological techniques, we noted that nearly 20 per cent of the fast twitch fibers stained as darkly as or slightly less than the slow twitch fibers in the oxidative NADH-TR stain, and are also positive for phosphorylase stain as shown in the figures (Figs. 7, 8). Because this variety of fast twitch fibers is rich in oxidative enzymes in addition to its glycolytic enzymes, it is both fast twitch oxidative glycolytic and fatigue resistant, being able to use both aerobic and anaerobic energy pathways. This same population could also be identified in ATP'ase preparations, inasmuch as the fibers appear intermediate in staining density between slow and fast twitch fatigable fibers (Figs. 9, 10).

Our work showed the external sphincter to be partly slow twitch fibers; the slow twitch oxidative fibers (as indicated before, only 35 per cent of the whole urethral striated musculature) decrease in proportion toward the distal external sphincter. It is this percentage of the striated external sphincter that contributes to the mecha-

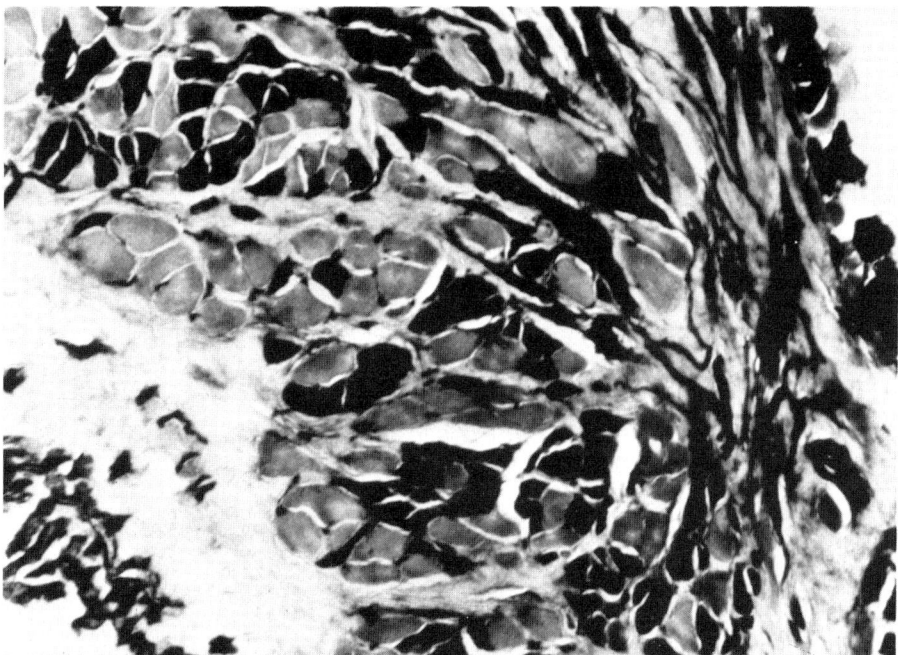

Fig. 6. Alkaline stain of the external striated sphincter at mid-urethra. Note the mixture of dark (fast-twitch) and light (slow-twitch) fibers

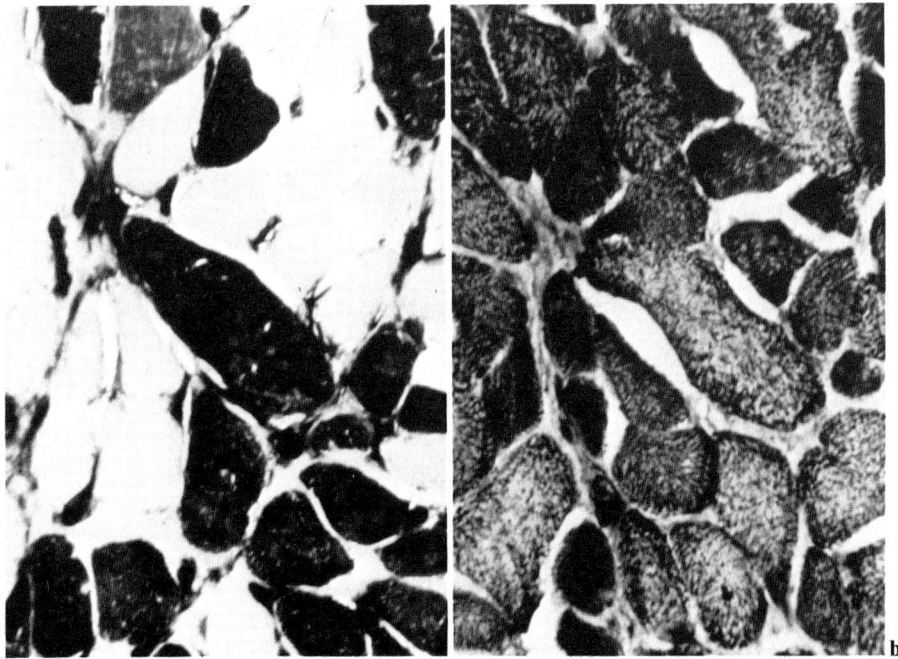

Fig. 7. The canine urethra: **a** alkaline ATP'ase stain; **b** oxidative stain

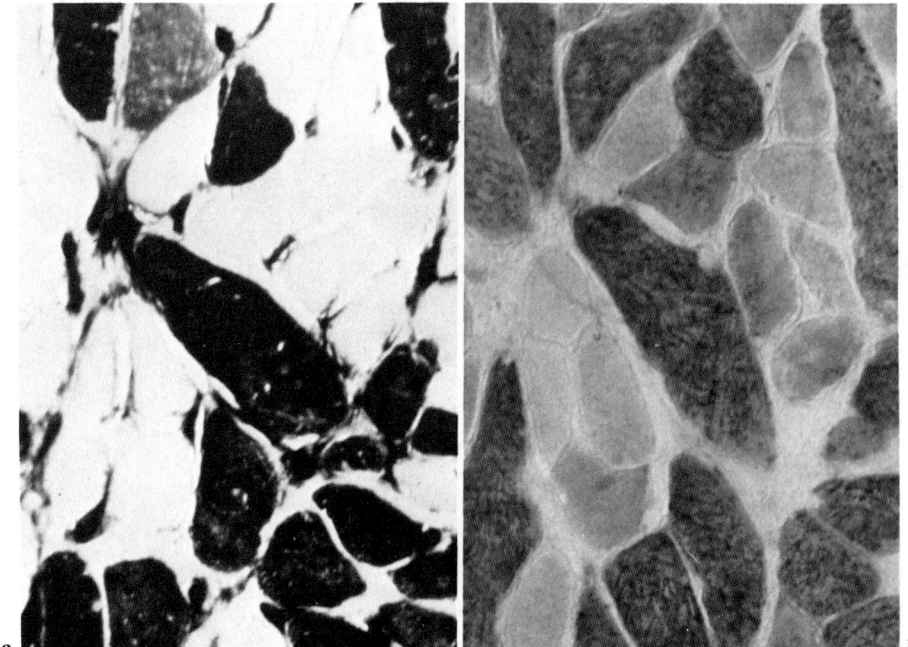

Fig. 8. Same section as in Fig. 7: **a** alkaline ATP'ase stain; **b** phosphorylase stain

nism of continence during resting conditions. On the other hand, the fast twitch fibers are the major elements called upon during emergency needs, to help increase the closure effectiveness of the external sphincter.

Our interest then centered on the small percentage of fibers that are fast twitch fibers, yet fatigue resistant. In an attempt to evaluate quantitatively their proportion in the striated external sphincter, we discovered that the 65 per cent of fast twitch fibers can be subdivided into 50 per cent glycolytic fast twitch fatigable fibers and 15 per cent oxidative glycolytic fatigue resistant fibers. The new understanding of the nature of the urinary external sphincter clearly suggests that the slow twitch fibers are probably constantly used to provide the functional tonus of the external sphincter, which adds to the sustained resistance of the bladder outlet. As far as emergency needs helping build up outlet resistance, it is specifically the fast twitch *fatigable* fibers that are called upon. The fast twitch fatigue resistant fibers are those that will lag behind in their relaxation; however, they are also capable of offering on command high magnitude closure pressure around the membranous urethra.

Sphincteric Function, Bladder Pacemaker, and Morphologic Changes of Musculature. What can be gained from this knowledge? We found ourselves in a unique situation inasmuch as we had done experimental studies to develop a bladder pacemaker, the major element of which was to control sphincteric function and maintain continence in neuropathic disorders. In our experimental model, we had chronically implanted

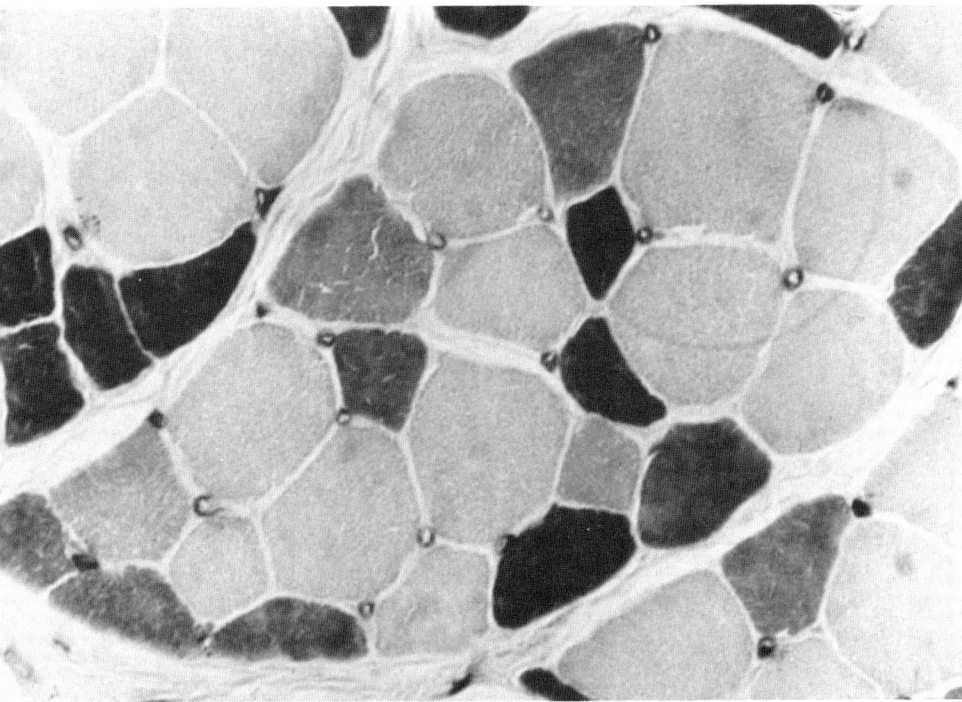

Fig. 9. Hypertrophied striated sphincter muscle. Note that the appearance is more rounded, with less space in between, after intermittent electrical stimulation

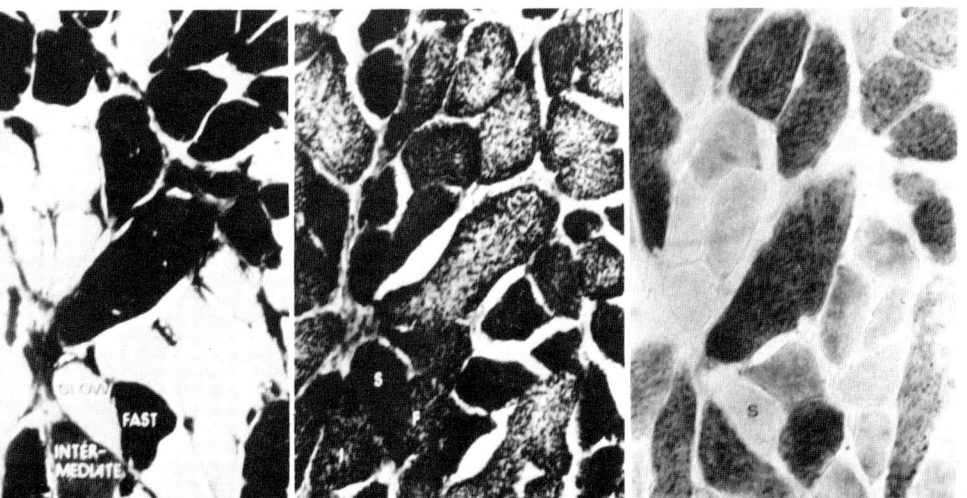

Fig. 10. Serial cross-sections of striated urethral musculature of the dog stained for the following reactions: **a** alkaline ATP'ase; **b** NADH-TR activity; **c** phosphorylase stain. Note that fast-twitch, fatigue-resistant or intermediate fibers are intermediate in staining density in alkaline ATP'ase, whereas slow-twitch fibers (*S*) are pale and fast-twitch fatigable fibers (*F*) dark. Intermediate fibers are dark in both oxidative and phosphorylase stain, indicating that they have both oxidative and glycolytic activities

electrodes around selected sacral roots for the purpose of continuous intermittent stimulation of the urinary sphincter in order to achieve control. We could electrostimulate a sacral root unilaterally for a prolonged period of time, which is probably the best exercise. Our stimulus parameters (between 50 ms on and 110 ms off, or 30 ms on and 70 ms off) could be carried on for several hours, repeatedly, day after day. The experimental model gave us the unique opportunity to study the effect of chronic stimulation or chronic exercise on the morphological structure of the striated urinary sphincter. After knowing the proportion of fast twitch fatigable fibers and fast twitch fatigue resistant fibers in the normal external sphincter, we started to study the chronic electrically stimulated external sphincter in the dog. We compared first the tail muscle, then urinary external sphincter of stimulated and control animals. We noticed with interest that chronic stimulation (chronic exercise) changed a high proportion of the fast twitch fatigable fibers into fast twitch fatigue resistant fibers. That increase in the number of fatigue resistant fibers was directly related to the duration of stimulation. When we stopped stimulation for a period of time (usually 4 weeks), most of those fatigue resistant fibers that had been transformed as a result of the stimulation reverted back to their previous status of fast twitch fatigable fibers. It appears from this experiment that exercise does change the morphology of the striated external sphincter or, to put it differently, *the morphology of the striated muscle fibers follows their physiological function.* When there is a need for a higher proportion of fast twitch fatigue resistant fibers, the muscle fibers can change their nature to assume these characteristics to provide for this function. A parallel is the fact that runners, after repeated exercise, eventually become fatigue resistant; the same is probably true of swimmers and tennis players and of all those who use a specific set of muscles over and over again: a higher proportion of their striated muscle fibers gradually becomes fatigue resistant so that physical exercise can be continued without actual fatigue. If these exercises are stopped for any length of time, the muscles revert to their previous condition.

This same phenomenon was noted in human clinical trials. By chronic electrical stimulation of the striated external sphincter, we could obtain a higher percentage of fast twitch fatigue resistant fibers, capable of providing constant control. If we stopped the stimulation, these muscles maintained their control for a certain period of time, but gradually lost it. When the stimulation was reactivated, some of these fibers were reconverted to fatigue resistant fibers and regained their control.

This new insight into the morphological structure of the urinary external sphincter provides extremely valuable information for the development of the bladder pacemaker in order to achieve complete continence and control. Clinical testing is supportive of these histological experimental studies. Probably in a few years, when we get together again, we will be presenting to you various experimental animal models and clinical findings in a series of humans who have been incontinent, and in whom, owing to chronic electrical stimulation, most of the striated external sphincter musculature was converted into fatigue resistant fibers and control of continence was regained.

The Scrotal Flap Technique as an Operative Method for the Treatment of Iatrogenic and Posttraumatic Male Incontinence

E. SCHMIEDT and W. WIELAND [1]

Introduction

Taking today's success rates of operative treatment of urinary incontinence in men, which fluctuate between 60 and 80%, all therapeutic efforts remain unsuccessful in about a quarter of these patients, whereby I and others think in particular of the operation methods of Tanagho et al. (1969, 1972), Leadbetter and Fraley (1967), Hauri (1981), Scott et al. (1973), Rosen (1981), Kaufman (1970, 1972) and Steffens (1981), and also of the Teflon injection into the bladder neck according to Politano et al. (1973). In my opinion, the reasons for the failures can be found partially in the frequently large-scaled and difficult operation technique, in the use of alloplastic cuffs and prosthetic material, which present a risk of infection and consequently rejection and are liable to produce pressure necrosis, and in the lack of experience of the individual surgeon, due to the relative small number of postoperative and posttraumatic urinary incontinences.

Although for example we could also achieve excellent and good permanent results in 67% (22 cases in total) (Mayer et al. 1983), using the Kaufman III method (1973), i.e. after perineal implantation of an oval silicone pad, we were, and are still searching for a method which is:
a) an operation technique that is not too difficult to apply, and by that
b) there is no necessity to use alloplastic material to restore continence.

The Scrotal Flap Technique

The list of the hitherto published methods for restoration of urinary incontinence in men is long (Table 1), which demonstrates that this problem despite much success still awaits a solution. Under this aspects I will add another operation method to the methods practiced up to now, which I published in 1969/1970 and 1975 (together with my assistant at that time, E. Elsaesser), and which in my opinion meets the two afore-mentioned demands: a simple operation technique, and the avoidance of the use of foreign body implants. All methods of restoration of continence depend upon an elevation of the urethral resistance, which means they depend upon the principle of creating an adequate urethral obstruction, whether by narrowing and lengthening

---

[1] Urologische Klinik, Klinikum Großhadern, Marchioninistr. 15, D-8000 München 70

Table 1. After Kaufman JJ, Raz S (1979) Treatment of male urinary incontinence. Campbell's Urology, vol 3, p 2262, table 74-4, Saunders, Philadelphia

I. Nonsurgical
   A. Expectant 9 months to 1 year
   B. Training
   C. Pharmacology
      1. Alpha-adrenergic stimulators
      2. Cholinolytic agents
   D. Electrical stimulation (+training) (Hopkinson and Lightwood 1967)
   E. Injection
      1. Sclerosing fluids (Sachse 1963)
      2. Paraffin (Quackels 1955)
      3. Supportive material – Teflon (Politano et al. 1971)

II. Surgical
   A. "Surrogate sphincter" formation
      1. Abdominal muscle and fascial slings
         a. Pyramidalis muscle (Goebell 1910)
         b. Rectus muscle or sheath (Cooney 1953; Frangenheim 1914; Milin 1969)
      2. Gracilis muscle slings
         a. Gracilis muscle (Deming 1926)
      3. Perineal muscles
         a. Ischiocavernosus (Lowsley 1936)
         b. Levator ani (Squier 1911)
         c. External sphincter ani (Mathiesen 1970; Verges-Flaque 1951)
      4. Bladder flaps
         a. Tube (Tanagho and Smith 1972)
         b. Spiral (Flocks and Boldus 1973)
      5. Prosthetic devices
         a. External (Foley 1947)
         b. Implanted (Scott 1973)
   B. Vesicourethral suspension + angulation
      1. Kelly 1928
      2. Marshall et al. 1949
   C. Posterior urethral lengthening
      1. Young 1919
      2. Thompson 1961
      3. Leadbetter and Fraley 1967
   D. Urethral plication and twists
      1. Young 1908
      2. Beneventi 1966
      3. Petersen 1967
   E. Urethral compression – passive
      1. Acrylic; Silastic (Berry 1961)
      2. Collagen (Girgis and Veenema 1965)
      3. Autologous rib (Hinman and Schmaelze 1970)
      4. Fascia lata (Milin 1969)
      5. Kaufman I (Crural cross); II (Crural); and III (Silicone-gel prosthesis (SGP)) (Kaufman 1973, 1972, 1970)
      6. Crural (Puigvert 1971)
      7. Marlex (Salcedo 1972)
      8. SGP + Marlex (Yarbrough 1975)

Table 1 (continued)

F. Electrical stimulation
  1. Caldwell 1963
  2. Merrill et al. 1971
G. Urinary diversion
  1. Ileal conduit
  2. Colon conduit
  3. Ureterosigmoidostomy
  4. Cutaneous ureterostomy
  5. Vesicostomy + BN closure
  6. Nephrostomy
---

the proximal urethra in the region of the bladder neck (Leadbetter and Fraley 1967; Tanagho et al. 1969), or by compression of the prostatic urethra from outside (Scott et al. 1973; Steffens 1981), respectively by compression of the bulbus urethrae by means of the Scott, Rosen or Kaufman cuffs or prostheses, and finally by the embedding of the bulbar urethra between the corpora cavernosa penis with transpubic pelvic floor musculature and prostatic capsule gathering (Hauri 1981).

While all the other operation techniques mentioned above are meant to produce an urethral occlusion by external pressure on the anterior or posterior urethra, we took into consideration to close the urethral lumen from inside with a type of "bottle cork", while this so-called "cork" expands and thereby releases the closed lumen, as soon as a detrusor contraction, i.e. the miction process, starts (Fig. 1). Initially, in 5 cases of posttraumatic incontinence with urethral strictures in the region of the pars membranacea urethrae we used the bulbus urethrae for the intermitting urethral closure which was divided and mobilised from the urogenital diaphragm, pulled through and fixed in the prostatic urethra, following the method of Solowow (1935) and Badenoch (1950).

In 2 cases we were able to achieve a nearly optimal continence. In 3 further patients this was only attainable after a second intervention, by which a perineal pendunculated scrotal skin flap, after Gil Vernet (1965) and Zoedler (1968) (Fig. 2), was pulled into the urethral lumen and fixed at the bladder exit.

Further cases showed frequent obstructions and difficulties in voiding the bladder after pulling-in the urethral bulbus into the prostatic urethra, and furthermore some perineal pendunculated scrotal skin flaps became necrotic due to disturbances in blood supply. So we decided to treat our patients with iatrogenic incontinence and urethral strictures in the pars membranacea with a lateral pendunculated scrotal skin flap, which was pulled into the prostatic urethra, as originally described by Michalowski and Modelski (1962) (Fig. 3), for the therapy of intradiaphragmatic urethral strictures.

Cross-cut in the region of the external sphincter

After a <u>bulbus-pull-through</u> operation

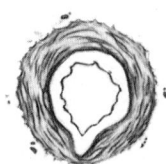

After a <u>scrotal-flap</u> operation

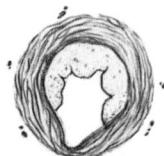

during miction

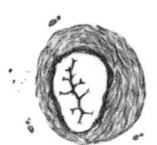

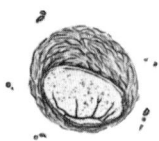

after miction

Fig. 1

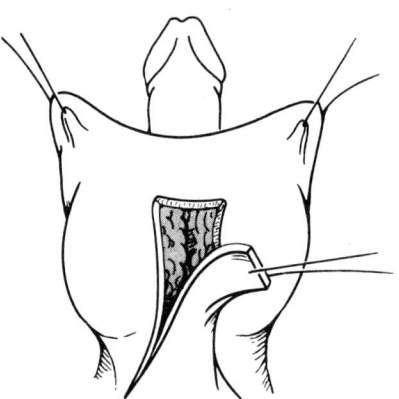
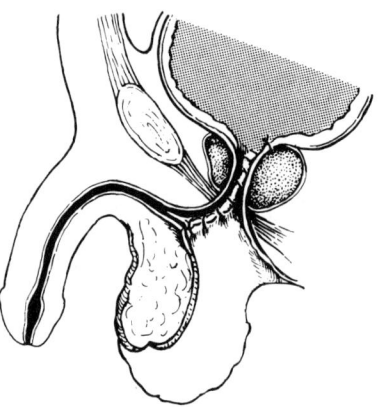

Fig. 2. Method Gil Vernet-Zoedler

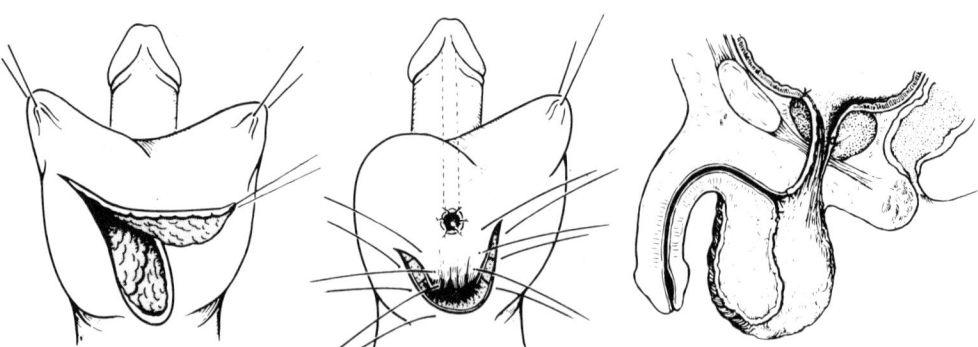

Fig. 3. Method Michalowski-Modelski

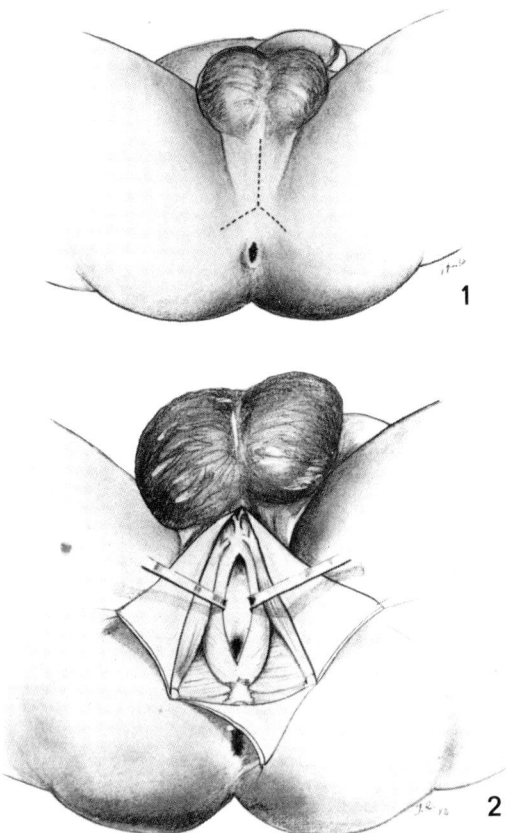

Fig. 4. Step 1 and 2

Method of the Scrotal Flap Technique

Before pulling-in the scrotal flap the mucosa of the prostatic urethra is transurethrally resected to the colliculus, to ensure a good healing of the flap. Then the preparation of the bulbus urethrae in lithotomy position follows. The urethra is opened longitudinally for 3–4 cm, directly distal to the urogenital diaphragm (Fig. 4, step 1 + 2). After mobilisation of the scrotal skin in the region of the right or left half of the scrotum, a laterally styled scrotal skin flap, about 5 cm wide and 12 cm long, is shaped, whereby this scrotal skin flap should only reach to the raphe scrotalis (Fig. 5, step 3), and both free corners of the rectangular scrotal skin flap are marked with differently coloured threads. The reason for this operation technique is to ensure the blood supply of the scrotal skin flap.

After that the bladder is opened suprapubically and with the aid of the marking threads the scrotal skin flap is drawn into the proximal urethra to the bladder exit, after a preceding rotation of 180 degrees (Fig. 6, step 4 + 5), and fixed with interrupted sutures at the dorsal circumference of the bladder exit.

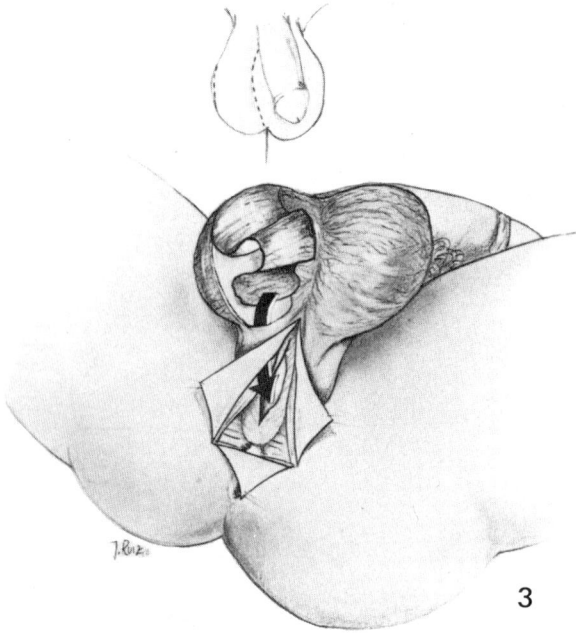

Fig. 5. Step 3

The urine is temporarily drained over a suprapubic bladder fistula and the urinary bladder is closed again. The scrotal edges are adapted with a continuous or interrupted suture and the scrotal skin is then joined to the edges of the previously resected prostatic urethra, so that a scrotal skin funnel is formed, through which one can pass a catheter both into the prostatic and distal urethra (Fig. 7, step 6 + 7). 8–12 weeks later the funnel is excised and the urethral lumen closed again.

Results

Since 1980 10 patients of ours were treated with the described operation method, because of an iatrogenic respectively posttraumatic urinary incontinence (ratio 8:2). In 9 cases this intervention led to a completely satisfactory continence for the patients, whereby merely by exertion a limited stress incontinence was observed by 1 patient, which demanded 1–2 urinary pads daily. All patients were pleased to be totally integrated in social life again (Table 2).

We had to register one failure, i.e. a patient who had an incontinence after a radical prostatectomy due to prostatic carcinoma. After pulling-in the scrotal flap there was a continuous 3rd grade stress incontinence. The reason for the failure of the scrotal flap method seems to be the resected prostatic capsule, which has to be a support for the scrotal flap. Therefore, the pulling-in of the scrotal flap does not seem to be an appropriate operation method for incontinence after radical prostatectomy.

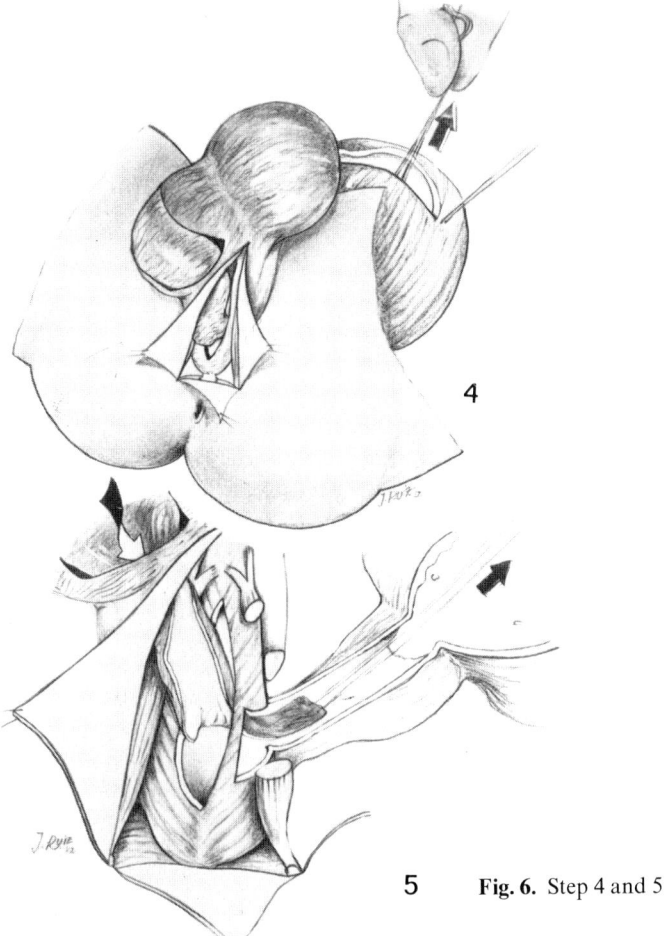

Fig. 6. Step 4 and 5

Table 2. Results of scrotal flap technique

Patient	Kind of lesion	Continent	Stressincontinent I–II	Stressincontinent III
1. B. M.	TUR	+		
2. A. P.	TUR	+		
3. R. G.	TUR	+		
4. S. L.	TUR		+	
5. N. F.	TUR	+		
6. T. M.	TUR	+		
7. L. G.	TUR	+		
8. Al. A.	Traumatic	+		
9. Al. D.	Traumatic	+		
10. R. K.	Radical Prostatectomy			+

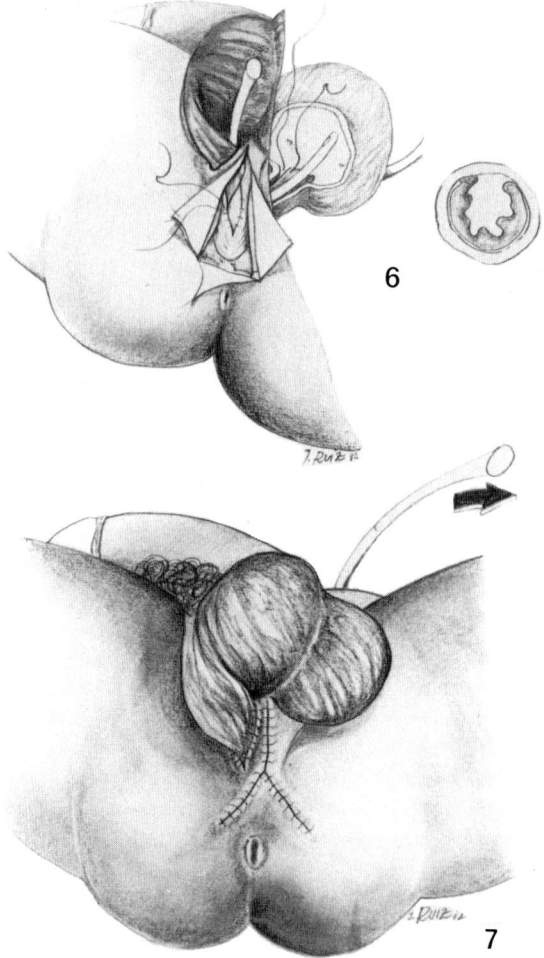

Fig. 7. Step 6 and 7

Although the number of patients with incontinence we have treated using the pulling-in of the scrotal flap technique is small, in our opinion the application of the operation method is justified and recommendable considering the relatively limited expense of this operation technique and the good healing prospects. Besides, this method does not demand any alloplastic material, which justifies the high success rate of 90%.

References

Badenoch AW (1950) A pull-through operation for impassable traumatic stricture of the urethra. Br J Urol 22:404
Elsaesser E, Schmiedt E (1970) Zur Behandlung der supra- und intradiaphragmalen posttraumatischen Harnröhrenstrikturen. Urol Int 25:563–570

Gil Vernet JM (1965) Un traitement des stenoses traumatiques et inflammatives de l'urètre postérieur. Nouvelle méthode d'uretéroplastie. J Urol Nephrol 72:97

Hauri D (1981) Unsere Methode der operativen Behandlung der Post-Prostatektomie-Inkontinenz. In: Weber W, Jonas D (eds) Die postoperative Harninkontinenz des Mannes. Thieme, Stuttgart, pp 70–80

Kaufman JJ (1970) A new operation for male incontinence. Surg Gynaecol Obstet 131:295

Kaufman JJ (1972) Surgical treatment of post-prostatectomy incontinence. Use of the penile crura to compress the bulbous urethra. J Urol 107:293

Kaufman JJ (1973) Treatment of post-prostatectomy incontinence using a silicone-gel-prothesis. Br J Urol 45:646

Leadbetter GW, Fraley EE (1967) Surgical correction of total urinary incontinence. Five years after. J Urol 97:896

Mayer P et al. (1983) Erfahrungen mit der Kaufmann-Prothese zur Behandlung der postoperativen Harninkontinenz des Mannes. Urologe A 22:113–115

Michalowski E, Modelski W (1962) Zur operativen Behandlung der Strikturen der hinteren Harnröhre. Urol Int 13:374

Politano VA et al. (1973) Periurethral teflon injection for urinary incontinence (Abstr. XVI). International Society of Urology, Amsterdam 1973, Trans Am Assoc Genito Urin Surg 65:54

Rosen M (1981) Die Harninkontinenz-Prothese nach Rosen. In: Weber W, Jonas D (eds) Die postoperative Harninkontinenz des Mannes. Thieme, Stuttgart, pp 116–124

Schmiedt E (1968) Beurteilung und Behandlung von Unfallverletzungen der Harnorgane. Arch Klin Chir 322:300

Schmiedt E (1969) Zur Behebung der posttraumatischen und postoperativen Harninkontinenz beim Mann. In: Verh.-Bericht 22. Tagung Dtsch. Ges. Urol. Springer, Berlin Heidelberg New York, p 329

Scott FB et al. (1973) The treatment of urinary incontinence by an implantable prosthetic sphincter. Urol 1:252

Solowow PD (1935) Wiestnik Chir 37:36

Steffens L (1981) Bisherige Erfahrungen mit dem Suspensionsband zur Behebung der postoperativen Harninkontinenz des Mannes. In: Weber W, Jonas D (eds) Die postoperative Harninkontinenz des Mannes. Thieme, Stuttgart, pp 80–95

Tanagho EA, Smith DR (1971, 1972) Clinical evaluation of a surgical technique for the correction of complete urinary incontinence. Trans Am Assoc Genito Urin Surg 63:103 (1971); J Urol 107:402 (1972)

Tanagho EA, Smith DR (1972) Clinical evaluation of a surgical technique for the correction of complete urinary incontinence. J Urol 107:791

Tanagho EA et al. (1969) Mechanism of urinary incontinence. II. Technique for surgical correction of incontinence. J Urol 101:305

Zoedler D (1968) Rekonstruktionsverfahren der proximalen Harnröhre. Z Urol 61:19

A Urodynamic Review of Bladder Outlet "Obstruction" in the Male and Its Treatment

R. TURNER-WARWICK [1]

The development of methods of objective urodynamic evaluation and their introduction into clinical urological practice has lead to a fundamental revision of both concept and treatment. However, while entirely new techniques such as percutaneous nephrolithotomy tend to be swiftly adopted, time honoured misconceptions and procedures are often slow to change; regrettably, some urologists still believe that they are able to evaluate urodynamic dysfunction with a cystoscope and many still treat an obstructive bladder neck mechanism by loop resection. Thus, in an update of our contribution to the First International Urodynamic Symposium held in Aachen 12 years ago, it is still necessary to include some of the fundamental facts and concepts that were introduced at that Meeting (Turner-Warwick 1973).

The Myth of 'Prostatism.' Unfortunately the symptom complex of frequency, nocturia, urgency and a 'poor' stream is still misconceptually referred to as 'prostatism' and is consequently regarded as indicative of bladder outflow obstruction when it occurs in men over middle age. This is both erroneous in concept and misleading in practice because:
1) The symptom complex is usually the result of unstable detrusor behaviour and is common in the *absence* of obstruction.
2) If obstruction is present it may be the result of a dyssynergic bladder neck mechanism or a urethral stricture and not the prostate.
3) The same symptom complex not referred to as 'prostatism' when it occurs in females.

The Symptoms Associated with Bladder Outflow Obstruction. Irrespective of its cause, the direct result of partial restriction of the outlet of the bladder is simply its effect on the voiding flow – a *slow start, a poor or intermittent stream* and a *terminal dribble* – no more.

The symptoms of frequency, nocturia and urgency only occur as a direct result of mechanical outflow obstruction in the occasional case of a large residual urine associated with borderline retention; they can sometimes result from hypersensitive conditions such as urine infection or vesical calculi but, very much more commonly, they are a result of unstable involuntary voiding detrusor contractions which create an erroneous premature sensation of fullness before the bladder is distended.

However, unstable detrusor dysfunction often occurs in men and women who void efficiently so these symptoms should never be regarded as diagnostic of outflow

---

[1] The London University Institute of Urology and 61 Harley House, Marylebone Road, GB-London NW1 5HL

obstruction; furthermore, as a result of the characteristically diminished voiding volumes many patients confusingly complain of a 'poor' stream, referring sometimes to its unsatisfactory volume and sometimes to its consequently diminished flow rate (Turner-Warwick and Whiteside 1977, 1979).

Thus, when a patient has both prostatic enlargement and the symptom complex of instability it is essential to determine objectively whether he has bladder outlet obstruction before advising a prostatectomy.

Detrusor Behaviour During Voluntary Retention. Although we do not fully understand its neurological mechanism we recognise that the bladder is unique in being the only smooth muscle that is normally under complete voluntary control. A normally functioning detrusor contracts only during volitional voiding and at no other time; this controlled behaviour is conveniently referred to as 'stable'. However, by definition, a detrusor cannot be designated as 'stable' without objective provocative urodynamic testing (Bates et al. 1970; Turner-Warwick 1979).

About 10–15 per cent of 'normal' males and females never achieve full inhibitory control over their sacro-vesical reflex mechanism so their bladders develop 'unstable' involuntary contractions between voidings; these contractions increase the intravesical pressure long before the bladder is fully distended and are usually, but not always, associated with a premature sensation of bladder-fullness – hence the symptoms of frequency, nocturia and urgency which they regard as normal for their 'weak' bladder.

In the absence of obstruction, the natural incidence of idiopathic unstable detrusor behaviour seems to increase with age to about 20 per cent in the 8th decade in both males and females; furthermore, a further 50–60 per cent of men with bladder outflow obstruction develop unstable detrusor behaviour. Thus, 70–80 per cent of men with proven outflow obstruction also have symptoms of frequency, nocturia and urgency and thus only about one in five is troubled only by mechanical symptoms of delay and a poor stream (Turner-Warwick 1979).

The Response of Unstable Detrusor Symptoms to the Relief of Obstruction. In men, the relief of bladder outflow obstruction may lead to the reversion of secondary detrusor instability to stability but, of course, idiopathic instability does not revert. Thus, about three out of four men with proven obstruction can expect a great improvement in their symptoms of frequency, urgency and nocturia. It is most important to explain to every patient presenting with proven outlet obstruction and symptoms of instability that although surgery should certainly resolve the obstruction the chances that the relief of this obstruction will result in resolution of their detrusor instability symptoms is only about 70 per cent (Turner-Warwick 1979). This is an important pre-operative communication because otherwise a patient who presented with symptoms of detrusor instability will return saying that he 'had the prostate operation but it failed'; he will not be satisfied with the restoration of his competitive voiding stream if he had been allowed to expect that his more troublesome symptoms would be resolved. Fortunately however, when instability persists after the relief of a proven obstruction the symptoms are usually less severe.

It is also important to appreciate that unstable detrusor behaviour may be asymptomatic. Routine pre-operative urodynamic evaluation shows that a pro-

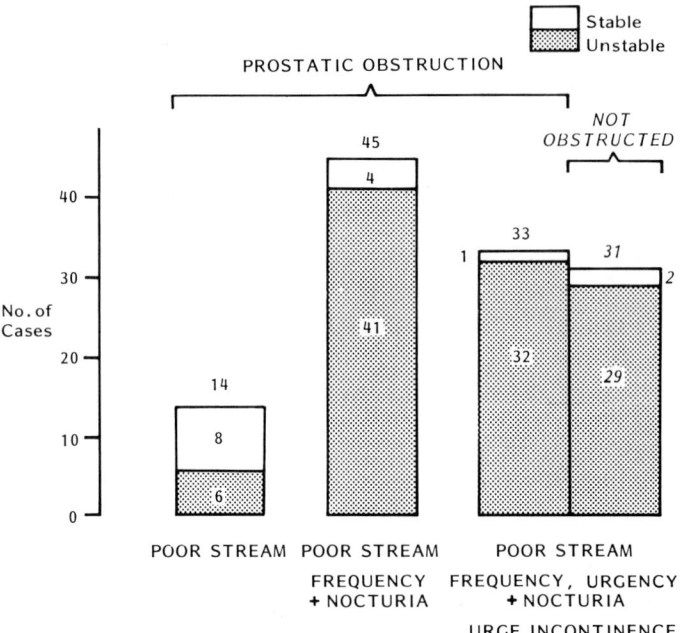

Fig. 1. The close relationship between symptoms and unstable detrusor behaviour: the poor relation between symptoms and the incidence of obstruction (Turner-Warwick et al. 1973)

portion of male patients presenting with proven outlet obstruction and simple flow reduction symptoms of slow-flow, poor stream, and terminal dribble, have *asymptomatic* involuntary unstable detrusor behaviour (Fig. 1) (Turner-Warwick 1979). After a prostatic resection, sensitivity sometimes seems to increase so that if detrusor instability persists, the patient may subsequently become aware of his involuntary contractions for the first time and develop the appropriate symptoms; if such a patient is investigated by cystometry for the first time postoperatively it should not be assumed that his bladder has become unstable as a result of the operation – in fact, this is rare (Turner-Warwick 1979).

The 'Cause' of Unstable Detrusor Behaviour in Male Bladder Outlet Obstruction. Stable detrusor function is fundamentally dependent upon a positive, centrally orientated, inhibition of the sacro-vesical reflex mechanism, however, although stability must be neurologically mediated, in the absence of demonstrable neuropathy it is not clinically helpful to conceive unstable detrusor dysfunction as essentially 'neurogenic'; furthermore, neuropathy may result in a variety of detrusor dysfunctions and it is irrational to use the word 'neurogenic bladder' to indicate any particular dysfunction such as instability (Thomas 1979; Turner-Warwick 1979).

For clinical purposes we recognise three types of unstable detrusor behaviour: idiopathic, neuropathic and obstructive, however it is rarely possible to distingush between these on the basis of detrusor response measurements alone hence if a patient with proven bladder outlet *obstruction* also has a mild *neuropathy,* such as a stroke or Parkinsonism we are, at present, unable to determine pre-operatively whether relief of the obstructive element is likely to result in reversion of an unstable detrusor dysfunction to stability.

We do not know exactly why bladder outlet obstruction in the male is associated with such a high incidence of detrusor instability: the common factor in most cases seems to be a high-resistance outlet obstruction, but why an obstruction during the voiding phase should be associated with an abnormality of detrusor function during the sphincter-contained 'storage' phase is not clear. However, 'obstruction instability' is unique in that it is the only type of unstable detrusor behaviour that can often be reverted to stability by a local operative procedure; this is clear proof that some local factors are involved and it should further dissuade us from assuming that the only significant aetiological factor is central mediation (Turner-Warwick 1974).

It has been suggested that an increase in afferent impulses, possibly 'tension arising in the prostatic capsule' may play an important role in the development of instability – however, in general, hypersensitive conditions such as cystitis and prostatitis, associated with a massive increase in afferent neurone activity, do not result in a significant increase in the natural incidence of instability.

There is a close correlation between the effective relief of bladder outlet obstruction and reversion to stability, irrespective of the actual operative procedure that is used: thus the removal of the bulk of a prostatic enlargement may not be sufficient if a small remnant of apical tissue causes persistent outlet obstruction. On the other hand the reversion rate after the simple selective endoscopic incision of a dyssynergic bladder neck obstruction in the absence of any prostatic enlargement approximates to that resulting from the extensive resection of large obstructive prostates. Furthermore, although the incidence of instability resulting from obstruction due to an anterior urethral stricture is, in fact, somewhat less than that due to a posterior urethral obstruction, it approximates to the natural incidence after the relief of the obstruction (Turner-Warwick 1979).

It might be reasonable to suppose that the likelihood of reversion to stability might diminish in patients who had had bladder outlet obstruction for a long time – however, Arnold (1980) found no evidence to support this; similarly he found little correlation between the severity of an obstruction, the incidence of instability and the incidence of its reversion after relief of the obstruction. However, this raises the interesting question – what degree of obstruction has to be present to offer a worthwhile chance of reversion to stability after the relief of marginally obstructive states? Our attention is currently focussed on this problem.

The Detrusor Behaviour and Obstructed Voiding. In the male, the voiding detrusor contraction reacts to outflow obstruction in a variety of ways – 'not all detrusors are equal' (Turner-Warwick et al. 1973).

Although most detrusors respond by developing an increased voiding contraction-pressure to overcome the increased outflow resistance, others do not.

In some the voiding contraction is normally sustained until the bladder is completely empty in spite of a significant outflow obstruction; in others it fades before the bladder is empty, leaving a residual urine. This prematurely fading contraction should be accurately described as an 'unsustained voiding contraction' – it should not be described as a 'de-compensated bladder' because this conceptual term is based on the supposition that an unsustained contraction is the result of 'failure of the bladder to compensate for obstruction' – although this may sometimes be true, it is often inaccurate because an unsustained detrusor contraction is also one of a number of characteristic types of *unobstructed* detrusor dysfunction.

Unobstructed Neuropathic Detrusor Dysfunction. This again emphasises the importance of describing all urodynamic findings accurately and objectively without prejudgement or conceptualisation. Occasionally a gradually increasing outflow obstruction evokes little or no detectable detrusor pressure-rise response – the bladder gradually becomes over-distended and progressively fails to empty.

However, irrespective of the detrusor response to chronic obstruction, acute retention commonly arises as a result of an episode of over-distension because overstretched muscle fibres cannot generate their maximum contraction force thus causing the important warning symptom of 'increased' difficulty in voiding when the bladder is overfull.

Should the Natural Age-Related Diminution of the Voiding Flow Be Regarded as 'Normal?' So well recognised is the age-related diminution of the voiding flow and the increase in diurnal and nocturnal frequency that men commonly accept this as their natural burden. The average flow pattern diminishes in each decade after the age of 50 (Abrams 1977); however, it is highly questionable whether this should be regarded as 'normal' because, in the majority of males, this 'natural' diminution of flow is the result of a significant increase in the outlet resistance, either as a result of a natural age-related increase in prostatic size or of a progressive increase in a subclinical dyssynergic bladder neck obstruction or a combination of both; the accuracy of this observation is self-evident from the fact that effective operative relief of the obstruction restores the flow pattern to normality and resolves the symptoms of frequency and urgency arising as a result of it (Turner-Warwick 1979).

While some men prefer to procrastinate and live with their increasing symptoms others are philosophically inclined towards an early resolution of their increasing symptomatic obstruction – it is unreasonable to dissuade them from this on the basis of the natural instance of age-related obstruction, supposing this to be 'normal.'

'Bladder Neck Obstruction'

The term 'bladder neck obstruction' is open to misinterpretation;
1) It can be used in a specific sense to indicate that the bladder neck mechanism itself is obstructive.
2) It can be used generally to indicate that the site of obstruction is located in the 'neck of the bladder' (i.e. the internal meatus): this, of course, includes all forms of obstruction at this level such as prostatic enlargement and carcinoma.
3) It is still sometimes used clinically to denote a bladder outlet obstruction in general, without any distinction between proximal and distal location but this is archaic.

Bladder Outflow 'Obstruction' and "Relative Obstruction"

Efficient voiding is fundamentally dependent on the balance between the detrusor and the abdominal components of the voiding pressures on the one hand (which are easy to quantify and evaluate), and the outlet resistance on the other (the functional components of which are difficult to measure individually).

Urodynamically, the term 'bladder outflow obstruction' should not be conceptually restricted to patients with a positive increase in outflow resistance, partly because, even when this is identifiable, there may be an additional bladder-deficiency component and partly because voiding inefficiency commonly proves to be a 'relative' imbalance in which the element of outlet resistance is not abnormally increased, as, for instance, after a bowel cystoplasty in which the sphincter mechanisms were, and remain, quite normal but require an adjustment to resolve the imbalance that results from the substitution of a normal detrusor with the functionally inappropriate characteristics of bowel peristalsis (Turner-Warwick and Handley Ashken 1967).

Voiding Inefficiency. Thus, there are two important factors in the evaluation of voiding inefficiency.
1) The identification of voiding inefficiency and its quantification.
2) The actual site of the outlet occlusion and its cause, which is fundamental to appropriate treatment.

A Urodynamic View of Inappropriate Diagnostic Methods and Misconceptions of Outflow Obstruction

Many outdated misconceptions of function and dysfunction still persist in both urological and gynaecological practice more than 10 years after the general introduction of objective urodynamic methods of evaluation (Bates et al. 1969; Turner-Warwick et al. 1973). This is a sad reflection upon the time that it takes to achieve significant changes in clinical practice (Turner-Warwick and Whiteside 1982).

Symptoms. Symptoms are often grossly misleading, whether they suggest normality or abnormality: patients often feel the bladder is full when it is empty and vice versa: appropriate investigation is necessary to determine whether 'urgency' is the result of a motor disorder, a sensory disorder or a rigid small-capacity bladder.

A man's claim that this stream is 'normal' often proves grossly inaccurate and diagnostically misleading, especially in life-long dyssynergic obstruction when he may regard his flow rate of less than 5 ml/s as 'normal', because he has never experienced a better one.

Clinical Examination and the Irrelevance of Prostatic Size. Clinical examination is generally unhelpful in the diagnosis of bladder outlet obstruction unless the bladder happens to be grossly distended.

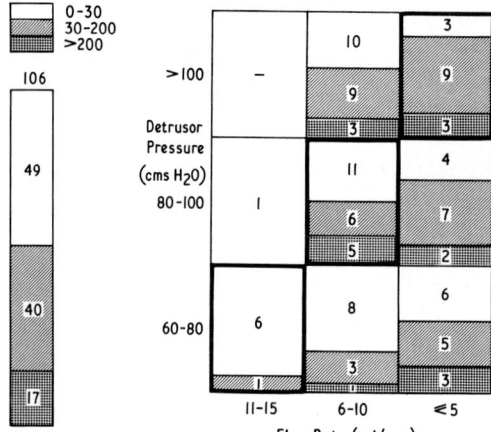

Fig. 2. The poor relationship between residual urine and the severity of bladder outlet obstruction (Turner-Warwick et al. 1973)

The size of the prostate is quite irrelevant to the diagnosis of obstruction: enlarged prostates do not create a proportionate obstruction, sometimes none at all – while many patients without any enlargement have severe obstruction. While this statement of fact is generally acknowledged patients presenting with so-called 'prostatism' whose prostates are found to be much enlarged, are still often erroneously advised to have them resected unless they are appropriately investigated, others with obstruction are often dismissed because their prostates are not 'enlarged'.

Post-Voiding Residual Urine. The demonstration of a residual urine on the post-voiding film of a standard urographic examination is not always representative because some patients cannot void normally, on request when their bladder is only partially distended 30 minutes after the preliminary voiding. This is one of several reasons for advocating the replacement of the standard intravenous urogram by the urodynamogram for the routine investiation of many clinical problems (Fig. 2) (Turner-Warwick et al. 1979).

A true-post-voiding residual indicates inefficient voiding and the need for further urodynamic evaluation to determine whether this is the result in the increase of bladder outlet resistance or an inefficient detrusor contraction or a combination of both. However, the absence of a post-voiding residual urine by no means excludes even the severest degree of bladder outlet obstruction in the male (Turner-Warwick et al. 1973) (Fig. 2): unfortunately this is often erroneously recorded on a urogram report as 'the bladder empties normally' instead of 'the bladder empties completely'.

Calibration. A rigid stricture of the urethra does not cause a significant diminution of the voiding stream until it calibrates to less than about 10 F (Smith 1966). The so-called 'meatal stenosis' of a female urethra calibrating to 16–18 F does not necessarily indicate an obstructive situation and, if outflow obstruction co-exists, it must be the result of a sphincter-dynamic or distortional failure of the urethra to achieve this potential calibre during voiding (Turner-Warwick 1979).

Endoscopy. The cystourethroscope is not a urodynamic instrument; a diagnosis of bladder outflow obstruction can neither be proven nor excluded with it unless it happens to reveal an impassable stricture; deductive conclusions made with it can be grossly inaccurate.

'Trabeculation'. The endoscopic appearance of trabeculation in the male is usually associated with a thick-walled bladder but neither is diagnostic of obstruction; their commonest correlation is with unstable detrusor dysfunction which may or may not be associated with obstruction (Turner-Warwick et al. 1973). Trabeculation is generally conceived as the result of muscular over-work and, insofar as this correlation is valid, it is perhaps to be expected that the frequent exercise of unstable contractions against a volitionally closed sphincter mechanism is a more potent cause of it than relatively infrequent voiding contractions against an increased outlet resistance. However, the rapid development of trabeculation in certain neuropathic conditions in the absence of large co-ordinated contraction pressure rises suggests that it may be the result of uncoordinated muscular activity.

Although hypertrophic trabeculation is generally associated with a great increase in the thickness of the bladder wall, Gosling and Dixon (1984) have shown that the bulk of this is due to the deposition of interstitial collagen and not to a significant increase in the size or the number of the muscle fibres: However, in general such bladders usually create abnormally high detrusor contraction pressures – or at least they did during the development stage.

Contrary to traditional thinking the appearance of trabeculation in the female generally suggests the bladder is *not* obstructed. The female bladder often proves to be unusually thin-walled and hypotrophic trabeculation due to aggregation of sparse muscle bands, is commonly associated with infrequent voiding and stable detrusor behaviour; a thick-walled female bladder is almost always associated with unobstructed instability because the high-resistance outlet obstruction sufficient to cause 'hypertrophic trabeculation', or indeed unstable detrusor behaviour, is extremely rare in females (Turner-Warwick et al. 1973; Farrar and Turner-Warwick 1979).

Hypertrophy of the Bladder Neck. The endoscopic appearance of 'hypertrophy' of the bladder neck is certainly not acceptable urodynamic evidence that it is obstructive although it is still commonly erroneously conceived and treated as such. Secondary 'hypertrophy' of a normally functioning bladder neck mechanism (resulting from unstable detrusor dysfunction or from a distal urethral stricture in the male) does not cause it to become obstructive and furthermore, many dyssynergic bladder neck mechanisms that are causing severe obstruction do not appear endoscopically abnormal in any way (Turner-Warwick 1970, 1979; Turner-Warwick et al. 1973).

Appropriate Methods of Urodynamic Evaluation

Uroflowmetry. A uroflowmetric record of a full-bladder voiding is the essential basic clinical screening test for outlet obstruction. It must be used routinely for the evaluation of male patients to avoid the *under-diagnosis* of clinically significant bladder neck obstruction and the *over-diagnosis* of prostatic obstruction. Indeed, in the author's opinion, except in retention, it should be a mandatory investigation in every case before advising an obstruction-relieving operation, furthermore, there is little doubt that surgeons who do not use it as a routine post-operative investigation considerably over estimate the success of their obstruction-relieving operations: endoscopic examination is an entirely unacceptable substitute for it.

The voiding flow pattern of some patients is greatly affected by their immediate environment and this may not be associated with a significant dysfunction; this emphasises the importance of ensuring a uroflow record of a full bladder voiding in privacy that the patient regards as reasonably representative of his usual performance.

Many patients with dyssynergic bladder neck obstruction complain of difficulty in voiding in the company of others or under strange circumstances. This emphasises the short-comings of trying to identify outlet obstruction by the traditional procedure of 'watching them void' which is often most difficult for the patient for whom it matters most – indeed, even when a uroflowmeter is easily available at all times, some patients find it quite difficult to achieve a flow record that they regard as reasonably representative of their normal.

Pressure Flow Studies. Many patients have equivocal flow patterns between 10 and 20 ml/s which require pressure studies to determine whether they are acceptably normal low-pressure/low-flow or obstructed high-pressure/low-flow systems (Turner-Warwick et al. 1973; Abrams and Torrens 1979; Turner-Warwick 1979).

The Intravenous Urodynamogram. Intravenous urography is, in fact, a dynamic procedure in which the natural passage of a bolus of contrast can be recorded as it concentrates in the kidney and passes along the urinary tract to the point of discharge from the urethra; the natural progress of this usually takes between 1–4 hours according to the bladder behaviour.

The standard intravenous urograph spot-film procedure fails to record all the valuable evidence that it can provide relating to the lower urinary tract function and dysfunction; this is a legacy of the long-standing urological misconception that this can be evaluated from the apparent residual urine (which may not be representative) and from endoscopy.

Thus for must routine investigations, the standard urographic series is better replaced by the more rational, clinically valuable and economical Intravenous Urodynamogram (I.V.U.D.) (Fig. 3) the details of which are described elsewhere (Turner-Warwick et al. 1973) but in principle:
1) After the preliminary and upper tract series (often modified to 5 and 15 min films), the lower urinary tract films are postponed until the patient feels the need to urinate as a matter of some urgency – whatever the time interval after the contrast injection.
2) A spot film is taken to outline the distended bladder.
3) A uroflow record of the natural full-bladder voiding is obtained in the privacy of an apparently conventional toilet adjacent to the X-ray facilities – the flow pattern/voided volume record is an essential component of an IVUD report.
4) A post voiding film shows the natural residual urine.

A Urodynamic Review of Bladder Outlet "Obstruction"

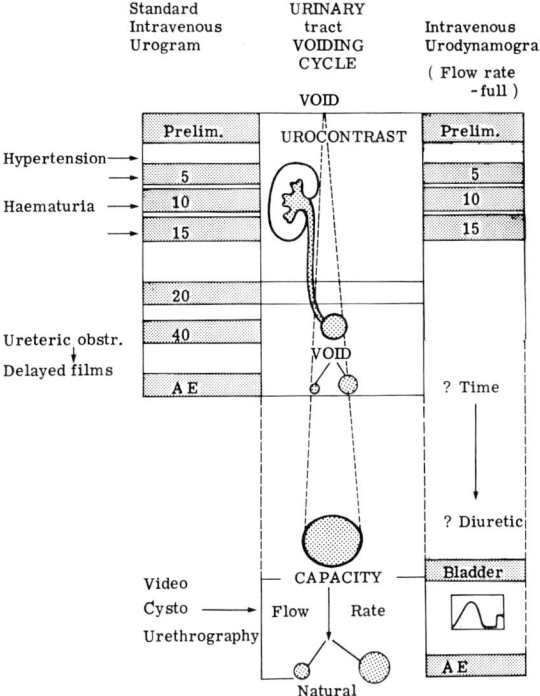

Fig. 3. The intravenous urodynamogram (Turner-Warwick et al. 1979)

The Intravenous and Ultrasound Cystodynamogram. It is sometimes appropriate to modify the principle of a urodynamogram to a simple lower tract series – for instance to evaluate the voiding efficiency after an operative procedure (Turner-Warwick and Pitfield-Marshall 1984); a simple ultrasound cystodynamogram is often sufficient – its advantages are self-evident, requiring no preparation or contrast injection, the patient merely presents with a full bladder and an ultra scan is obtained before and after uroflowmetry.

Voiding Cystourethrography. Simple image-intensified urographic evaluation of the bladder outlet and sphincter function during cystographic voiding is a most important and much under-used *urodynamic* procedure, the equipment for which is standard in the radiological service that is available to every urologist. No combination of electronic-pressure-flow measurements can substitute adequately for it, and without it, many urodynamic investigations are 'blind' (Video = I see, non-video = I do not see – Turner-Warwick 1979). The fluoroscopic image of a urodynamic voiding cystourethrogram should always be *video-recorded* because much urodynamic information is lost in the still-film records; furthermore, synchronous *audio-record* much improves the recall information available during playback, especially during the evaluation of the sphincter function by the voiding 'stop-test.'
1) In both males and females the voiding cystourethrogram provides the most accurate method of identifying the actual site of the bladder outlet obstruction that has been urodynamically proven by flow or pressure-flow measurements.

2) Video studies of the sphincter mechanisms during voluntary interruption of the voiding stream – the 'stop-test' (Turner-Warwick 1979) provides detailed information about the function and dysfunction of individual sphincter mechanisms, many of which are exceedingly difficult to obtain in any other way (Turner-Warwick and Whiteside 1982).
3) *Synchronous* video-pressure studies are particularly important for evaluation of bladder neck and urethral sphincter function and dysfunction in certain disorders but they require special equipment that is only appropriate in major referral centres: however, the absence of synchronous facilities is no excuse for failure to use simple video voiding cystourography in appropriate cases to obtain valuable urodynamic evidence – this is particularly important in: a) The accurate identification of the actual level of a urodynamically proven outlet obstruction when there is any possible doubt about this; b) in neuropathic bladder dysfunction; c) urinary incontinence in females.

When an obstruction is video-located distally, simple calibration will distinguish between a sphincter-dyssynergia and a sphincter-stricture. However, to identify the true cause of a residual urine in a patient whose bladder neck is seen initially to open widely, it is important to observe the conclusion of the voiding phase, otherwise a bladder neck obstruction due to premature closure of its mechanism, due to an unsustained voiding detrusor contraction, may be misdiagnosed. Furthermore, it is important to appreciate that apparently inappropriate electromyographic activity in the region of the distal mechanism, does not always indicate that it is causing a significant functional obstruction, even when it is associated with a mild neuropathy.

Voided-Volume Records. The diagnostic and therapeutic value of a simple 24–48 hour voided-volume chart is often overlooked – it is, in fact, a natural volumetric, cystometric record (Turner-Warwick 1979). It is of special value in the clinical management of a patient with unstable detrusor behaviour both before and after the relief of the obstruction. Not only does it identify unstable detrusor behaviour with remarkable accuracy as a result of characteristically wide variations in the voided volume resulting from involuntary contractions at widely varying degrees of distension, but the unequivocal evidence that this provides will convince all but the most obtuse patient that their bladder sensation of distension is quite untruthful; this is the fundamental basis of overcoming unstable detrusor symptoms by bladder training.

The Endoscopic Identification of the Cause of a Video-Located Outlet Obstruction. Although endoscopy can neither prove nor exclude a bladder outlet obstruction it is essential to identify the actual cause of a proven obstruction that is proven to be located at the internal meatus – i.e. whether it is due to a dyssynergic bladder neck, simple prostatic enlargement or a 'double' obstruction created by incidental combination of these two common conditions (Fig. 8).

The Use and Limitations of Some Special Urodynamic Tests and the Identification of Outflow Obstruction in the Male. The clinical value of simple urethral profilometry in the evaluation of outlet obstruction in the male is strictly limited and is not ad-

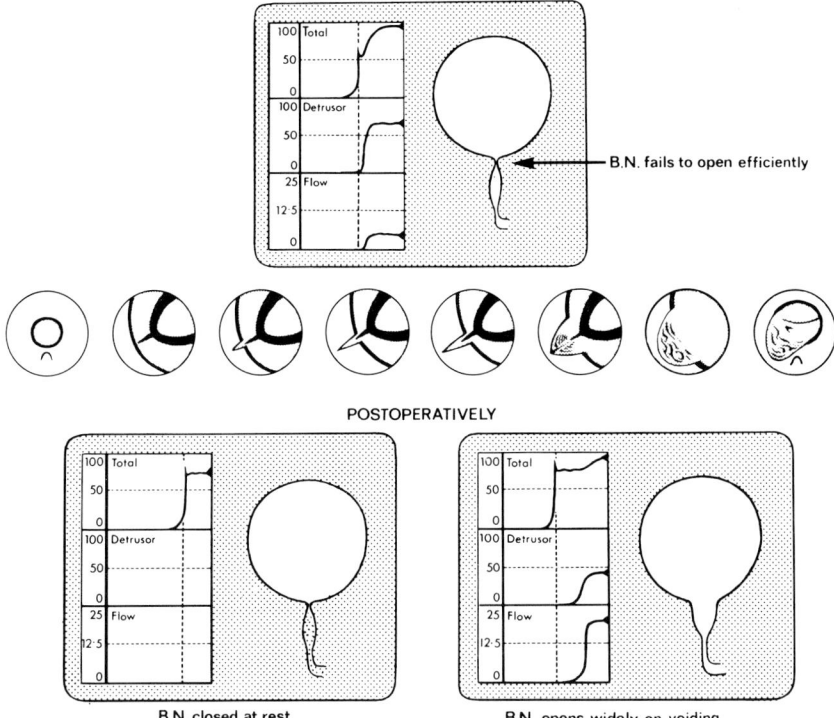

Fig. 4. The video-pressure-flow appearances of dyssynergic bladder neck obstruction before and after its relief by a single full-thickness endoscopic incision from bladder base to verumontanum (Turner-Warwick et al. 1973)

vocated for routine use. A particular short-coming of urethral pressure profile studies is that it identifies bladder neck function and dysfunction very poorly. Without synchronous video studies the initial pressure rise shown on a profile study cannot be assumed to be located at the bladder neck and when it is, simple profile studies are generally insufficient to determine whether its mechanism is competent or incompetent (although this is usually entirely obvious on a simple videocystogram). Furthermore, if it is occlusive, pressure profile studies cannot readily determine whether it is normal or dyssynergically obstructive because the resting closure pressures are not dissimilar.

Synchronous electromyographic records of the activity of the perianal musculature is sometimes used in conjunction with pressure-flow studies. This may be important in the evaluation of patients who have associated neuropathy but it is of limited value and open to serious misinterpretation when it is used as an office substitute for radiographic evaluation of sphincter behaviour in patients without neuropathy. Synchronous detrusor and pelvic floor muscle activity during the filling phase is sometimes misinterpreted as 'detrusor-sphincter dyssynergia' when it is in reality an entirely normal and appropriate leak-preventing sphincter response to an involuntarily unstable detrusor contraction when the patient is trying to hold on.

Normal electromyographic activity of the pelvic floor musculature virtually ceases during a volitional voiding detrusor contraction; however, under the strange circumstances of urodynamic evaluation it is not unusual for a patient to develop an involuntary contraction of the sphincter mechanism which prevents voiding on request. While it is not considered surprising that some patients fail to void when standing in front of a video-screen and consequently, this is not regarded as 'abnormal'; when similar voiding difficulties occur during electromyographic studies, they are sometimes misinterpreted as detrusor/sphincter dyssynergia. Thus, although accurate electromyography may be important in neuro/urological research, in the absence of neuropathy, it contributes little and is not advocated as a routine study reserving it for the evaluation of patients when:
1) Bladder outlet obstruction has already been proven by pressure-flow studies.
2) The functional obstruction has proven to be located at the distal sphincter mechanism by voiding cystourethrography.
3) It is relevant to determine whether the functional distal obstruction is the result of striated muscle over-activity.

Normal Detrusor Function and Dysfunction. Thus if a detrusor is functionally normal
1) It only contracts during volitional voiding.
2) Its voiding contraction is volitionally initiated.
3) Its voiding contraction is sustained till evacuation is complete.

Any of these elements may be abnormal, singly, or in any combination and they are often highly relevant both to a voiding inefficiency and to the identification of the cause of frequency and urgency when it is important to be certain whether a detrusor is stable or unstable. Therefore, subtracted detrusor studies during both the filling and the emptying phase are often important to the urodynamic evaluation of complicated voiding disorders and a report of these should describe the individual elements of detrusor behaviour or misbehaviour accurately, i.e. an unstable detrusor with a volitional but unsustained voiding bladder contraction.

The procedure of provocative cystometry, pioneered by Hodgkinson for clinical purposes is designed to reproduce within a short period of testing an approximation of the stresses and strains to which the bladder is normally subjected during daily life. The technique of continuous monitoring of subtracted intravesical detrusor pressures are used to study bladder behaviour under circumstances which are closer to those of daily life (James 1979), however such testing is naturally time consuming and rarely essential for evaluation of voiding disorders in the male.

Normal Bladder Neck Function

The bladder neck sphincter mechanism is formed by a concentration of detrusor smooth muscle around the internal meatus extending down to the level of the verumontanum. It is easy to show, by synchronous video-pressure studies, that it creates an occlusive cough-competent sphincter mechanism while the detrusor is at rest – however, its competence is dependent upon stable detrusor behaviour because it funnels open in association with a detrusor contraction.

The actual mechanism of normal bladder neck opening is also incompletely understood but certainly, it is not explained by Hutch's over-simplistic base-plate concept. Tanagho (1979) has shown that bladder-neck-opening slightly preceeds detrusor contraction and that it is reflex mediated.

Dyssynergic Bladder Neck Dysfunction

Varying degrees of failure of the bladder neck to open normally in association with a voiding detrusor contraction are not uncommon in the male although this is exceedingly rare in the female (Turner-Warwick 1972, 1979; Turner-Warwick et al. 1973); they range from inefficient opening associated with a marginally poor flow rate to grossly self-obstructive dyssynergic contraction. The fact that a clinically significant dyssynergic bladder neck obstruction in the male is caused by progressive positive contraction of the bladder neck rather than by a simple failure of its opening is shown by the simple observation of Bates and Arnold (1973) that although the resting closing pressure of a dyssynergic mechanism on a simple profile study is not abnormally elevated (about 10 cm H_2O) it can be seen on synchronous video-pressure studies to maintain an effective closure that progressively exceeds the intravesical pressures created by a voiding detrusor contraction and we have examples of this greater than 100 cm H_2O.

The mechanism of dyssynergic contraction of the bladder neck muscle is presently as poorly understood as the mechanism of its normal synergic opening, however, a number of relevant facts emerge:

1) Although the smooth muscle fibres of the concentric bladder neck sphincter mechanism of the female and the proximal part of the male bladder neck are morphological extensions of the cholinergically innervated detrusor fibres, Gosling (1979) has shown that the innervation of the male bladder neck mechanism, like seminal vesicles, is adrenergic, whereas that of the female, like the detrusor of both the male and the female, is cholinergic.

The smooth muscle fibres of the distal part of the male bladder neck are morphologically distinct from the detrusor fibres being smaller, aggregated into smaller muscle bundles and separated by a greater proportion of collagen than detrusor bundles. They are derived from the 'prostatic capsule' and form a proximal sex orientated procreative mechanism which prevents reflux seminal emission by orgasmic contraction synchronous with that of the seminal vesicles (Booth et al. 1983). It is probably that this differential innervation and function explains why dyssynergic bladder neck dysfunction is common in the male but virtually never occurs in the female; certainly it explains why sympathetic blockading phenoxybenzamine relaxes dyssynergic bladder neck obstruction in the male.

2) Although opening of the bladder neck mechanism is almost always *associated* with a voiding detrusor contraction and vice versa, Tanagho (1979) has shown that it is not only reflex-mediated, but that it marginally preceeds the detrusor pressure rise – thus it is most unlikely that either a normal synergic opening or an abnormal

dyssynergic closure are the simple result of a 'normal' or 'abnormal' morphological arrangement of the component fibre-bundles.

3) Although the bladder neck mechanism is reflex-mediated, dyssynergic dysfunction of this should not be regarded as 'neuropathic'; indeed it is interesting that dyssynergic contraction of the neck mechanism is a dysfunction which very rarely develops as a result of overt neuropathy (Turner-Warwick 1979).

4) Although opening and closing of the bladder neck is associated with detrusor contraction, they are not directly related to the actual contraction pressure; synchronous video-pressure voiding studies often show that the detrusor pressure at the time of its opening is often quite different from that at the time of its closing (Turner-Warwick and Whiteside 1982).

5) The weight of evidence suggests that the characteristic behaviour of a particular bladder neck mechanism rarely changes. Although the self-obstruction caused by a dyssynergic mechanism may increase somewhat with age, its characteristic dysfunction can usually be traced back to childhood. The unequivocal conversion of an overtly synergic mechanism to dyssynergia is exceedingly rare except, possibly, in diabetes (Turner-Warwick and Whiteside 1982), and its behaviour is not significantly affected by a generalised hypertrophy in response to a distal obstruction.

The Symptoms and Presentation of Dyssynergic Bladder Neck Obstruction. There are wide variations in the degree of obstruction that dyssynergic bladder neck behavior causes – the most severe require treatment in childhood and moderate degrees are much the most common cause of obstruction up to the age of 50: after this the apparent incidence appears to fall because outflow obstruction is then commonly ascribed solely to coincidental prostatic enlargement, however minimal, and the significance of a tight circular bladder neck, proximal to it, suggestive that it is dyssynergic, is still not generally recognised (Turner-Warwick 1973, 1979, 1982).

Because dyssynergic bladder neck obstruction is usually a life-long condition, few patients complain of the classic symptoms of outlet restriction, slow-start, poor-flow and terminal dribble; even a detailed enquiry can be a misleading substitute for uroflowmetry because many patients regard their pathetically poor flow as 'normal for them' and commonly report as 'good'. The most common feature is an admission that their voiding flow has always been 'non-competitive' – they 'could never play that game at school' but this information has to be sought, it is seldom uttered. Some patients complain of being unable to void in the company of others at a public urinal. This particular symptom sometimes causes considerable distress: it is not unusual for patients to have consulted a psychiatrist (without avail) and some have embarrassing memories, such as missing the last act of an opera because they could not urinate in the crowded toilet during the interval. Such symptoms should never be regarded as functional until an organic cause has been excluded urodynamically. A few patients primarily complain of hesitancy bordering upon retention when the bladder is overdistended. The development of unexpected retention of urine after an incidental operative procedure such as a hernia repair in a younger age group is commonly the result of unsuspected long-standing dyssynergic bladder neck obstruction; however, unlike retention due to large prostates, natural voiding is usually restored by a short period of catheter drainage.

Secondary Symptoms. The majority of patients with dyssynergic bladder neck obstruction develop unstable detrusor behavior sooner or later and most of these then have the characteristic symptoms of frequency, urgency and nocturia with the usual incidence of reversion after effective relief of the obstruction. Urinary infection in the male always suggests outflow obstruction and a dyssynergic bladder neck is much the commonest cause of this before the age of 50 (Turner-Warwick 1979; Booth et al. 1981).

'Prostatitis' and the Dyssynergic Bladder Neck. Overlap of somewhat non-specific symptoms sometimes makes it difficult to differentiate clinically between dyssynergic bladder neck obstruction and 'hypersensitive prostatitis', furthermore when the two conditions coexist, it is virtually impossible to apportion them.

Thus, the flow rate of every patient with suspected prostatitis should be recorded to avoid failure to identify a treatable element of obstruction which, in an average series, may be found in about 1 in 10 cases (Turner-Warwick 1979); however, in the case of infected prostatitis, it is important that the flow rate should be checked between exacerbations of inflammation which may themselves create a mild obstruction.

When an element of dyssynergic bladder neck obstruction is identified in a patient with equivocal 'prostatitis' symptoms, treatment should be discussed on the basis that the relief of the obstruction may improve matters to some extent, and possibly to a considerable extent, but, by the nature of things, it may not. If the result is satisfactory then the patient is only marginally more delighted that he is relieved of the burden than his urologist.

Synergic 'Bladder Neck Obstruction' – Detrusor Dysfunction

As already discussed, bladder neck opening is not a *direct* effect of detrusor contraction, it is closely associated with it; thus a detrusor contraction failure is generally associated with failure of opening of a normal occlusive *synergic* mechanism, urodynamically this can be regarded as a voiding imbalance in which the outlet is occluded at the bladder neck.

A variety of detrusor dysfunctions may result in failure or inadequacy of bladder-neck-opening:

1) The detrusor may be acontractile.

2) The patient may be unable to volitionally initiate a contraction of an otherwise functional detrusor and this disability may be occasional or complete.

3) An unsustained voiding detrusor contraction commonly results in premature closure of a synergic bladder neck which initially opened widely, thus results in a residual urine due to terminal bladder neck occlusion – this is a common neuropathic dysfunction but it is not unusual in the absence of neuropathy.

4) An indifferent low-pressure detrusor contraction may be associated with an indifferent opening of the bladder neck mechanism. Synchronous video-pressure studies may be required to distinguish this from dyssynergic bladder neck ob-

struction in the male because both conditions are characterised by a prolonged poor flow rate and a poorly opening bladder neck mechanism on cystography with a considerable symptom overlap. However, a true dyssynergic bladder neck obstruction usually results in the development of an elevated detrusor pressure before the third decade.

5) The results of treating 'relative outlet obstruction' associated with low-pressure detrusor dysfunction by endoscopic bladder neck incision are relatively poor, particularly when this is the result of neuropathy such as Progressive Autonomic Failure (PAF) of which the Shy-Drager Syndrome is but one variety (Bannister 1983) [this condition may present as a urodynamic dysfunction and its accurate diagnosis in the early stages depends upon a high index of suspicion and appropriate investigation (Kirby et al. 1983)].

6) Dyssynergic bladder neck obstruction almost never occurs in females: not only is outlet obstruction located at the bladder neck itself relatively rare but, when present, it is almost invariably associated with a primary detrusor contraction failure that is rarely the result of overt neuropathy (Brown and Turner-Warwick 1979).

The Diagnosis of Dyssynergic Bladder Neck Obstruction. Whether they recognise it or not the great majority of patients with dyssynergic bladder neck obstruction have a grossly impaired voiding flow pattern. The fact that many have difficulty in voiding in the company of others or under strange circumstances, emphasises the shortcomings of trying to identify it by the classic exercise of watching them void; this often most difficult to achieve for those for whom it matters most. The importance of routine uroflowmetry cannot be over-emphasised because, without it, the condition is inevitably under-diagnosed.

Many patients are referred for a second opinion on troublesome symptoms that prove to be the result of a severe and easily relieved dyssynergic bladder neck obstruction when obstruction supposedly had been excluded by previous routine urological findings of a prostate that is not enlarged, the absence of a residual urine and normal appearances on endoscopy: more than 10 years after the unequivocal demonstration of the importance of objective urodynamic evaluation in the accurate diagnosis and treatment of disorders of lower urinary tract function this simply should not happen – it is virtually impossible to justify the treatment of voiding disorders in the male without routine pre- and post-operative uroflow records.

Many patients present with a reasonable flow pattern and a peak flow which appears within the equivocal range of 10–20 ml/sec; as previously emphasised, pressure studies are required to identify those that are the result of elevated pressure obstruction.

Occasional patients present with a peak flow of over 20 ml which is nevertheless the obstructed result of a grossly elevated detrusor contraction pressure of over 100 cm H_2O; the identification of these is easily missed and is dependent upon a particularly high index of suspicion.

It is fundamentally important to appreciate that there are *no* endoscopic appearances by which a dyssynergic bladder neck can be unequivocally identified or excluded. Hypertrophy of a dyssynergic bladder neck mechanism itself is a late event and many bladder necks that are causing severe outlet obstruction do not appear abnormal in any way – so much so, that having observed them endoscopically one feels the need to double-check the patients identity with that of the pressure flow record before proceeding to endoscopic surgery.

Global hypertrophy is more often the result of unobstructed unstable detrusor dysfunction and such a secondary hypertrophy of a synergic bladder neck does not compromise its opening mechanism or result in obstruction thus the endoscopic appearances of hypertrophy of the bladder neck and bladder wall trabeculation are certainly not diagnostic of 'bladder neck obstruction' (Fig. 8) (Turner-Warwick et al. 1973).

Unfortunately the erroneous ablation of a normally functioning bladder neck sphincter, undertaken as a result of its hypertrophic appearance, is still all too common. A synergic bladder neck sphincter is opened and rendered incompetent by a detrusor contraction, so, fortunately, its erroneous ablation does not compromise the continence of a patient with unstable detrusor behaviour because this is essentially dependent upon the distal sphincter mechanism; however, the erroneous ablation of a competent bladder neck that is hypertrophied as a result of a posterior bulbar stricture may be disastrous if a definitive repair is consequently contra-indicated because it is bordering upon the only residual sphincter mechanism (Turner-Warwick 1973).

Thus, in summary the diagnosis of dyssynergic bladder neck obstruction depends upon:

1) Objective evidence of outlet obstruction by uroflowmetry, pressure uroflowmetry, or a significant residual urine.

2) Evidence that the thus-proven outlet obstruction is located at the internal meatus.

Although incontravertible evidence of this is provided by voiding cystourethrography, in practice, in the adult, the diagnosis of an obstructive bladder neck mechanism is usually confirmed deductively, having excluded a distal stricture and prostatic enlargement endoscopically; this is because obstructive distal sphincter dyssynergia is exceedingly rare in the adult in the absence of an overt neuropathy (Turner-Warwick 1979).

The Indications for the Treatment of Dyssynergic Bladder Neck Obstruction. A proven dyssynergic bladder neck obstruction does not necessarily require treatment. This depends upon the extent of the trouble that it is causing, the degree of obstruction, the exclusion of pre-existing damage to the distal sphincter mechanism upon which continence will depend, and the importance of ejaculation. Every case requires individual consideration. The decision is often simplified by a strong indication such as recurrent infection or episodes of retention: it is also facilitated if the prospect of a possible failure of ejaculation is unimportant to the patient.

Many patients with moderate obstruction are reassured by the identification of the cause of their problem and prefer live with their symptoms and to postpone definitive treatment until their family is established. Medication with alpha-blocking agents is sometimes used as a confirmatory diagnostic test and for short-term treatment but side effects are common, particularly in the adult, and this drug is occupationally contraindicated when postural hypotension might be critical such as scaffolding workers or augmented in aircrew.

The Effective Relaxation of the Dyssynergic Bladder Neck by Endoscopic Incision.
Dyssynergic bladder neck obstruction is definitively and reliably treated by transecting the full thickness of its ring with an endoscopic knife electrode; a single full-thickness incision in one position is quite sufficient unless there is a coincidental element of prostatic enlargement (Fig. 4) (Turner-Warwick 1973, 1979; Turner-Warwick et al. 1973). The incision should extend from the bladder base down to the level of the verumontanum; as the initial cut is deepened progressively, its V-shape springs open to a U-shape defect, the appearances of which suggest that several loop-fulls of tissue have been removed; the incision is further deepened until minute interstitial fat globules are revealed between the latticework of the residual prostatic capsule fibres by pin-points of reflected light. Haemostasis is achieved by electro-coagulation using the flat of the knife-electrode.

The functional results of single endoscopic relaxation of a dyssynergic bladder neck obstruction are both urodynamically reliable and relatively uncomplicated compared with treatment by loop resection.

There has been no case of recurrent dyssynergic obstruction or secondary bladder neck contracture in our series of more than 200 cases. The incidence of a diminished volume of ejaculate has been in the region of 10% and in less than 5% has it been absent altogether. However, if necessary, the ejaculate can be retrieved from the posterior urethra by postcoital self-catheterisation wash-out for artificial insemination.

Videocystourethrography after incisional relaxation usually shows the bladder neck to be closed while the detrusor is at rest during stable bladder filling but it opens widely in association with a voiding detrusor contraction giving the appearance that an extensive loop-resection has been performed (Fig. 4) (Turner-Warwick 1973, 1979).

Partial thickness incisions are somewhat unreliable and generally inadvisable unless a patient requiring urgent treatment particularly wishes to further reduce the small incidence of ejaculation failure, in which case he must accept the possibility of the need to repeat the relaxation procedure.

Because the thickness of a dyssynergic bladder neck is so variable, the proportional depth of a partial incision cannot be judged accurately and thus it is necessary to accept an arbitrary limit such as the point at which the V-shaped cleft first opens into a U-shape: however, from this point the thickness of the residual bladder neck mechanism that remains uncut varies considerably and, of course, the potential of its residual dyssynergic occlusion is quite unpredictable.

Thus it is difficult to justify the treatment of dyssynergic bladder neck obstruction by loop-resection, there are no advantages and potential complications involved in removing lumps of dyssynergic bladder neck muscle, particularly when this does not involve transection of the full-thickness of the bladder neck ring at any point.

1) More blood vessels are exposed which inevitably carries an increased risk of secondary bleeding.

2) The first loop-cut resects 50% of the urothelial lining of the bladder neck and subsequent loop-fulls increase the area of the urothelial defect and the potential for secondary scar formation.

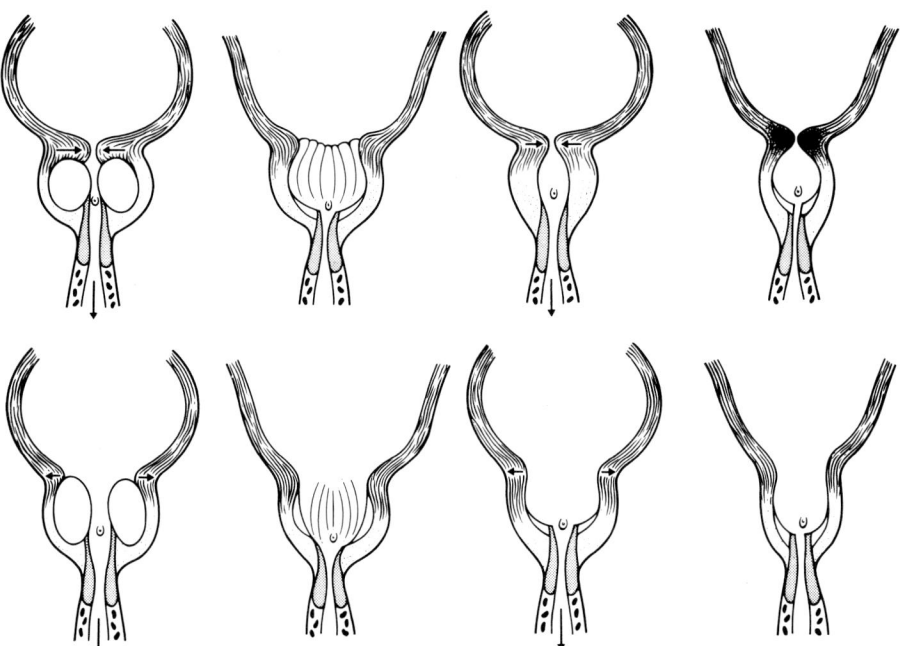

Fig. 5. In the case of proven outlet obstruction, failure to recognise the dyssynergic significance of the appearance of a circular bladder neck above a prostatic enlargement, and consequent failure to resect the full thickness of its ring in at least one position, is a common cause of secondary bladder neck contracture (Turner-Warwick 1979, 1982). The uncut thickness of such a bladder neck continues to contract dyssynergically and tends to heal in a contracted state – the residual thickness of a partially resected normal bladder neck continues to open and heals open. Hence for simple urodynamic reasons, secondary bladder neck contracture almost never results from the resection of a triangulated prostatic internal meatus

3) The functional occlusion of the bladder neck is almost invariably destroyed by an effective loop resection so that the incidence of ejaculation failure is relatively high.

4) The incidence of secondary bladder neck contracture after the loop resection of a dyssynergic mechanism is significant. Unless the full-thickness of the dyssynergic bladder neck ring is completely transected at at least one point, the residual dyssynergic occlusion created by its residual thickness, which is not apparent at the time of resection, continues to create an occlusion post-operatively and, because it never opens widely, it heals in a contracted state with extensive scar formation associated with excessive resected tissue deficiency (Fig. 5).

Thus most functionally orientated urologists who understand the dysfunctional nature of obstruction by the bladder neck mechanism have thankfully abandoned the old method of treating it by loop resection.

The Relationship of 'Prostatic Enlargement' to the Normal Bladder Neck Mechanism

McNeal (1973) has shown that the origin of the so-called 'lateral' and 'middle lobes' do not represent areas of the normal prostate but develop by hypertrophy of small paraurethral glands; they naturally tend to enlarge into the lumen of the upper prostatic urethra. Initially a small enlargement is of no urodynamic significance, later however there are wide variations in size of a 'prostatic enlargement' and the degree of outlet obstruction associated with it; remarkably little consideration seems to have been given to the reason for this but it must in fact relate to the confines of the surrounding bladder neck and prostatic 'capsule' (Turner-Warwick 1969, 1973, 1979).

The bladder neck mechanism is integral with the so-called 'prostatic capsule' which is formed by the expansion of the normal prostatic tissue by the grossly hypertrophic paraurethral glands nodules which are conveniently, but erroneously, referred to by surgeons as 'adenomata'.

The enlarging 'lobes' naturally expand into the prostatic urethra and, presumably because the normal bladder neck mechanism funnels widely open during a voiding detrusor contraction, they are normal free to extend upwards through the internal meatus into the base of the bladder, widely expanding the bladder neck mechanism and the upper prostatic capsule (Turner-Warwick 1983); thus, essentially as a result of normal urodynamic function, the 'lateral' and 'middle' 'lobes' come to form the margins of a new 'triangulated' internal meatus. Occasionally an enormous enlargement of over 100 g of hypertrophic prostatic tissue causes only a minimal outlet obstruction, presumably because it escapes almost completely from the confines of the prostatic tissue to half-fill the bladder.

The Relationship of 'Prostatic Enlargement' to a Dyssynergic Bladder Neck Mechanism: The Trapped Prostate

The functional and mechanical situation is quite different when the hypertrophic elements of the prostate enlarge below a tight bladder neck/capsule, especially when the bladder neck mechanism is dyssynergic, because this not only remains closed between voidings but closes even tighter during voiding contractions. Furthermore, the bulk of the secondary 'hypertrophy' of the bladder and bladder neck associated with outlet obstruction results from a deposition of interstitial collagen (Gosling 1978) and while this does not significantly affect its functional behaviour, it probably increases its resistance to expansion. Under these circumstances the 'lateral lobes' expand into the mid-prostatic urethra but failing to expand the bladder neck and its integral capsular ring, they become 'trapped' in the restricted space below it so that a relatively small enlargement causes a significant obstruction and, furthermore, augments any pre-existing bladder outlet obstruction caused by a dyssynergic bladder neck (Turner-Warwick 1973, 1983; Turner-Warwick et al. 1973) (Fig. 6).

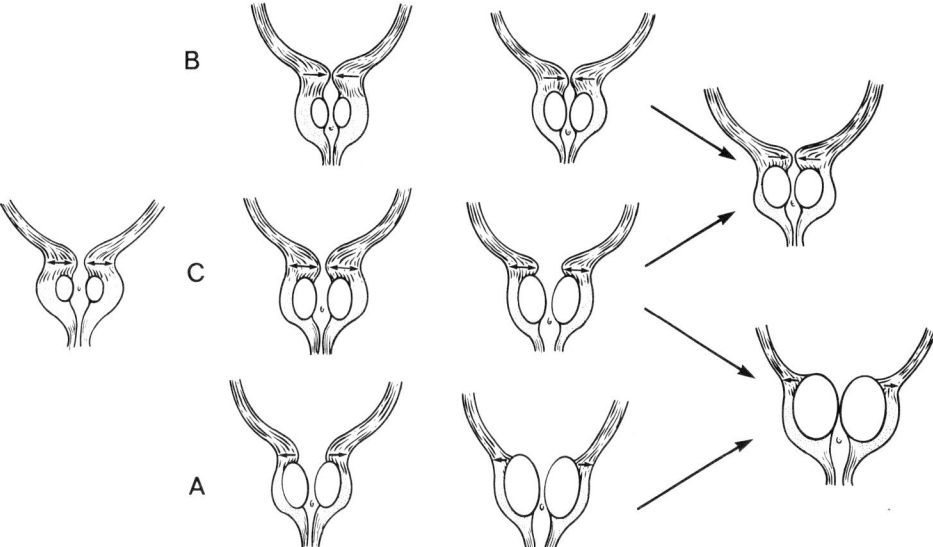

Fig. 6. *A* When the bladder neck opens normally the lateral and middle 'lobes' expand widely as they enlarge upwards into the base of the bladder: the internal meatus is formed by prostatic tissue and appears triangulated. *B* A dyssynergic bladder neck never opens widely and positively closes during detrusor contraction so that a relatively small enlargement of the prostatic 'lobes' 'trapped' beneath a ring-shaped bladder neck causes a disproportionate obstruction – 'Double Obstruction' (Turner-Warwick 1970). *C* Equivocal degrees of bladder neck opening are not uncommon and result in intermediate appearances of the internal meatus, however, this does not invalidate the significance of 'Double Obstruction'

The characteristic endoscopic appearance of this situation is a relatively small enlargement of the 'lateral lobes' meeting in the midline with a ring-shaped bladder neck mechanism above. In such cases no 'middle lobe' is seen; this originates from a group of para-urethral glands in the midline posteriorly just above the verumontanum meatus and when it enlarges in relation to a tight bladder neck mechanism, it tends to burrow outwards to expand behind it under the trigone (Turner-Warwick 1978, 1983) (Fig. 7).

However, while the endoscopic appearances of an intraurethral prostatic enlargement beneath a bladder neck ring are quite *characteristic* of a 'double' obstruction, they are not *diagnostic* of it, unless a significant bladder outlet obstruction has been proven urodynamically (Fig. 8). Identical endoscopic appearances are seen in the early stages of prostatic enlargement in patients who have no outlet obstruction whatsoever because their normally functioning bladder neck, which has not yet been expanded by the enlarging prostate, funnels widely open during a voiding detrusor contraction.

This emphasises once again the fact that the cystourethroscope is not a valid urodynamic instrument and that it is impossible to evaluate, with any degree of accuracy, the functional behaviour of the bladder neck mechanism with it.

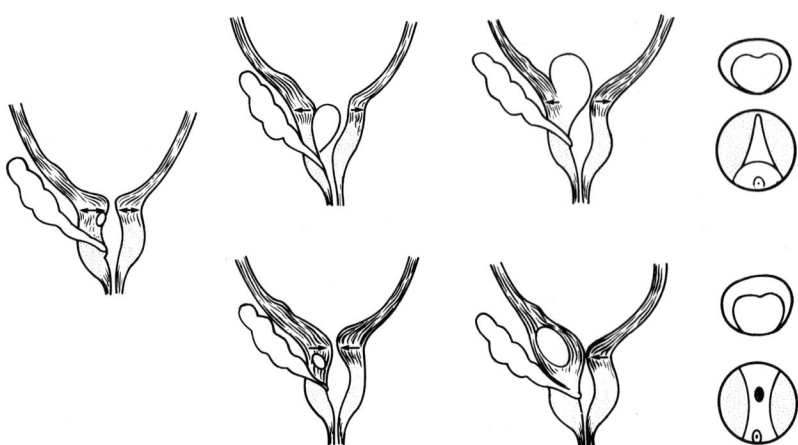

Fig. 7. When a 'middle lobe' enlarges below a synergically opening bladder neck it expands upwards through it into the base of the bladder to create the posterior element of the triangulated internal meatus; when it enlarges below a dyssynergic bladder neck it tends to burrow under it, into a sub-trigonal position (Turner-Warwick 1982)

'Double Obstruction: The Combination of Prostatic and Dyssynergic Bladder Neck Obstruction' – the 'Trapped Prostate'. Thus in general, minor degrees of prostatic enlargement do not seem to create a significant outlet obstruction unless they are 'trapped' below a tight ring-shaped bladder neck and much the commonest cause of this, outside areas of endemic schistosomiasis, is a dyssynergic mechanism.

Prostatic enlargement and dyssynergic bladder neck dysfunction are both common conditions so their coincidence by no means uncommon; it should be suspected whenever a patient with a relatively minor degree of prostatic enlargement develops symptoms of bladder outlet obstruction (Turner-Warwick 1969, 1973; Turner-Warwick et al. 1973).

In such cases the patient commonly gives a history of a recent on-set of symptoms relating to the relatively short period of his prostatic enlargement, because he accepted his previous life-long slow-flow as normal. Thus the existence of 'double obstruction' is often strikingly obvious after its relief because, while the patient with a simple prostatic obstruction is grateful for the 'restoration of his stream to its former state', patients with a 'double obstruction' like those with a simple dyssynergic bladder neck obstruction, often declare with delight, that they have 'never voided so well'.

It follows that in most cases in which an outflow obstruction has been relieved by the resection of less than about 10 G of prostatic tissue, either the enlarged element has been incompletely resected or it was 'trapped' by a tight bladder neck with the high probability of an additional element of dyssynergic obstruction (Turner-Warwick 1979, 1983).

Because there is a wide variation in the degree of dyssynergic obstruction associated with bladder neck dysfunction there are also gradations between the triangulated internal meatus associated with a simple trilobar prostatic enlargement on the one hand and the tight dyssynergic bladder neck ring that is unequivocally

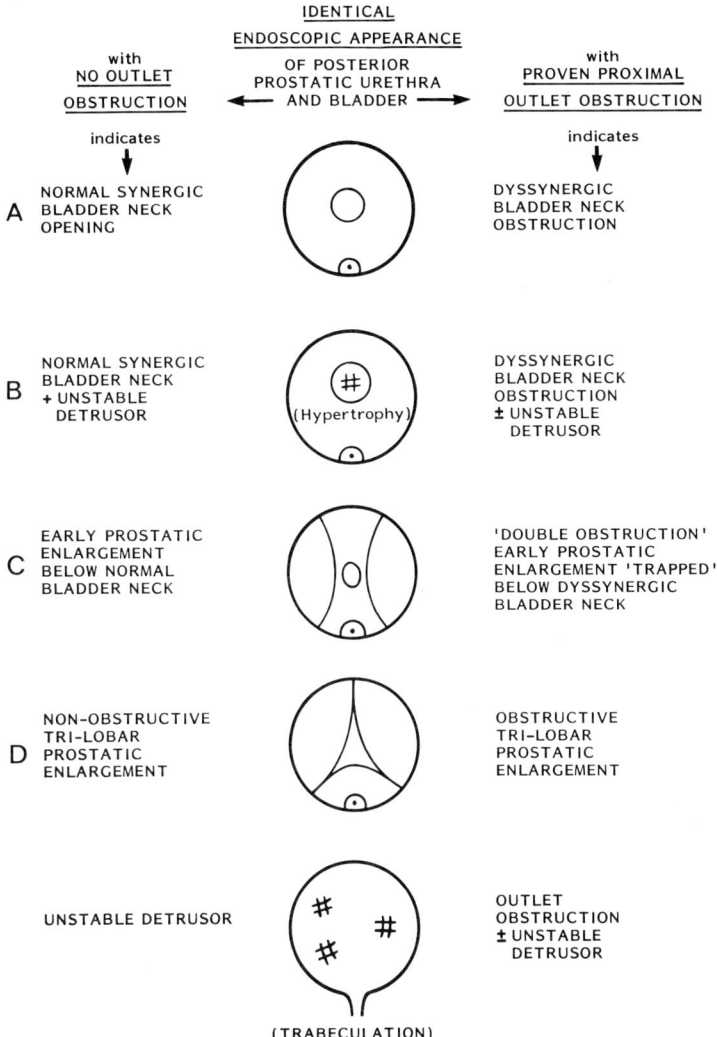

Fig. 8. The fallacies of 'endoscopic guestimation' of obstruction. Each of the four basic endoscopic appearances of the proximal posterior urethra may or may not be associated with obstruction. *A* It is impossible to determine endoscopically whether a ring-shaped bladder neck mechanism is functionally normal, i.e. opens synergically during detrusor contraction, or whether it contracts dyssynergically. *B* Hypertrophy of the bladder neck associated with trabeculation does not necessarily indicate obstruction – it commonly results from non-obstructive unstable detrusor exercise. Global hypertrophy does not affect bladder neck function. *C* The endoscopic appearances of early prostatic enlargement beneath a ring-shaped bladder neck is only diagnostic of 'Double Obstruction' due to a trapped prostate if outlet obstruction has been urodynamically proven – otherwise it is simply the normal appearance of early prostatic enlargement beneath a synergic bladder neck. *D* The degree of outlet obstruction is not proportionate to the size of the prostate. Gross intravesical enlargement may be associated with minimal obstruction, insufficient to create unstable detrusor behaviour. When a patient with an enlarged prostate presents with symptoms of unstable detrusor behaviour, failure to verify a diagnosis of outlet obstruction objectively may result in unavailing prostatic resections, dissatisfied patients and diminished urological reputations (Turner-Warwick 1979)

'trapping' the prostate on the other; within the middle area an enlargement of prostatic element may gradually stretch open and expand a moderately tight bladder neck (Fig. 5). However, these natural intermediates do not invalidate the practical value of the distinction between obstruction due to pure prostatic enlargement with those due to double-obstruction.

The Development of Secondary Bladder Neck Contracture After Loop Resection of a 'Double Obstruction'. The mechanism of the development of secondary bladder neck contracture after loop resection of a combination obstruction is precisely similar to that following loop resection of a simple dyssynergic bladder neck (Turner-Warwick 1983); however, for conceptual reasons it is potentially commoner because the dyssynergic significance of the ring-shaped bladder neck is commonly unrecognised and although its margin is removed as an incidental to a resection that is primarily directed at the prostatic element, there is a considerable risk that a significant circumferential thickness of the bladder neck will remain; unless it is completely transected its continued dyssynergic contraction may result in secondary scarring contracture during the healing process. Secondary bladder neck contracture rarely occurs after the endoscopic resection of a large prostate in which the normal bladder neck mechanism has been widely expanded neither does it occur after even a circumferential partial thickness resection of a normal synergic bladder neck mechanism, the remnants of which continue to open widely during every voiding detrusor contraction throughout the healing period.

Thus, it is fundamentally important to recognise the potential urodynamic significance of the endoscopic appearance of a ring-shaped bladder neck mechanism above an early prostatic enlargement and to treat it appropriately.

The Treatment of 'Double Obstruction' by Combined Endoscopic Incision and Loop Resection. The author's preferred procedure for resolving a double-obstruction is to start with a full-thickness incision of the bladder neck ring in the 5, 7, 11 and 1 o'clock positions (Fig. 9); if, after this, the element of prostatic enlargement appears rather insignificant, it may not be necessary to proceed to its resection because the efficient relaxation of the bladder neck ring may have provided space for its further enlargement. Otherwise the initial full-thickness four-quadrant relaxation of the bladder neck ring seems to facilitate the complete loop-resection of the prostatic element (Turner-Warwick 1983).

Conservative Surgery of 'Double Obstruction'. Naturally 'double obstruction' tends to present at an earlier age than pure prostatic enlargement so it is not unusual that a patient in his early fifties requires treatment when he has recently married or remarried and wishes to have children. While no definitive surgical treatment involving the bladder neck mechanism can guarantee the preservation of ejaculation, the effective loop-resection of both obstructing elements virtually guarantees the failure of ejaculation.

The temporising options that reduce this risk are:

1) The incisional relaxation of the dyssynergic bladder neck ring at 5 o'clock and 7 o'clock, without any resection of prostatic tissue or anterior incision. This is certainly the easiest option.

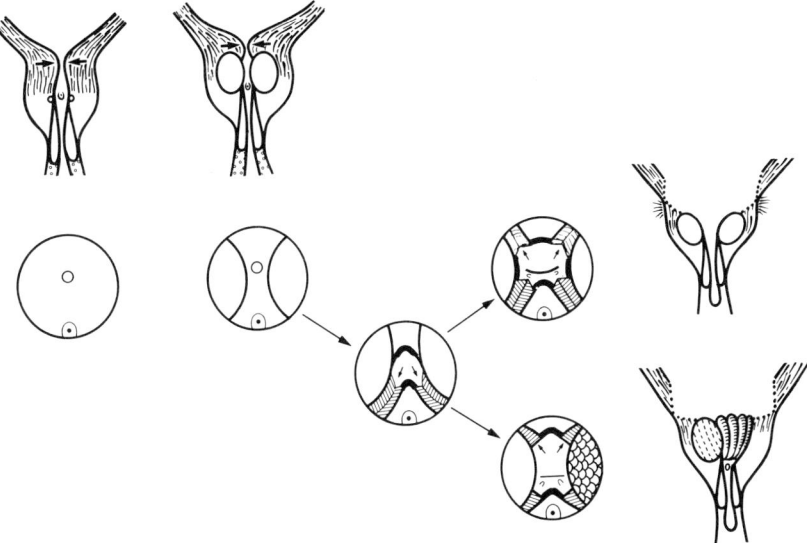

Fig. 9. Proven 'Double Obstruction' can be simply treated by an initial endoscopic transection of the dyssynergic bladder neck element. Because secondary smooth muscle hypertrophy is associated with the extensive deposition of interstitial collagen (Gosling 1980) a four-quadrant incision is advised to overcome secondary rigidity of the bladder neck ring – if procedure to a loop resection of prostatic tissue is also required, it is in fact facilitated by the initial incisions (Turner-Warwick 1979, 1982)

2) Resection of the prostatic element with maximal preservation of the bladder neck and the distal sphincter mechanisms. The accurate transurethral resection of the element of enlargement without compromising the function of the bladder neck mechanism is by no means as simple or as uncomplicated as it is sometimes thought to be. When preservation of either the bladder neck or the distal sphincter is particularly critical, for instance when a prostatectomy is required after the impairment of the function of the distal mechanism due to a pelvic fracture injury or to neuropathy, in the author's opinion this is probably best achieved by a conservative transcapsular intraurethral mid-prostatic dissection-reconstruction (Turner-Warwick 1979, 1983).

Before undertaking a compromise conservative procedure, it is important that patients should understand that there is nothing experimental about a conservative approach, it is simply a question of a trial of a limited procedure to see whether it is sufficient; subsequently one can always proceed to a definitive procedure and, by the nature of both underlying conditions, it is likely that both the appropriate definitive procedures will indeed become necessary in the course of time.

The 'Small Fibrous Prostate'. Strictly speaking, with the possible exception of specific conditions such as schistosomiasis, tuberculosis and carcinoma, there is no such entity as bladder outlet obstruction caused by a 'small fibrous prostate'.

The term has been used as a synonym for Marion's Disease or 'sclerose du col' (Turner-Warwick 1973); however, this condition is simply the end result of a life-long dyssynergic bladder neck obstruction without a significant element of prostatic enlargement and the secondary collagen deposit seen in the histological sections is quite unrelated to the development of the obstruction.

The situation most commonly referred to as a 'small fibrous prostate' is that of double obstruction (Turner-Warwick et al. 1973); resectionists have used the term somewhat phantasmagorically because of its tendency to develop secondary bladder neck contracture after a routine loop-resection and enucleationists used it when they found difficulty in enucleating the small element of prostatic enlargement.

Summary: The Three Endoscopic Appearances of the Proximal Posterior Urethra and Their Appropriate Treatment in Proven Outlet Obstruction

In summary, endoscopic examination of the proximal posterior urethra will generally reveal one of three appearances each of which may or may not be associated with obstruction; *when obstruction is urodynamically proven*, the principles of the appropriate treatment of each is different:

1) *A ring-shaped bladder neck with no prostatic enlargement* indicating, in the absence of schistosomiasis, a dyssynergic dysfunction which is more appropriately treated by endoscopic incision than by loop-resection.

2) *A triangulated internal meatus*, the margins of which are created by a large bulk of hypertrophic prostatic tissue. The resolution of this requires a formal loop-resection or an enucleation procedure. The use of an endoscopic prostatotomy incision is manifestly inappropriate because there is no tendency for the cleft of such an incision into the solid tissue to 'open out' into a U-shaped channel.

3) *A relatively small intraurethral 'prostatic' enlargement with a proximal ring-shaped internal meatus – 'Double Obstruction':* An initial bilateral full-thickness incision of the bladder neck element of this, down to the level of the verumontanum, may be all that it is required to relieve the obstruction but if not, a significant residual intrusion of prostatic tissue is treated definitively by an additional loop-resection. To suppose that the effect of this endoscopic incision is the result of incising the prostate and to refer to this as 'prostatotomy' is conceptually erroneous and this has tarnished the reputation of the excellent procedure of bladder neck relaxation.

Conclusion

The development of methods of objective urodynamic evaluation of bladder outlet obstruction in the male have led to a fundamental revision of many functional concepts relating to symptomatology, radiographic findings, endoscopic appearances and consequently, to treatment.

There can be no doubt that the fundamental basis of appropriate treatment of male outlet obstruction is uroflowmetry – without this, inevitably, prostatic obstruction is overdiagnosed, dyssynergic bladder neck obstruction is underdiagnosed and furthermore, a surgeon may overestimate the reliability of his obstruction relieving procedures.

It is highly questionable whether surgical treatment for male bladder outlet obstruction is justifiable without, at least, pre- and post-operative uroflow records: the cystourethroscope is certainly an unacceptable substitute for a flowmeter. The evidence of need for this relatively inexpensive basic equipment is overwhelming, furthermore, it is most certainly cost-effective in terms of patient care and the avoidance of unnecessary operations.

Simple videocystourethrography is also important to the urodynamic evaluation of many patients and although it is still sometimes under-used, this radiographic facility is, in fact, readily available to every practising urologist in this country. Facilities for pressure-flow studies should be available in appropriate centres; synchronous video-pressure study facilities are essential in urodynamic referral units.

References

Abrams PH (1977) Investigation of bladder outflow obstruction in the male. PhD Thesis University of Bristol
Abrams P, Torrens M (1979) Clinical urodynamics. Urol Clin North Am 6:71–79, 103–109
Arnold EP (1980) Bladder outlet obstruction in the male – a urological analysis of the detrusor response. PhD Thesis, London University
Bannister R (1983) Disorders of the autonomic system. A text book of clinical disorder. Oxford University Press
Bates CP, Whiteside CG, Turner-Warwick R (1970) Synchronous cine pressure-flow cystourethrography. Br J Urol 42:714–723
Bates CP, Arnold EP, Griffiths DG (1973) The progressive dyssynergetic contraction of the bladder neck. Br J Urol 45:58–59
Booth C, Whiteside CG, Milroy EJG, Turner-Warwick R (1981) Unheralded urinary tract infection in the male – a clinical and urodynamic assessment. Br J Urol 53:270
Booth C, Shah J, Gosling J, Milroy EJG, Turner-Warwick R (1983) The structure of the bladder neck in the male. Br J Urol (to be published)
Brown AG, Turner-Warwick R (1979) A urodynamic evaluation of urinary incontinence in the female and its treatment. Urol Clin North Am 6:31–38
Farrar D, Turner-Warwick R (1979) Outflow obstruction in the female. Urol Clin North Am 6:217–227
Gosling JA, Dixon JS (1981) Structural changes associated with obstruction. Prog Clin Med 78:283–284
Kirby RS (1983) Non-obstructive detrusor failure – a fresh look. Br Assoc Urol Surg Meeting
Kirby RS, Fowler C, Milroy EJG, Bannister R, Gosling JA, Turner-Warwick R (1983) Vesico urethral dysfunction in progressive autonomic failure (Shy Drager Syndrome). Proc Internat Continence Soc
McNeal JE (1972) The prostate and prostatic urethra – a morphological synthesis. J Urol 107:1008
Smith J (1966) The measurement and significance of urinary flow. Br J Urol 30:701–705
Tanagho EA (1978) The anatomy and physiology of micturition. Clin Obstet Gynaecol 5:101–119
Thomas D (1979) Neurogenic bladder dysfunction. Urol Clin North Am 6:237–253
Turner-Warwick R (1970) Clinical problems associated with urodynamic abnormalities. In: Lutzeyer W, Melchior H (eds) Urodynamics. Springer, Berlin Heidelberg New York, pp 237–263
Turner-Warwick R (1979) Clinical urodynamics. Urol Clin North Am 6:13–30, 171–190

Turner-Warwick R (1983) The relationship of prostatic enlargement to the distal sphincter mechanism, the bladder neck mechanism – dyssynergic bladder neck obstruction. In: Hinman F, Chisholm G (eds) Benign Prostatic Hypertrophy. Springer, Berlin Heidelberg New York, pp 809–828

Turner-Warwick R, Handley Ashken M (1967) The functional results of partial, subtotal and total cystoplasty. Br J Urol 39:3

Turner-Warwick R, Pitfield-Marshall J (1984) Outpatient evaluation of lower urinary tract function and dysfunction. In: Kaye KW (ed) Outpatient urologic investigation. Lea & Febiger, Philadelphia, pp 92–108

Turner-Warwick R, Whiteside CG (1982) Scientific foundations of urology, 2nd edn. Heinemann, London

Turner-Warwick R, Whiteside CG, Arnold EP, Bates EP, Worth PHL, Milroy EJG, Webster JR, Weir J (1973) A urodynamic view of prostatic obstruction and the results of prostatectomy. Br J Urol 45:631–645

Turner-Warwick R, Whiteside CG, Worth PHL, Milroy EJG, Bates CP (1973) A urodynamic review of clinical problems associated with bladder neck dysfunction and its treatment by endoscopic incision – trans-trigonal posterior prostatectomy. Br J Urol 45:44–59

Turner-Warwick R, Whiteside CG, Milroy EJG, Pengelly AW, Thompson DT (1979) The intravenous urodynamogram. Br J Urol 15:15–19

Surface Factors in Recurrent Infection

F. HINMAN JR.[1]

Abstract. Twelve years ago, our research was directed toward those hydrodynamic factors influencing the establishment of bacteriuria. Their importance in initiating and perpetuating infection was found in further studies, looking at midurethral pressure, spontaneous urethral peristalsis, washout of residual bacteria versus trapping, and the effects of overdistention on bladder function.

Of equal importance are reactions between bacteria and the urothelium (which include adherence factors between bacteria and the cell surface), as seen in observations on aging and desquamation of luminal cells, reaction of the wall to bacteria and surface antibacterial activity.

The bladder urine remains sterile in normal males and females, and bacterial entry is prevented by extrinsic urodynamic functions aided by intrinsic antibacterial activity of the mucosa. This was shown some years ago (Cox and Hinman 1961) when it was observed that bacteria were not eliminated from an inoculated flask but were rapidly cleared from the bladders of human volunteers. The bladder defenses are important, not because the presence of bacteria in the urine is itself harmful, but because the resulting cystitis is distressing and is the precursor of damaging upper tract infection when the bacteria ascend during transient reflux.

Extrinsic Defenses

Bacteria are prohibited access to the bladder principally by the effects of mechanical washout, by the so-called extrinsic defenses constituting the primary bladder defense mechanism. Flushing of the urethra and bladder emptying are the principal mechanisms involved.

Urethral flushing of any unattached bacteria that might be present occurs with each voiding, because of the turbulent flow involved and the forced separation of the folded mucosa. Relative narrowing at the meatus (distal urethral stenosis) or at the external sphincter in females during intermittent voiding may allow recirculation of bacteria within the canal and their entry into the bladder when micturition is incomplete (Hinman 1966).

Since our report to the 1971 meeting in Aachen (Hinman 1972), we have determined that the urethral washout mechanism is assisted by a high pressure zone in mid-urethra (Mayo and Hinman 1973), which tends to limit the ascent of bacteria in the resting state (Fig. 1). A further contribution is made by intrinsic urethral peristalsis (Mayo and Hinman 1974), which milks residual secretions toward the meatus (Fig. 2).

---

1 Department of Urology, U-518, University of California, San Francisco, CA 94143, USA

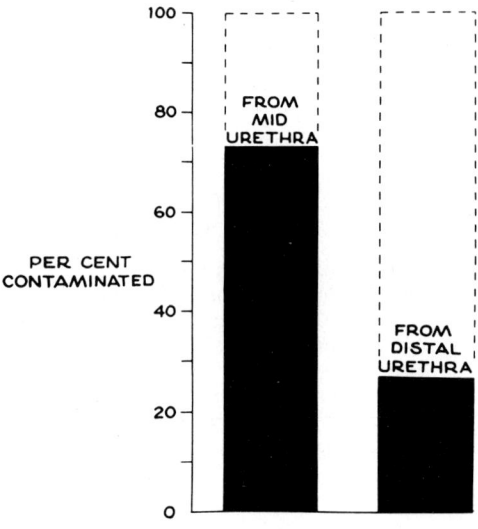

Fig. 1. Contamination of bladder urine after distal (15 dogs) and midurethral (15 dogs) inoculation with ^{125}I labelled E. coli. (From Mayo and Hinman 1973)

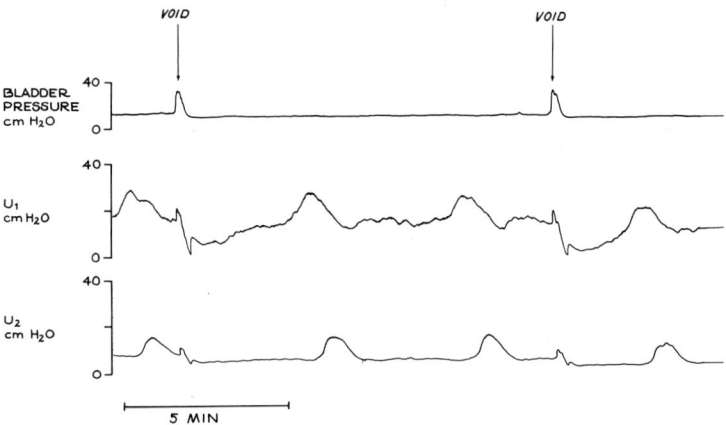

Fig. 2. Pressure tracings from bladder, proximal and midurethra, showing progression of wave down urethra

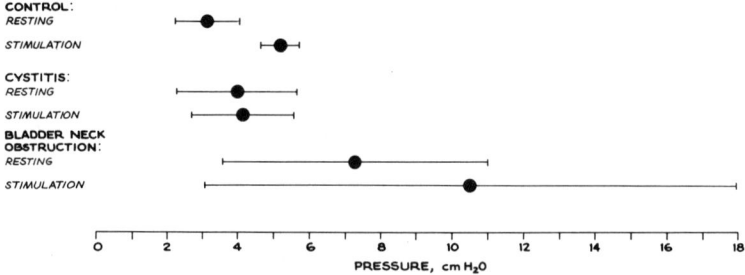

Fig. 3. Intravesical pressure in control, chronically infected and obstructed bladders, before and after nerve stimulation. (From Mayo and Hinman 1976)

Bladder emptying, the other extrinsic defense, is effective if the volume, frequency and completeness of evacuation is sufficient to overcome the doubling rate of bacteria (Hinman and Cox 1966). The amount of residual urine that could be present to keep the level of bacteria constant is related to the voiding volumes and frequencies. Large residues are tolerated if the voiding volume is adequate and especially if the interval between voidings is short, since frequent emptying reduces the time for the geometrical progression of bacteria. Since residual urine so adversely affects the extrinsic, washout defenses, disorders reducing detrusor contractility would be expected to increase susceptibility to infection. It was shown that acute overdistention of male rabbit bladders not only alters the structure of the detrusor muscle (Lloyd-Davies and Hinman 1970) but also fosters chronic bacteriuria (Mayo and Hinman 1976). Infection alone did not affect the muscle histologically but did reduce its response to pelvic nerve stimulation (Fig. 3).

In summary, the extrinsic mechanisms are the first line of defense; if they are breached, the efforts of the intrinsic, surface defenses may be nullified.

Intrinsic Defenses

Even if the extrinsic defense mechanism is intact, as determined by all radiological and urodynamic tests, infection may occur owing to defects in the intrinsic surface defenses. A caveat here is that the common recurrent infections in female children and adults probably require some initiating extrinsic disturbance (delayed voiding, occasional incomplete emptying, or coitus). In males, some defect in emptying or established infection in the prostate is usually found.

Bacterial attachment to the urothelium is the initial break in the intrinsic defenses. The bacteria must become established at least at the meatus to begin the infective process. Years ago by monitoring the flora of the meatus in normal women and in those with recurrent infection (Cox et al. 1968), we were able to predict the organism that would be in the urine at the next episode by finding it weeks earlier colonizing the meatus. This observation has been confirmed and extended by others (Stamey et al. 1971; Fowler and Stamey 1977; Schaeffer et al. 1981). The finding that mucus has a protective effect (Parsons and Mulholland 1978) and that pathogenic bacteria have adapted their glycocalyx and fimbria to achieve adherence (Svanborg et al. 1976) has opened a new line of research and increases the potential for effective prevention. This area, however, is not a subject for review at a urodynamic forum.

Trapping of bacteria occurs, since the urothelial surface is mechanically active when defending against infection. Normally, when not distended, the surface cells are thrown into microvilli, initially seen by scanning electron microscopy (Lloyd-Davies et al. 1971a). When the urethra is distended, as during free voiding, the surface is smooth. With the initiation of infection, it becomes very irregular (Lloyd-Davies et al. 1971b), presenting an ideal contour for holding bacteria. Moreover, bladder contraction produces microplicae capable of trapping bacteria and non-adhesive latex spheres alike (Hinman et al. 1976). In fact, as expected, inoculated bacteria were more difficult to wash from the canine urethra than from a smooth latex model (Hinman 1974) (Fig. 4).

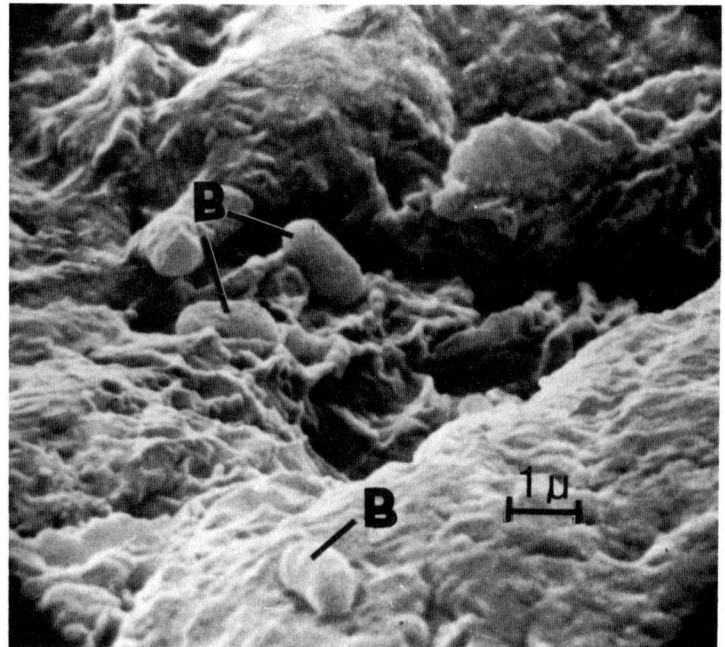

Fig. 4. Microplicae trapping bacteria, SEM. (From Mooney et al. 1976)

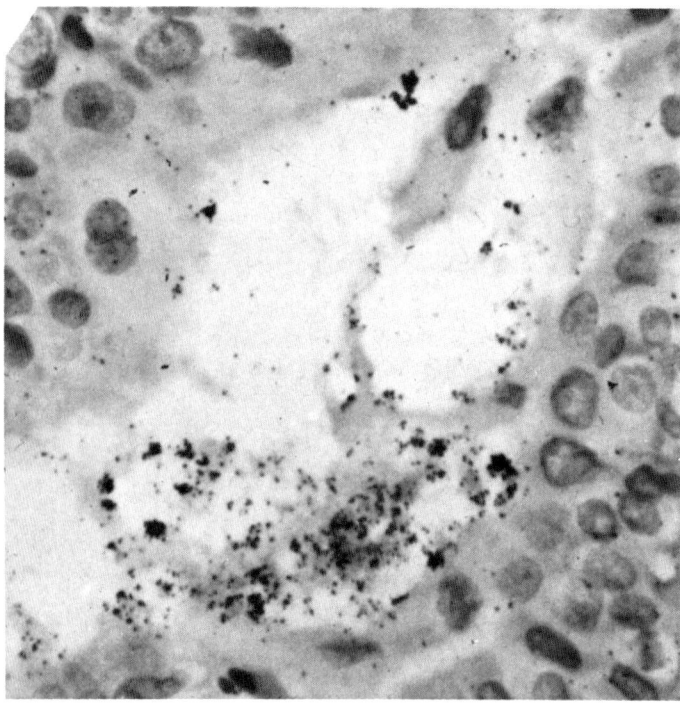

Fig. 5. Surface cells, penetrated by bacteria, being sloughed away into the bladder lumen. (From Orikasa and Hinman 1977)

Desquamation of the surface cells acts to rid the urothelium of adherent bacteria. Cells are replaced progressively (Mooney and Hinman 1974) and, when penetrated by bacteria, they are sloughed and voided, carrying the adherent, trapped bacteria with them (Orikasa and Hinman 1977) (Fig. 5). The bacteria in those cells not desquamated are phagocytized or enter the lymphatics to be carried away.

In summary, the intrinsic defenses act first by inhibiting adherence by agents on the surface. If that fails, then trapping and desquamation of the surface cells may eliminate the bacteria before they can invade the bladder wall.

References

Cox CE, Hinman F Jr (1961) Experiments with induced bacteriuria, vesical emptying and bacterial growth on the mechanism of bladder defense to infection. J Urol 86:739–748

Cox CE, Lacy SS, Hinman F Jr (1968) The urethra and its relationship to urinary tract infection. II. Urethral flora of the female with recurrent urinary infection. J Urol 99:632–638

Fowler JE, Stamey TW (1977) Studies of introital colonization in women with recurrent urinary infections. VII. The role of bacterial adherence. J Urol 117:472–476

Hinman F Jr (1966) Mechanisms for the entry of bacteria and the establishment of urinary infection in female children. J Urol 96:546–550

Hinman F Jr (1972) Hydrodynamic aspects of urinary tract infection. In: Lutzeyer W (ed) First International Symposium on Hydrodynamics – Aachen, 1971. Thieme, Stuttgart

Hinman F Jr (1974) Washout of resident and introduced bacteria by constant flow through the intact and modified canine urethra and latex tubing. J Urol 111:114

Hinman F Jr, Cox CE (1966) The voiding vesical defense mechanism: The mathematical effect of residual urine, voiding interval and volume on bacteriuria. J Urol 96:491–498

Hinman F Jr, Mooney JK, Mooney JS (1976) The antibacterial effect of the bladder surface: An electron microscopic study. J Urol 115:381

Lloyd-Davies RW, Hinman F Jr (1970) Structural alterations and functional changes after overdistension of the rabbit bladder. Surg Forum 542–543

Lloyd-Davies RW, Hayes TL, Hinman F Jr (1971a) Urothelial microcontour. I. Scanning electron microscopy of normal resting and stretched urethra and bladder. J Urol 105:236

Lloyd-Davies RW, Hayes TL, Hinman F Jr (1971b) Urothelial microcontour. III. Mucosal alteration by infection. J Urol 106:81

Mayo ME, Hinman F Jr (1973) Role of midurethral high pressure zone in spontaneous bacterial ascent. J Urol 109:263

Mayo ME, Hinman F Jr (1974) Intrinsic urethral peristalsis. Invest Urol 12:1

Mayo ME, Hinman F Jr (1976) Structure and function of the rabbit bladder altered by chronic obstruction or cystitis. Invest Urol 14:6

Mooney JK, Hinman F Jr (1974) Aging and replacement of the luminal cells in the mammalian bladder studied by electron microscopy. Invest Urol 11:396

Mooney JK, Mooney JS, Hinman F Jr (1976) The antibacterial effect of the bladder surface: an electron microscopic study. J Urol 115:381

Orikasa S, Hinman F Jr (1977) Reaction of the vesical wall to bacterial penetration: Resistance to attachment, desquamation and leukocytic activity. Invest Urol 15:185

Parsons CL, Mulholland SG (1978) Bladder surface mucin: Its antibacterial effect against various bacterial species. Am J Pathol 93:423

Schaeffer AJ, Jones JM, Dunn JK (1981) Association of in vitro Escherichia coli adherence to vaginal and buccal epithelial cells with suspectibility of women to recurrent urinary tract infections. N Engl J Med 304:1062

Stamey TA, Timothy M, Millar M et al. (1971) Recurrent urinary infections in adult women: The role of introital enterobacteria. Calif Med 115:1

Svanborg EC, Hanson LA, Jodal U et al. (1976) Variable adhesion to normal urinary tract epithelial cells of Escherichia coli strains associated with various forms of urinary tract infection. Lancet 2:490–492

Causes and Consequences of Bladder Neck Obstruction

H. MARBERGER[1]

Causes and consequences of bladder neck obstruction are only partly understood and up to now subject under discussion. There is a great number of causes, reflecting a variety of symptoms, clinical and pathoanatomical findings.

Let us have a look at a few of them: Bladder neck and posterior urethra are anatomically and functionally a unit (Marberger 1958). Simultaneously with the contraction of the detrusor muscle, the bladder neck opens and shapes up to a streamlined funnel, which provides the best urodynamic condition for quick expulsion of the urine. Disturbances of these mechanisms are the main cause of bladder neck obstruction. Due to the double function as a part of the genital and urinary tract the posterior urethra and its adnexa are a common site of disease, such as benign prostatic hypertrophy, carcinomatous and inflammatory disease of the prostate and seminal vesicles change the physical properties of the prostatic urethra and the bladder neck and make ideal funneling of the bladder outlet impossible, thus increasing resistance (Marberger 1957). This is probably the most common cause of obstruction.

Although it is known that a median lobe of an adenomatous prostate may act as a closing valve, the majority of patients with prostatic hypertrophy do not have real narrowing or closure of the urethra or the bladder outlet during micturition. Usually the cross section of the urethra remains of the same size or becomes only a bit smaller, but the transverse and the longitudinal contour of the urethra is changed. The hyperplastic prostate expands in diameter and length. From clinical experience we know that neither the size of the prostate nor the minimal diameter of the outlet is decisive for the degree of obstruction (Marberger 1964). Clinical observation, X-rays, cine studies and urodynamic investigations show very clearly that other factors, for example the contour and surface conditions of the prostatic urethra are of great importance in regard to flow (Marberger 1957).

We wanted to study a few of those factors more in detail in the experiment (Marberger 1973). Anatomical changes of the prostatic urethra and the bladder neck, as seen in common prostatic disease, were simulated by using rigid glass models or semi-elastic plastic tubes (Marberger 1969). We perfused them under controlled conditions and studied the flow (Marberger 1976). A motion picture was made to document our findings and to make them more comprehensive.

The experiments were performed at the Institute of Hydrology of the University in Graz with the help of Dr. Ziegler and Dr. Holl, and also the cooperation of Prof. Madersbacher was of great help.

---

[1] Universitäts-Klinik für Urologie, A-6020 Innsbruck

Causes and Consequences of Bladder Neck Obstruction

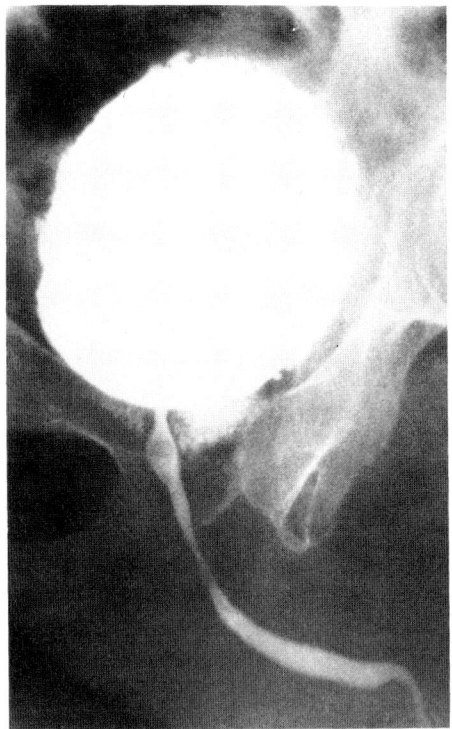

Fig. 1. Bladder neck sclerosis due to chronic prostatitis (the bladder neck does not take on funnel-shape during micturition

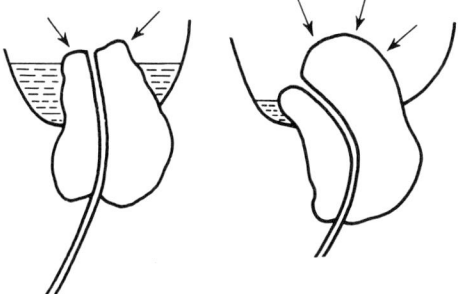

Fig. 2. Median lobe and large intravesical portion of adenomatous prostate

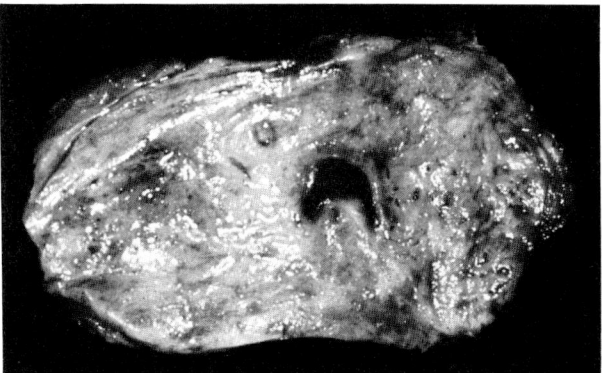

Fig. 3. U-shape form of the urethra in prostatic hyperplasia

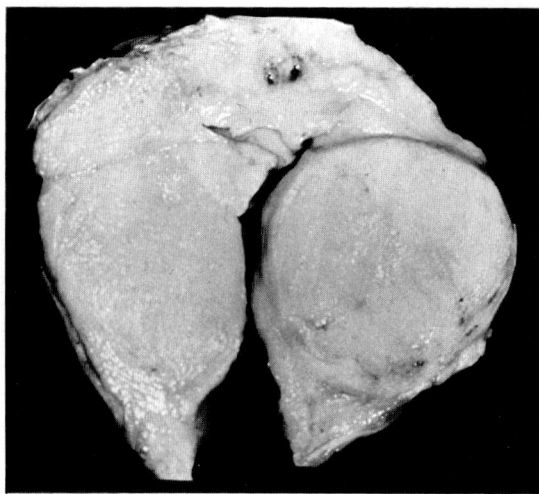

Fig. 4. T-bar contour in prostatic adenoma

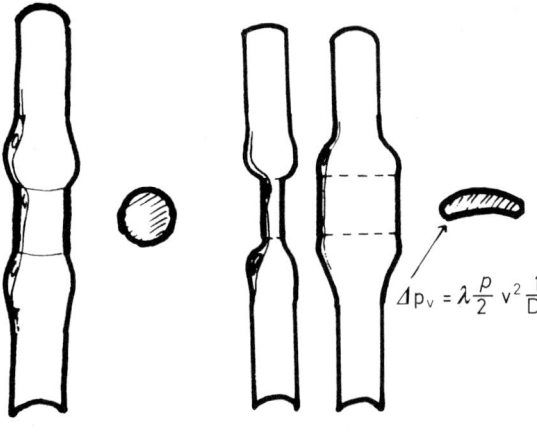

Fig. 5. Sketch of a semirigid model with a rigid section transforming the round lumen of a tube into a semilunar one. The impact of this transformation can be calculated by the given formula

$$\Delta p_v = \lambda \frac{p}{2} v^2 \frac{1}{D_h}$$

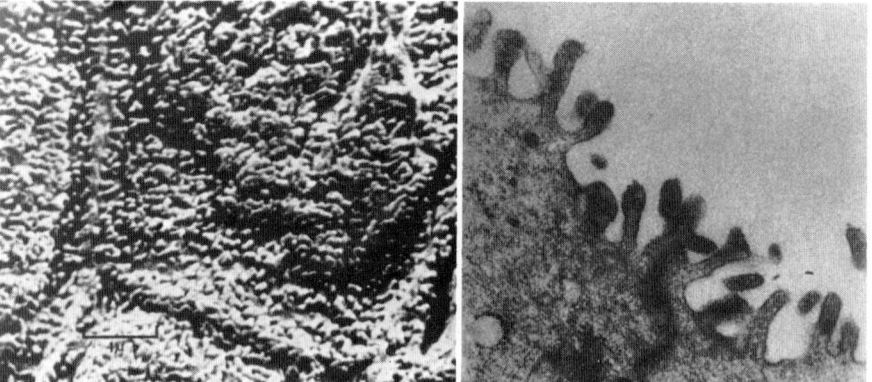

Fig. 6. High magnification picture of the surface of the posterior urethra

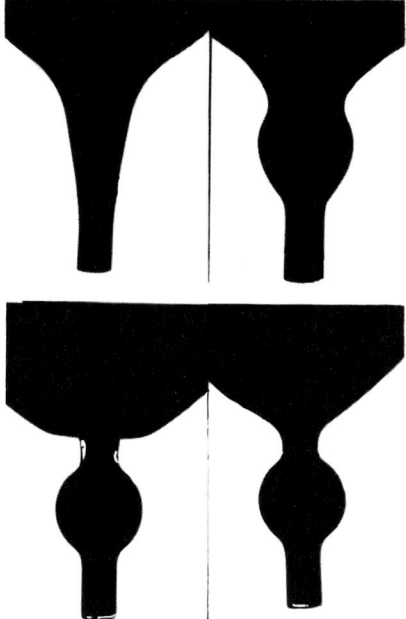

Fig. 7. Glass models of bladder outlets used in experiment to study the impact of the contour and shape on flow

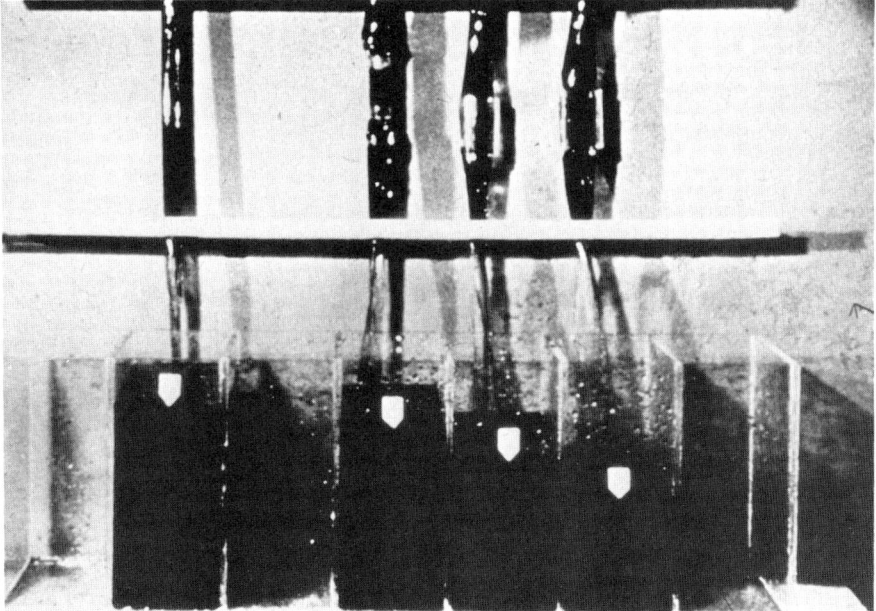

Fig. 8. Reduction of flow due to transformation of the lumen of various perfused tubes

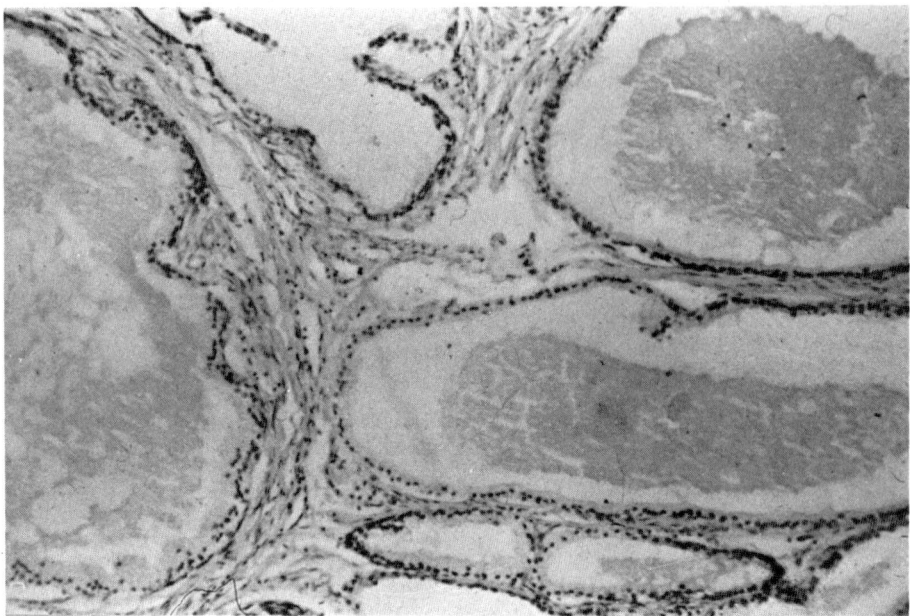
Fig. 9. Dilated acinar space in the periphery of the prostatic gland

Parameters which determine flow are partly subject to fluctuation, size and shape of the prostate and the seminal vesicles which vary with sexual stimulation and activity. Prostatic fluid accumulated between production and emptying of the secretion, as it can result from discrepancy between sexual stimulation and ejaculation, may cause congestion of the canalicular space and result in a true increase in size of the gland. Roughness of the surface of the posterior urethra as seen in prostatitis and cancer of the prostate increases obstruction.

The second part of my paper deals with the consequences of bladder neck obstruction.

> Here lies Mattias Spies – who died of a bladder disease. His end was full of pain and distress. Lord give him eternal rest.

The most common consequence of chronic obstruction was renal failure and death as the inscription on the tombstone of this poor Tyrolean man says.

Even today death from bladder neck obstruction is not rare, although it could have been avoided in most cases. The course of the disease is not very dramatic, the symptoms are taken for symptoms of old age or are misdiagnosed by the patient or the doctor.

A 72 year old patient, who was in good general health, woke up in the morning and found himself blind on one eye. The eye-doctor diagnosed a hemorrhage in the retina due to severe hypertension. The patient was referred to an internal specialist who confirmed the hypertension, found a large blood clot in the abdomen and pus cells and proteine in the urine. By catheterism only a few milliliter of bladder urine had been obtained, blood test and BUN were borderline. Excretory pyelograms showed bilateral dilated ureters, poor filling of the bladder. Suspicion arose of an obstructive tumor in the lower abdomen. The patient was in good general condition and stated that he was urinating well. He was referred to a surgeon who again palpated the mass expanding from the pelvis. Before an exploratory operation was considered, the urologist was called. I found a furious patient who refused to have his prostate and bladder reexamined. Finally I could persuade him, passed a catheter into the bladder and drained 1200 cc bladder urine. The patient was shocked when his tumor disappeared and he realized that his bladder had not been emptying properly for years. The man recovered quickly after catheter drainage, the prostate was removed by TUR. Within a year the blood pressure sank almost to normal. 4 years later he died of a bronchial carcinoma.

Everybody assumes that in a case like this there could not be any doubt in regard to diagnosis. We have to admit that all of us have made errors in the interpretation of unusual clinical symptoms, particularly in noncooperative, dissimulating patients.

Consequences of bladder neck obstruction are better understood if we remind ourselves of a few well known factors. With increasing bladder neck obstruction the detrusor muscle varies from case to case and so do the symptoms. Some people do not notice any difference from normal, if micturition pressure rises, doubles and/or triples. In others intravesical pressure remains almost the same but the flow is reduced. Old patients consider a change in cast distance and flow to be normal in these years.

Another way of compensation is incomplete emptying or voiding in fraction. It appears that the detrusor muscle needs to recuperate, to take another deep breath to do the whole job. Sometimes bladder emptying is only possible if optimal stretching conditions due to residual urine provide optimal force. In those cases residual urine facilitates urination.

In some patients the compensatory capacity is very limited, they show complete retention before irreversible damage occurs. Compensatory hypertrophy of the bladder muscle gives a typical endoscopic picture, trabeculation. Between prominent muscle network one can see deep diverticula as a result of high bladder pressure. Trabeculae and diverticulae formation are usually taken as a sign, better as a complication of bladder neck obstruction. Many clinical observations, however, have brought us to the conclusion that diverticulae formation may act also as a safety valve which protects the upper GU. Urodynamic studies and simple experiments show that the diverticulae or extreme distensibility act as an energy destroyer. They consume so much energy that intravesical pressure cannot exceed a certain limit.

There is an example: A patient, aged 81, came to our department and asked the doctor to drain his residual urine. The resident told him that he should have a complete work-up and then probably a prostate operation. The patient answered that he had already had his prostate removed four times and in spite of that the bladder would not empty completely. The patient was not complaining of any pain whatsoever, nor did he show symptoms of illness except for a slow stream and a mild recurrent infection. His i.V.P. was normal and his blood chemistry was within normal limits. He came to see the urologist because his physician had recommended to drain the bladder completely once a month and to clean out the reservoir. The only change the patient felt after emptying the bladder by catheterization was that he did not have to urinate for twelve hours.

The patient died 7 years later on a nonurological disease. He continued to come once a month to be catheterized, otherwise he lived very well without any problems. There is no doubt that the low bladder pressure saved the patients life and allowed him many more years to live a life without real health problems.

However, we also believe that an overdistended bladder should have further treatment after prostatectomy and that self-catherism may be very helpful and effective.

In the majority of cases, however, chronic bladder neck obstruction had its implication on the upper urinary tract and its function. The ureter has to work harder in order to compensate high bladder pressure, intraureteral and intrarenal pressure increases and the very complex renal function is endangered, the patient becomes ill. Compensatory increase in blood pressure compensates to some degree and keeps diuresis going.

Hypertension with all its risks is a very common consequence of bladder neck obstruction in old men, however, it seems to be a compatible or avoidable hazard.

The release of bladder neck obstruction helps to control hypertension and to avoid progress of vascular disease.

Summary

Our knowledge of causes and consequences of bladder neck obstruction did improve within the last 10 years, the urodynamic studies became a wide field in research and an important diagnostic tool in urological practice. By simple means we can determine whether the detrusor muscle works too hard or too little and very often that knowledge is decisive for the plan of treatment and prognoses.

We could prove that residual urine may help to keep micturition going and an abnormally large bladder capacity may prevent renal damage.

By the proper use of the diagnostic armentarium available today, based on knowledge of normal and abnormal function of the urinary tract, gives a good guideline for combatting bladder neck obstruction effectively and to save our patients from an unpleasant fate.

References

Marberger H (1957) Dringliche Harnröhrenchirurgie. Chir Praxis 2:229–246
Marberger H (1958) Die Kontrastdarstellung der Harnröhre. Chir Praxis 2:237–243
Marberger H (1964) Bladder neck obstruction in childhood. Acta Urol Belg 4:492–504
Marberger H (1969) Hydrodynamics and urinary infection (Motion Picture). Trans Am Assoc Genitourin Surg 61:77
Marberger H (1973) Energy destroyer in urology. In: Lutzeyer W, Melchior H (eds) Urodynamics, upper and lower urinary tract. Springer, Berlin Heidelberg New York, p 23
Marberger H (1976) Causes and consequences of bladder neck obstruction. 31 Prostatic disease. Liss, New York, pp 31–47

Urinary Velocity: Twelve Years Later

M. R. Bottaccini[1], D. M. Gleason[2] and H. H. Meyhoff[3]

Introduction

In 1971 we proposed to measure the total energy generated in the urinary bladder and to compare it with the total energy contained in the voided urine (Bottaccini et al. 1973; Gleason et al. 1972). From ordinary hydrodynamic practice we expected the difference between the two energies to be a function of viscous dissipation, turbulence, inertial impedance and energy storage in elastic tissues (Streeter and Wylie 1979). Given that turbulence generation, the primary energy conversion mechanism affecting the movement of liquids in steady flow, is highly dependent on internal geometry, we hoped that the energy difference could be correlated with obstructive pathology.

The measurement technique was simple enough; bladder energy was to be measured directly from intravesical pressure and the energy of the voided urine would be calculated indirectly from the force generated by the urine as it struck a vertically mounted disc. There was great hope that the procedure would yield simple, clinically useful correlations. Sufficient evidence was adduced to show the probable validity of the method (appendix). Examination of clinical data reported in the literature and a short series of tests conducted by the authors showed that correlation between energy loss and pathology existed in practice (Byrne et al. 1972).

In the twelve years since the publication of the tentative report discussed above, the methodology has been validated by hundreds of clinical tests (Bottaccini and Gleason 1980; Gleason et al. 1976; Gleason and Bottacini 1982; Gleason et al. 1982). The theory, somewhat shaky at the start, is now established beyond argument. The urodynamometer and the paddlewheel velocimeter have been used routinely so that energy measurements in the male are sufficiently well established to make them useful to the clinician (Gleason et al. 1982). It was also shown that obstructive diseases are not common in the female and that in most instances energy measurements are not too valuable in the diagnosis of ordinary female urinary disorders.

A Review of the Theory

It must be understood, at this point, that within the context of the first law of thermodynamics the phrase "energy loss" has no meaning; energy may be transformed,

---

1 The University of Wisconsin, Platteville, WI 53818, USA
2 The University of Arizona, Tucson, AZ 85724, USA
3 The University of Copenhagen, DK-2730 Herlev

stored or rearranged but it can never be lost. In the relevant form of the first law of thermodynamics it is stated that the rate of work being done on a fluid system added to the heat transferred to the system must always equal the rate of change of energy within the system plus the rate of energy being transported by the fluid through the boundaries of the system (Wark 1983). All energy must be accounted for and none is permitted to be "lost". It is true, however, that mechanical engineers who are concerned with pumping liquids or with designing heat engines agree that some of the energy applied to a fluid cannot be recovered in the form of useful work. Although it is understood that the energy has been changed, rather than lost, it is, nevertheless, called "lost" because unavailable.

Two methods have been proposed for the analysis of energy loss in engineering fluid mechanics. The oldest procedure involves the set of "bernouillian theorems" which, although originally developed for steady, non-viscous, incompressible and uniform flows, was later modified empirically to encompass a wide variety of practical applications (Bottaccini and Gleason 1979; Streeter and Wylie 1979). The second technique involves the use of the first and second laws of thermodynamics in a straightforward energy accounting procedure. Energy methods ultimately lead to the same algebraic results as the bernouillian equations but are mathematically and conceptually more natural.

In the early days of urodynamics bernouillian theorems were used with great abandon without much concern for applicability or scientific validity, thereby leading some urodynamicists to declare the methods invalid (Schafer 1983). It seems best, therefore, to avoid further use of the modified principle of Bernouilli and to restrict all demonstrations with respect to energy transfer in the urinary tract to the laws of thermodynamics.

We are concerned with discerning the effects of disease on the motion of urine in the lower urinary tract and with determining if there exists a term definable as "loss" which can be connected with clinically defined obstruction. We begin by measuring the bladder pressure, an indicator of energy, through a superpubic canula and the exit velocity and flow rate with the urodynamometer. The power generated in the bladder can then be calculated by multiplying the intravesical pressure by the flow rate (appendix). For a typical male patient (Fig. 1) the power rises to approximately 0.10 watts and oscillates around that value for approximately 15 seconds before declining to zero watts during the last 7 seconds of the micturition. The power remaining in the voided stream, calculated by multiplying the latent kinetic energy of the stream by the flow rate (appendix), follows a similar pattern but reaches only a quasi-stable maximum of 0.02 watts. During the middle 15 seconds of the voiding approximately 80.0% of the power produced in the bladder is "lost". We can determine the loss more accurately if it is remembered that the area under the curve is the work done on the urine by the detrusor and that the area under the exit power curve is the latent capacity for doing work of the voided urine. The two areas can be calculated by a routine application of Simpson's rule for numerical integration (Gerald 1980). During the micturition 5.238 watt-s of work are generated in the bladder and 0.934 watt-s of latent work remain in the voided urine. 82.2% of the work is lost in transit.

The experiment described above is a straightforward application of the first law of thermodynamics. If we apply the symbolic operations discussed in the appendix

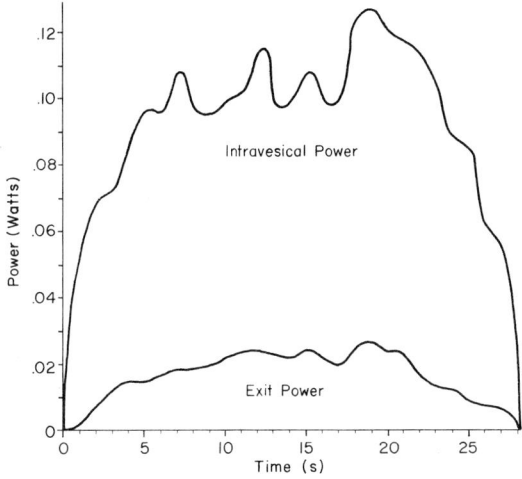

Fig. 1. Comparison of intravesical power to the power remaining in the voided stream

we obtain the customary loss parameter (Bottaccini and Gleason 1979):

$$K = \frac{p_I - 0.5\,\varrho\,V_E^2}{0.5\,\varrho\,V_E^2},$$

a theoretically valid, but much maligned construct which is quite general and is not derived from rigid pipe considerations as some urodynamicists would have it (Schafer 1983). When the values of K before and after a satisfactory transurethral resection of the prostate are plotted together as a function of time for a single patient it becomes obvious that the pre-operative tracing remains always above the postoperative graph (Fig. 2).

In the case documented in Fig. 2 and in most cases measured by the authors, K stabilized to an approximately constant value during the mid-third of the micturition and the two curves remained approximately parallel. As a consequence of the above observation it seemed a reasonable alternative to calculating the entire power curve to simply choose a well defined point in the middle of the micturition record and to use the value of K at that reference point as a clinical index of loss. A few tests convinced us that the point of maximum flow rate in a micturition usually lies within the region of stable loss coefficient and is, therefore, a reasonably repeatable point of reference.

That the procedures discussed above are applicable to the detection of obstructive pathology in the male urethra can be confirmed by appeal to independently gathered data published in the European literature long before the urodynamometer was invented. Bryndorf and Sandøe (1960) diagnosed the degree of urinary obstruction in a group of males by customary urologic office techniques and then determined the bladder pressure through a superpubic canula whilst measuring the urinary exit velocity by the cast distance method (Schwartz and Brenner 1921). Using the published data we calculated the loss coefficient K and its equivalent, L, the fractional loss coefficient (appendix). It is doubtful that a more

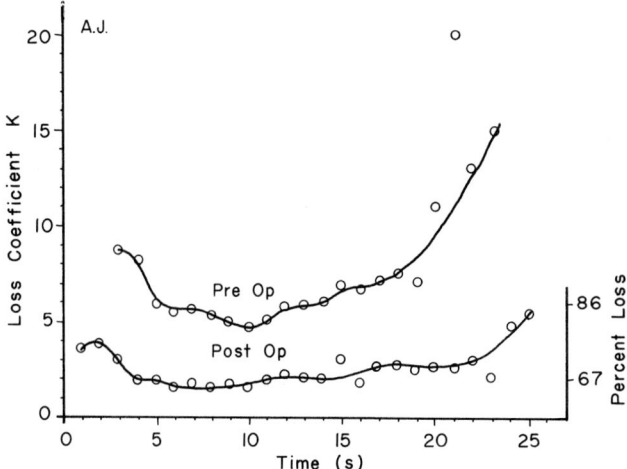

Fig. 2. Comparison of the loss coefficient K before and after resection of the prostate. Before the procedure the urethra is moderately obstructed (86% energy dissipation). After the procedure the urethra is nearly unobstructed

convincing demonstration can be given; K and L match the clinical categories perfectly (Table 1). The parameter L is interesting because it shows that a normal male urethra uses nearly 60 percent of the bladder power in maintaining flow against obstruction whereas the severely constricted urethra expends more than 90 percent of the original energy. We are dealing with the sort of losses noticed in hydraulic systems near places in which the fluid is first forced to accelerate through a severe narrowing of the pipe and is then permitted to decelerate to a much larger size in a very short segment of pipe. A gate valve ¾ open, for example, will induce a 50 percent kinetic energy loss whereas the valve ¼ open will cause 96 percent of the local kinetic energy to be consumed. If we grant that the male urethra is quite narrow in the neighborhood of the membranous urethra, we need no other information to explain the origins of loss.

The parameter K is a much more sensitive discriminator of energy loss and of pathology than is L. Whereas L varies from 49.9% to 99.8%, a rather narrow range, K changes from 0.996 to 499, thereby allowing a refined distinction among degrees of obstruction. K is the parameter of choice in the clinic. The effectiveness of K as a parameter for the documentation of successful treatment can be demonstrated by a set of data submitted for our analysis by Hans Henrik Meyhoff, M.D. of the Department of Urology, Herlev Hospital, Copenhagen, Denmark. From copies of Meyhoff's original tracing of tests accomplished with the DISA version of the urodynamometer we calculated the parameter K for a group of 11 patients before and after resection of the prostate (Table 2). The urethras varied from the extremely obstructed (K = 100) to the slightly obstructed (K = 5.11). The treatment reduced the degree of obstruction below the K = 9 level, that is, below the moderate obstruction point. At least four patients voided normally after the procedure (K < 4).

Table 1. Loss coefficient K and fractional loss coefficient L calculated from the clinical data reported in Bryndorf and Sandøe (1960)

Patient	K	L
	Normal	
P. C.	0.996	0.499
E. L.	1.994	0.666
H. L.	2.802	0.737
B. I.	1.299	0.565
B. A.	0.992	0.498
S. M.	1.625	0.619
	Slight Stricture	
J. S.	6.194	0.861
J. P.	5.329	0.842
O. P.	8.000	0.889
	Severe Stricture	
J. F.	61.5	0.984
V. P.	15.39	0.939
H. N.	19.40	0.951
J. K.	499.0	0.998

Table 2. Loss coefficient K before and after resection of the prostate. Tests conducted at the Herlev Hospital, Copenhagen. Test records provided to the authors through the courtesy of Hans-Henrik Meyhoff, Copenhagen

Patient	Pre-operative K	Post-operative K
G. C.	100	3.58
P. M.	94.2	5.47
B. N.	57.1	8.18
S. H.	18.1	6.20
B. B.	15.0	9.52
L. D.	12.1	4.85
V. H.	11.6	3.74
T. A.	7.45	3.38
H. A.	7.11	3.80
H. F.	5.99	1.98
F. J.	5.11	2.29

A Further Note About Energy Loss

It has been proposed by Griffiths and others (Griffiths 1980) to explain energy loss in the urethra by a "hydraulic jump", that is by a local collapse of the urethral lumen followed by a rapid jump to a fully expanded urethra. In this model the urine is assumed to leave the prostatic urethra as a high speed jet that expands to a low-velocity, low kinetic energy stream in the penile urethra. This phenomenon is not inconsistent with our energy findings and is certainly possible in long flaccid tubes (Kececioglu et al. 1981). We have tried to find clinical evidence of this jump radiologically and with urethral pressure profilometry and have expended considerable mathematical and hydraulic laboratory effort in the attempt, but have found no evidence in its favor. At this moment we prefer to believe that the urethra flows fully distended at all times and that energy loss comes from boundary separation just distal to the bulbous urethra.

Recent Investigations

Obstruction in the Female Urethra

Delighted with our success in the determination of urinary obstruction in the male, we subsequently attempted to apply the methodology to female urethras (Bottaccini and Gleason 1980; Gleason et al. 1982). The results were disappointing. Although we developed a good method for accurate measurement of exit velocity in the female, we found little or no correlation between energy-loss and disease. In the majority of cases studied by us we discovered that urinary exit energy for a human female appears to be independent of pathology and that flow rate is the sole discriminator between normal subjects and patients. To date we have found no energy dependent diagnostic technique in the human female probably because obstructive pathology is rare in the female.

We discovered that in females with stress incontinence and voiding dysfunction the reduction of flow rate was mediated almost entirely through a reduction of the cross-sectional area of the voided stream. We pursued the subject in depth and concluded that there must exist a zone of active neuromuscular control within the urethra and that surgical intervention in this "flow modulation zone" tends to compromise voiding function and to affect flow rate adversely (Gleason and Bottacini 1982).

Non-Intrusive Testing in the Male

One of the inherent problems of energy-loss testing is the need to introduce a catheter in the bladder to measure intravesical pressure. Both superpubic canulation of the bladder and intraluminal urethral catheterization are invasive, uncomfortable for the patient and carry a small chance of morbidity. In an attempt to avoid catheterization we proceeded to study the correlation between exit energy and obstructive disease in the male. A two year prospective study of 584 male patients was conducted with the aid of a new device, the paddlewheel velocimeter (Gleason et al. 1982). We compared normal subjects to patients with prostatitis, benign prostatic hypertrophy and strictures of the bulbous and membranous urethra before and after treatment. The results were very gratifying. We discovered that if the maximum flow

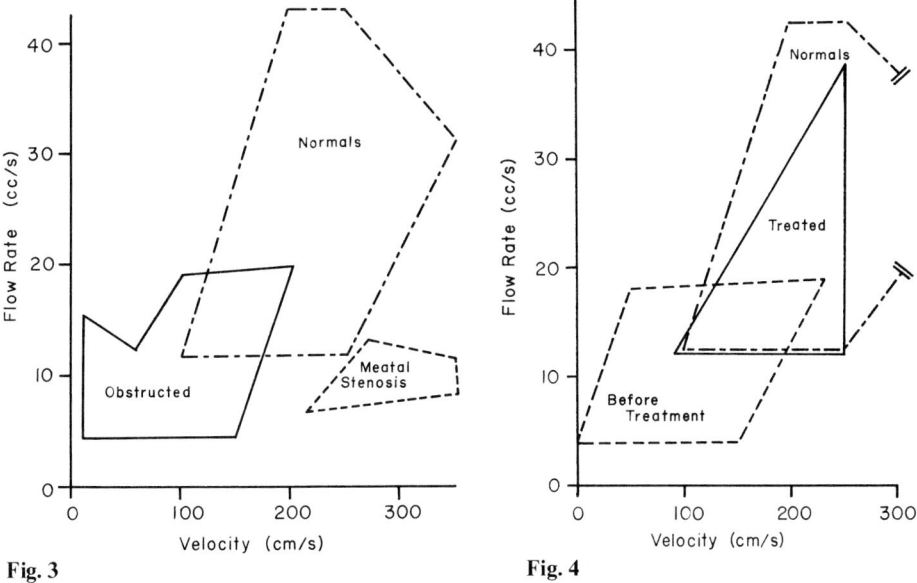

Fig. 3. Flow rate versus velocity for 399 male subjects. The solid line encloses data from 278 patients with diagnosed obstruction of the proximal urethra. The normal region includes 121 subjects. The meatal stenosis region includes only 12 subjects and is, consequently, poorly defined

Fig. 4. Effect of surgical treatment of the prostate. Before treatment: 208 subjects; after treatment: 121 subjects. Note how the post-operative patient population is moved almost completely into the normal region

rate and the velocity were plotted as single points on a graph (Fig. 3) the normal subjects and the patients would fall into distinct regions that could not be separated by flow rate alone. Each disease had its own region in the flow versus velocity diagram and the effectiveness of treatment could be documented clearly (Fig. 4).

Conclusions

Energy measurements lead to novel urodynamic interpretations; we have demonstrated that energy loss, exit energy and velocity give additional information not usually extracted from flow rate alone. For example, a patient with severe prostatic hypertrophy may void with a low normal flow by developing high bladder pressures and several months after resection of the prostate would produce the same flow rate. Such a patient could be listed as not responding to treatment whereas he can be shown objectively to have a much reduced urethral obstruction and a much lower bladder pressure. A patient whose urine flows with a higher velocity after treatment has had his urethral outflow resistance reduced. A patient with low flow rate and high velocity is probably suffering from meatal stenosis, whereas a patient with moderate to low flow-rate coupled with low velocity is suffering from proximal obstruction. A patient who voids with a flow-rate below 5 ml/s and a velocity below 5 cm/s is not only highly obstructed: he most likely suffers from a decompensated detrusor. In the clinic and in the research hospital additional information is always welcome; although we agree that bladder pressure and flow rate will continue to be the primary voiding parameters, we are now convinced that velocity and energy measurements will add an absolutely necessary refinement to urodynamic investigation.

Appendix

Theory of Energy Measurement

In the lower urinary tract a small amount of the local kinetic energy is transferred out of the urethra by work on the boundaries and by heat transfer, but the majority of the available energy is retained in the urethra in two forms, the useful kinetic energy of linear motion and the unusable rotational energy carried by turbulence. Any reduction of flow rate with respect to the normal is the result of degradation of linear kinetic energy into turbulence, that is, a lower "quality" form of energy within the context of the second law of thermodynamics (Wark 1983).

Two theories have been proposed to explain the generation of turbulence within the urethra. The "rigid boundary" model and the "elastic boundary", or hydraulic jump, model. The trigger mechanism is the same in both theories; velocity is increased by a constriction of the urethra; adaptation of the high speed urine to the larger urethra distal to the constriction causes a large local increase of turbulence. In the elastic boundary theory it is proposed that the narrow, high speed jet leaving the stricture is carried for some distance in a partially collapsed urethra and that adaptation to the larger lumen occurs a considerable distance downstream from the stricture. The proposers of the rigid wall theory posit a similar mechanism but believe that the rapid expansion occurs immediately downstream of the narrowing. The two theories are not in opposition because the rigid boundary theory is merely the special case of the elastic theory in which the "jump" has moved as far proximally as is possible.

Let it be understood that in both theories it is assumed that the loss does not occur at the point of obstruction but that the amount of loss is a function of the degree of constriction. The greater the narrowing of the urethra the greater is the loss. It follows, therefore, that measurement of energy loss in the urethra should correlate with mechanical obstruction.

The Loss Coefficient

To avoid excessive mathematical apparatus we shall outline the theory and refer the interested reader to the literature.

The applicable energy transfer theorem is a special form of the first law of thermodynamics

$$\frac{DE}{Dt} = \frac{DW}{Dt} + \frac{DH}{Dt}$$

in which E is the energy content within a predefined control volume, W is the work done on the control volume during a process and H is the heat energy in the process of being transferred to the volume. The symbol D refers to the material derivative (Truesdel and Toupin 1960).

Four assumptions are made:
1) The intravesical pressure is uniform throughout the bladder and is representable by a single variable p_I.
2) The urinary velocity within the bladder is small in comparison to the velocity of the voided stream.
3) The velocity of the voided stream is uniform and is representable by a single variable V_E, the exit velocity.
4. Most of the power is generated within the bladder.

We skip much calculus and write the final result

$$\frac{dE}{dt} = (p_I - 0.5 \varrho V_E^2) Q. \tag{1}$$

The derivative dE/dt is the "power" not available to propel urine. Our equation states that the power loss is equal to the power generated within the bladder minus the power remaining in the voided urine. The expression can be made dimensionless by dividing by $0.5 \varrho Q V_E^2$ a customary and legitimate procedure (Streeter 1979), to yield the "loss coefficient"

$$K = \frac{p_I - 0.5 \varrho V_E^2}{0.5 \varrho V_E^2}. \tag{2}$$

An equivalent parameter is the fractional loss L

$$L = \frac{p_I - 0.5 \varrho V_E^2}{p_I} = \frac{K}{1 + K}. \tag{3}$$

Measurement

The measurement of loss is done most precisely with Eq. (1) although Eqs. (2) and (3) can be shown to be as useful and a little easier to calculate. We need, therefore, bladder pressure, flow rate and exit velocity. Pressure and flow rate are measured routinely in the clinic, but velocity is harder to obtain.

Four methods have been proposed for the measurement of exit velocity, the cast distance procedure (Schwartz and Brenner 1921), the drop spectrometer (Zinner and Harding 1971), the urodynamometer (Byrne et al. 1972) and the paddlewheel velocimeter (Gleason and Bottacini 1982). All four methods give good results but we have found that the urodynamometer meets our needs best. The principle of operation is simple. It is known that the impact force exerted by a fluid stream striking a vertically mounted disk at an angle θ is

$$F = \varrho \, Q \, V_E \, \beta \cos \theta.$$

F and Q can be measured and $\cos \theta$ can be made nearly equal to 1 by keeping the voided stream as horizontal as possible. The kinetic energy and velocity of the voided stream can be calculated

$$E = 0.5 \, \varrho \, \alpha \, V_E^2 = \frac{0.5}{\varrho} \, \frac{\alpha}{\beta^2} \left(\frac{F}{Q} \right).$$

The angle θ and the quantities α and β are the principal sources of error. α and β are introduced into the equations to eliminate the effects of non-uniformity. Since it is known that for fully developed flow $\alpha = 1.058$ and $\beta = 1.017$ (Massey 1957), we feel confident in neglecting them. If, on the other hand, the flow is not fully developed, the ratio α/β^2 can be as high as 1.5.

References

Bottaccini MR, Gleason DM (1979) Fluid mechanics of micturition. In: Krane RJ, Siroky B (eds) Clinical neuro-urology. Little-Brown, Boston, pp 35–43
Bottaccini MR, Gleason DM (1980) Urodynamic norms in women. I Normals versus stress incontinents. J Urol 124:659–662
Bottaccini MR, Gleason DM, Byrne JC (1973) Resistance measurements in the human urethra. In: Lutzeyer W, Melchior H (eds) Urodynamics. Upper and lower urinary tract. Springer, Berlin Heidelberg New York, pp 301–316
Bryndorf J, Sandøe E (1960) The hydrodynamics of micturition. Dan Med Bull 7:65–71
Byrne JC, Bottaccini MR, Gleason DM (1972) Energy loss during micturition. Inv Urol 10:221–225
Gerald CF (1980) Applied numerical analysis, 2nd edn. Addison-Wesley, Reading, pp 214–217
Gleason DM, Bottaccini MR (1982) Urodynamic norms in female voiding. II. The flow modulation zone and voiding dysfunction. J Urol 127:495–500
Gleason DM, Bottaccini MR, Reilly RJ, Byrne JC (1972) The residual stream energy is a diagnostic index of male urinary outflow obstruction. Inv Urol 10:72–77
Gleason DM, Bottaccini MR, Drach GW (1976) Urodynamics. J Urol 115:356–361
Gleason DM, Bottaccini MR, Drach GW, Latyon TN (1982) Urinary flow velocity as an index of male voiding function. J Urol 128:1363–1367
Griffiths DJ (1980) Urodynamics. Hilger, Bristol
Kececioglu I, McLuren ME, Kamm RD, Schapiro AH (1981) Steady supercritical flow in collapsible tubes. Part 1. Experimental observations. J Fluid Mech 109:367–389
Massey BS (1957) Mechanics of fluids. Van Nostrand, London, pp 102–105
Schafer W (1983) The contribution of the bladder outlet to the relation between pressure and flow rate during micturition. In: Hinman F (ed) Benign prostatic hypertrophy. Springer, Berlin Heidelberg New York pp 470–496
Schwartz O, Brenner A (1921) Untersuchungen über die Physiologie und Pathologie der Blasenfunktion. Z Urol Chir 1/2:32–61
Streeter VL, Wylie EB (1979) Fluid mechanics, 7th edn. McGraw-Hill, New York, pp 182–228
Truesdell C, Toupin RA (1960) The classical field theories. In: Flügge S (ed) Handbuch der Physik, Bd III/1. Springer, Berlin Göttingen Heidelberg, pp 337–344
Wark K (1983) Thermodynamics. McGraw-Hill, New York, pp 42–45
Zinner NR, Harding DG (1971) Velocity of the urinary stream, its significance and a method for its measurement. In: Hinman F (ed) Hydrodynamics of micturition. Thomas, Springfield, pp 186–203

Review of Techniques to Evaluate Micturitional Performance. Promises of 1971 Revisited

N. R. ZINNER[1]

It will be difficult to reconstruct the mood and experience of the marvellous meeting in Aachen held in 1971 but I will try to bring some of the flavor to the reader, and to review subsequent events with a view towards examining what progress has occurred since that time.

This presentation will concentrate on micturition performance and cover the subjects of hydromechanics, pressure, flow, and "resistance" which were more fashionable in 1971. It will not encompass the outstanding newer research in pharmacology, neurophysiology and anatomy which has grown in interest since that time.

What were the events that lead up to 1971?

In the main, there was no one item but rather, a series of discoveries coming from broadly dispersed researchers throughout the world. To my knowledge, bladder pressure was first measured by Mosso and Pellicani in Italy in 1882, and Reyfish, in Germany in 1897. Rose developed the first practical clinical cystometer in 1927. This cystometer has been in wide use until relatively recently. Denny-Brown and Robertson combined pressure and flow measurements in 1933 followed by the pioneer work of Langworthy, Kolb and Lewis in 1940.

The role of first in the new era of electromanometric measurement was claimed by von Garrelts of Stockholm (1956). Doctor von Garrelts used the then modern technology of electromanometrics and analyzed micturition in a relatively large series of patients. He standardized his techniques, proved the accuracy of his methods and then demonstrated the distinctions in pressures and flows of patients with strictures and with benign prostatic hypertrophy (1957).

He introduced data concerning the relationship of flow to voided volume in males. My own entry to the field concerned pressure measurements in normal female volunteers (1963). This series, taken from student nurses and prisoner volunteers in Virginia examines intravesical pressures as a function of body position and bladder volume and studies the effects of cough and strain on intravesical pressures. Flow rate is also investigated. The 1963 manuscript, *Clinical Urodynamics I: Studies of Intravesical Pressure in Normal Female Subjects,* introduces for the first time, the word "urodynamics". My reasoning for use of this term derived from the then new work of cardiovascular physiologists. If they could speak of "Cardiovascular Dynamics", we in urology could speak of "Urodynamics". Our work was followed by a major advance by Miller and Hinman first presented at Duke University in 1965 and again before this learned society in 1971. At that time, they demonstrated simultaneous bladder and

---

1 Adult and Pediatric Urology, Urodynamics, 23451 Madison Street, Torrance, CA 90505, USA

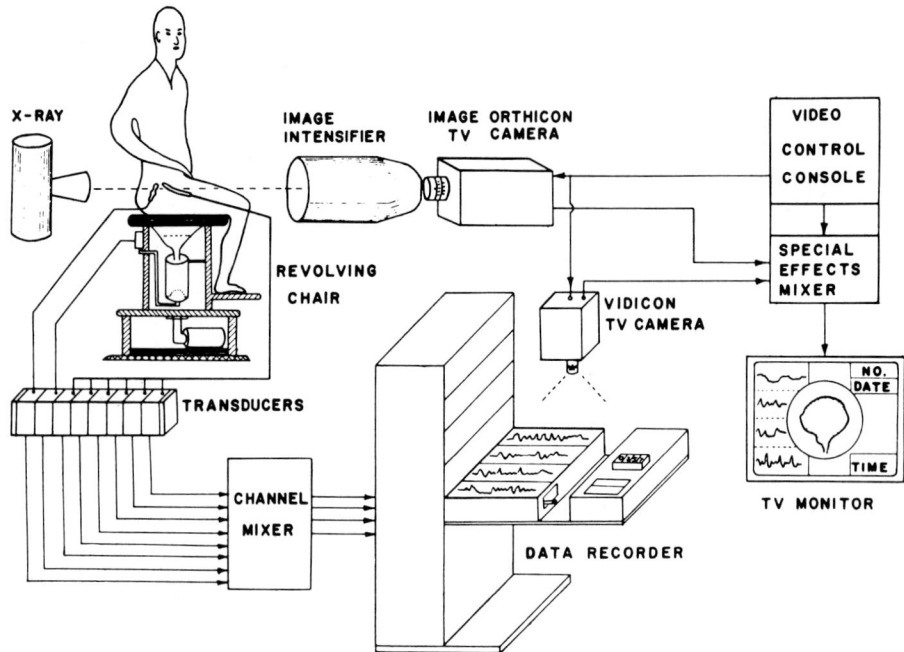

Fig. 1. Scheme of Miller-Hinman system for simultaneous recording of electromanometric information and fluoroscopy of voiding function using television recording equipment

rectal pressure with flow rate on a video screen together with video fluororadiography of the entire micturition process. Their outstanding contributions have stood the test of time. I believe that during this period, these workers also modified the detrusor pressure concept of von Garrelts who, in 1957, measured gastric and intravesical pressures in an attempt to estimate true detrusor pressure. Hinman and Miller introduced the concept of subtracted rectal pressure. Figure 1 illustrates the Miller-Hinman system which, for the most part, is still in use today.

Clearly, the period surrounding 1971 was a particularly innovative one fostered by imaginative people paving new ground. While others were doing their work, my own interest focused more towards noncontact evaluation. My associates and I believed that one interfered with the process of urination by making the types of measurements which were being made – both by physical interference of the probes and by psychological interference of a process which is normally done in private (Fig. 2). Straub, Ripley and Wolf showed this as long ago as 1950 when they performed a cystometrogram in a patient who was simultaneously undergoing a stressful psychiatric interview (Fig. 3). In view of this, it seemed to our group that we would not only have to deal with the external stream which could be measured without physical contact but we would also have to avoid conscious awareness by the subject that a test was being made.

In the beginning, strides by many in the field were directed toward study of the external stream which at least required no internal probes. In 1971, in Aachen, Tam-

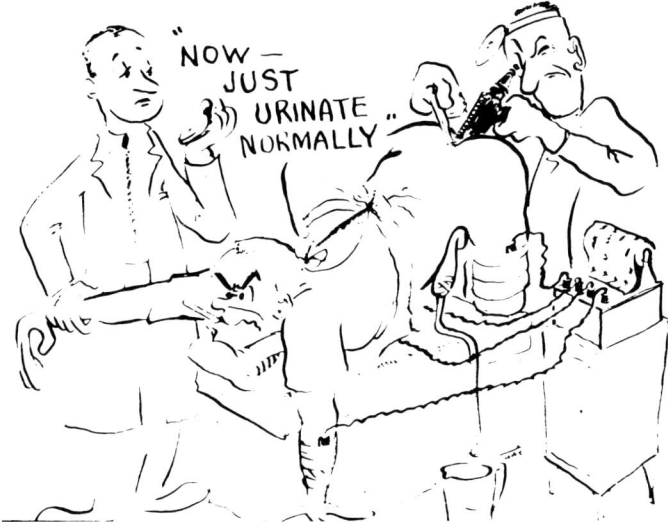

Fig. 2. Depiction of clinical urodynamics study circa 1968

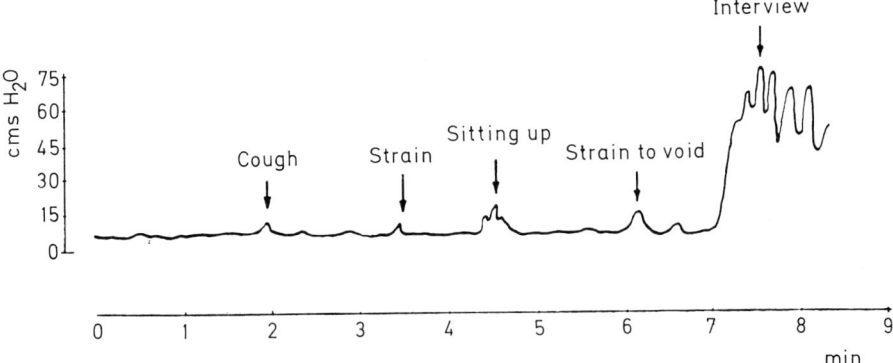

Fig. 3. Cystometrogram showing effect of stressful psychiatric interview upon intravesical pressure

men developed what has become, I believe, the Disa Uroflow meter. Also in 1971, at the Aachen meeting, Scott presented his work on flow. He demonstrated as had von Garrelts before him, the characteristic flow curves of prostatism and strictures and again showed that there is a certain type of flow curve for each condition. Scott made some additional comments which were of note. He stated that no one could really make diagnostic use of the instant or average flow rate or of the numerical value of intravesical pressure alone. One must analyze the curve shape as well. His reasoning was that there is considerable overlap in numerical values even though there are categories of pressures and flow rates which are used to segregate normal from abnormal. Scott elaborated upon relationships between pressure and volume extending previous understandings of this behavior. By 1971, our group had also

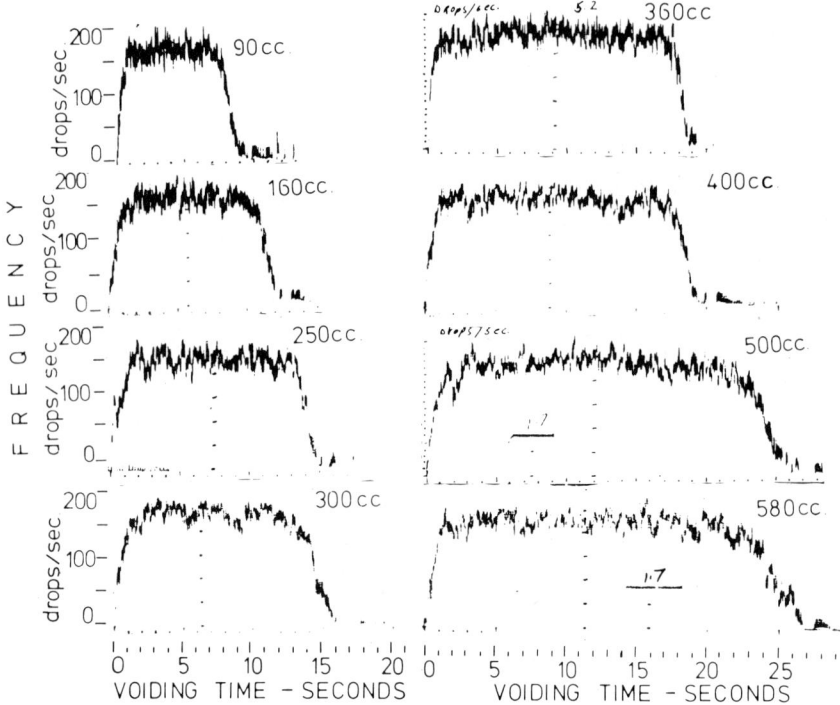

Fig. 4. Eight different voidings from one male using the urinary drop spectrometer for measurement. Note range of volumes voided (90–580 cc). Despite this broad range, pattern and peak frequency are quite consistent

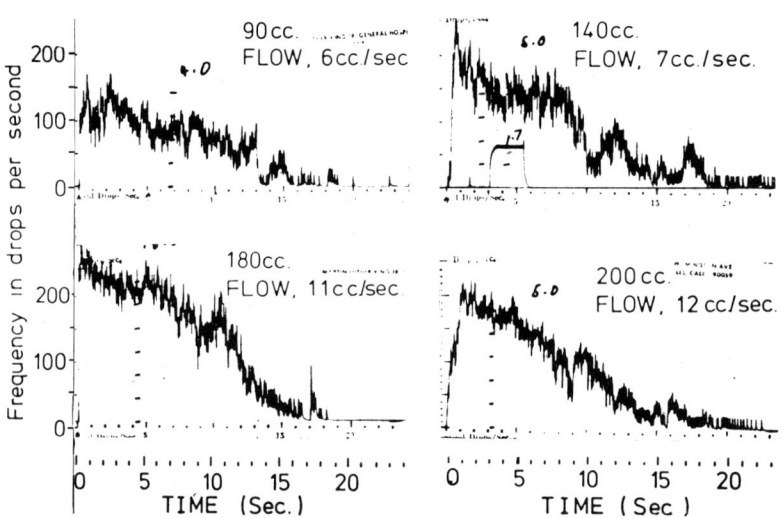

Fig. 5. Urinary drop spectrometer measurement of urinary drop frequency for four voidings from 60 year old male with benign prostatic hypertrophy. Note consistent pattern in this male over wide range of voided volumes. Compare patterns to those of subject in Fig. 4

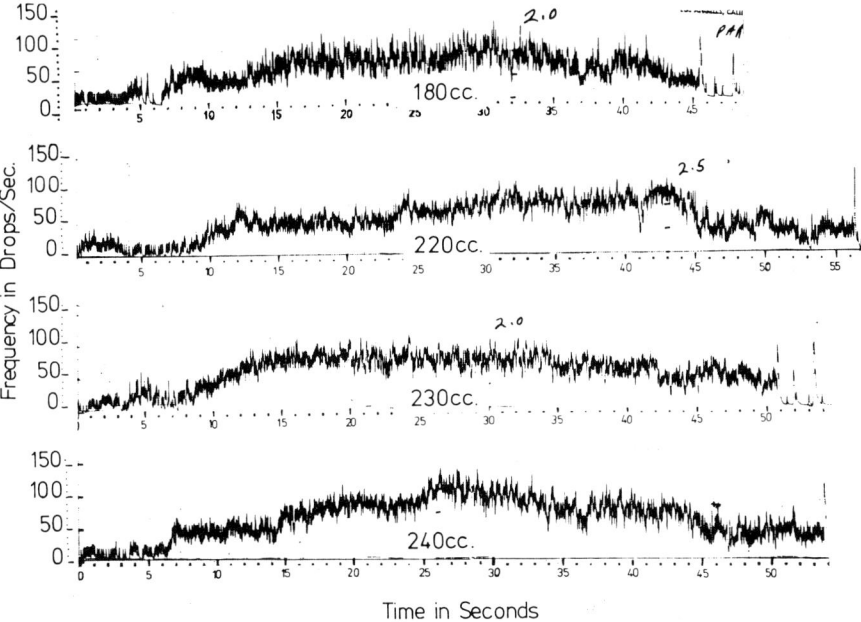

Fig. 6. Urinary drop spectrometer measurements of urinary drop frequency for four voidings from 58 year old male with benign prostatic hypertrophy. Note consistent pattern in this male also. However, compare pattern to patient in Fig. 5 who also has benign prostatic hypertrophy. Note each patient is different from each other and both from normal but each is internally consistent

shown that there is a consistency in flow for micturition from subject to subject despite different flow rates (Figs. 4–6). Platenkamp, using our joint data pool of 4,447 urinations calculated the relationship between flow and volume and confirmed von Garrelts' earlier findings that there are specific mathematical relationships between flow and volume. He added also that these predictable hyperbolic relationships exist for both average flow rate and peak flow rate measurements. Von Garrelts had demonstrated that the flow functions do not apply only to normal subjects. They exist also in patients with benign prostatic hypertrophy. The difference between normal and benign prostatic hypertrophy, is the extent of the slope. He also revealed that in cases of urethral stricture, such mathematical functions are not present and the slope is more nearly flat. Backman demonstrated flow-volume relationships for women in 1965. The reader can see that much of our information on flow comes from very well-controlled research performed in the 1950's and 1960's. This subject is reviewed in great detail by Siroky and Krane (1983).

Despite the proliferation of information in uroflowmetry, our group has always been concerned about unavoidable errors in flow measurement as now performed. Although it is possible for a patient to be studied without internal instrumentation, there are the physical and psychological factors which may limit the usefulness of the measurement. The physical problem is that flow assessment is not accurate no matter how well it is measured by the flow meter. The instrument may be perfect

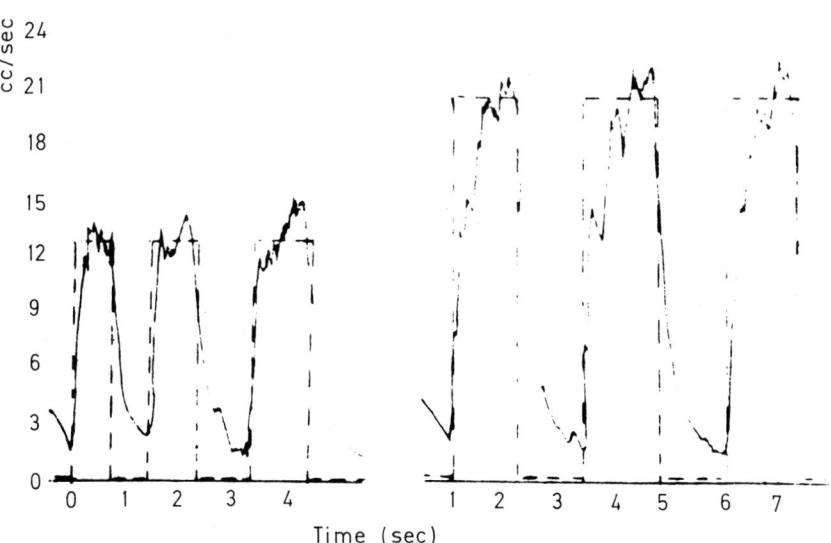

Fig. 7. *Dashed lines* represent actual flow rate; *solid lines* represent measured flow rate. Discrepancy owes to lag in measurement because of use of a funnel to guide urine to transducer location. Note that there appears to be measured flow occurring even when actual flow is completely stopped

but the actual urethral flow rate which is occurring is altered unpredictably by the measuring instrument simply because it comes into physical contact with the flowing stream (Zinner 1971) (Fig. 7). We also had concern regarding the clinical usefulness of a single flow measurement which is obtained in the office and not performed naturally at home. How would the physician assess an "observed" measurement performed "publicly" and on command? To be useful, it is necessary for the examiner to know that the flow which is measured in the office represents the usual performance of that patient when performed under more normal circumstances. I am not speaking here about expected variations between flow and volume but the variations between what is found on a command performance and that which would be found if the measurement were performed privately at home. Because of these concerns, we felt it would be necessary to develop instruments which were physically accurate but also could be used without being detected by the subject who is voiding into these instruments. Initially, our efforts were directed toward modification of existing flow meters and development of new ones. During this one or two-year period, we developed four or five novel and quite accurate flow meters some of which were described in 1971. All were unsatisfactory for our purposes because of artifacts they produced even though each was quite accurate in terms of actual flow evaluation. The evaluation, once the flow hits the meter is different than the flow which exits from the urethra prior to hitting the meter itself. This experience provoked Rogers Ritter to suggest a closer look at urination and later for him to suggest development of the urinary drop spectrometer (Zinner 1969 and Ritter 1974). The instrument was developed and found to outperform the standard flow meter (Fig. 8) because it was inherently more sensitive as a measurement device and because it did

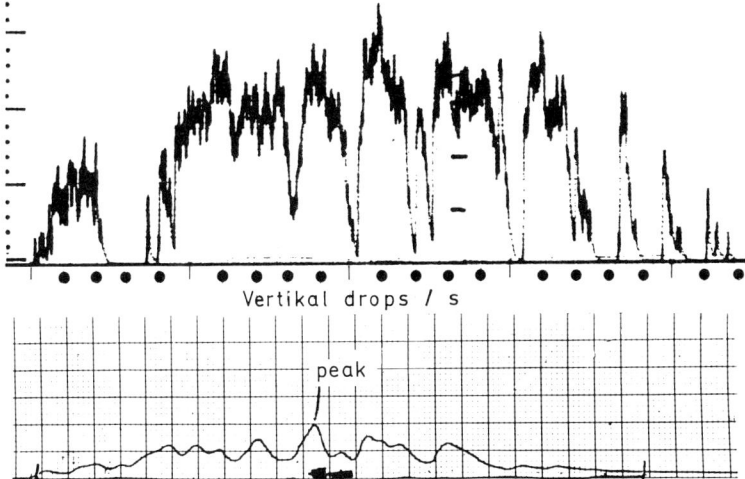

Fig. 8. *Top* illustration represents urinary drop spectrometery drop frequency measurement of voiding in nervous patient who had multiple flow interruptions. *Bottom* illustration is flow rate recording of the same urination made at the same time using the Scott flowmeter. Stream passed through beam of spectrometer into Scott flowmeter. Note greater sensitivity of spectrometer to stream variations

not touch the stream. Also, it could be hidden in a normal-appearing commode. However, at that time, the device was too expensive to produce and could not be made to be fiscally practical. Modern microcomputer technology and other engineering developments have changed this and I would personally like to see us try once again to enhance our ability to interpret flow rates and patterns.

In 1972, at Leiden, much work and testing was done using the urinary drop spectrometer. To evaluate the consistency of urination, three subjects were studied (Sterling et al. 1979). Each urinated over 150 times, data were subject to discriminant analysis to see whether an individual could be identified from a single voiding. By using three UDS parameters, it was found that 95% of the voidings could be classified correctly and the subjects identified from the characteristics of one voiding (Fig. 9). If just one parameter was used, the chances of identification was 50/50. This increased to 93% accuracy when a two-parameter analysis was performed. From this evaluation, we concluded that there is a consistency in voiding just as there is a consistency in a voice print. This is an important observation because it validates the usefulness of a single clinical test – at least if performed with the UDS. Another way of judging consistency is by visual analysis of the shape of the flow patterns obtained with the UDS. Figure 5 shows four tracings of drop frequency patterns obtained from the UDS for a patient with benign prostatic hypertrophy (BPH). Note that while volumes range from between 90 and 200 cc, the patterns are similar. Thus, there is visual as well as mathematical consistency. Figure 6 shows the drop frequency patterns in another patient who also has BPH. While the flow rate varies according to the volume as would be expected, the patterns themselves are quite consistent. Note also that the patterns from the patient shown in figure 5, while simi-

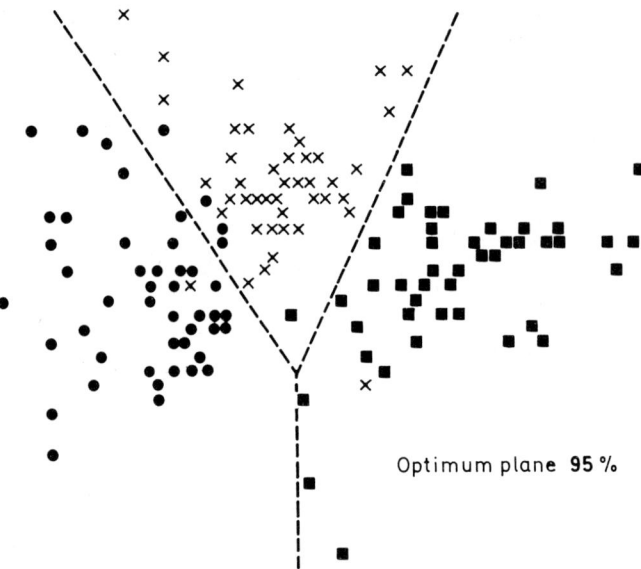

Fig. 9. Multidimensional analysis of multiple voidings from each of three normal adult males. Note that there is little overlap among the three males and that voiding analysis identifies male with 95% accuracy. *Dots* subject R.R., *Squares* subject N.Z., *crosses* subject A.S.

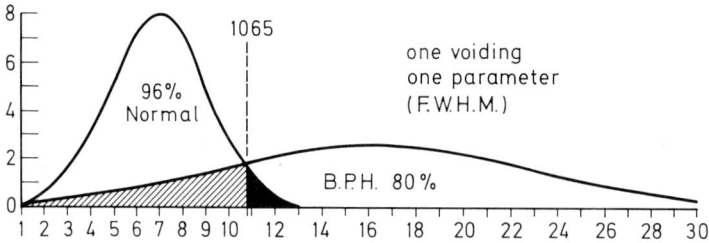

Fig. 10. Diagnosis of BPH from normal based upon one parameter analysis of urination. See text for discussion

lar to each other, are generally different than the drop frequency patterns from the patient shown in Fig. 6. However, both patients have the same disease, BPH.

Once it could be established that there is a within-subject consistency of voiding properties, we turned attention to the possibility of there being a between-subject consistency if the subjects share a particular voiding disorder. In examining BPH, we ask the question – "Is it possible to analyze statistically, the voiding from a patient with BPH and distinguish this patient from a normal subject based on the results of a single urination?" (Recall that at first glance, the voiding from subjects shown in Fig. 5 and 6 are quite different from each other). As it turns out, subjects in

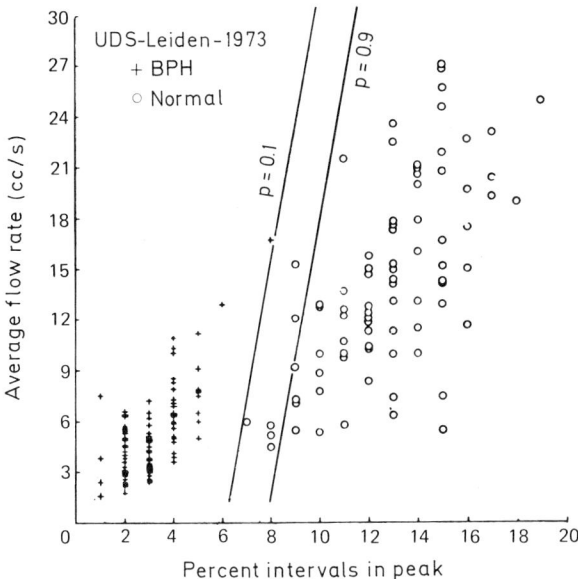

Fig. 11. Multiparameter drop spectrometry analysis of same subjects' voidings as shown in Fig. 10

Table 1. Numerical depiction of graph shown in Fig. 11. Note that only one patient (a normal male) was mislabeled. Of 109 voidings from patients with BPH, 107 were diagnostic; two could not be labeled but were not misclassified. Of 87 voidings from normal patients, 79 were correctly classified; seven were not diagnostic, and one was misclassified as BPH. (From Zinner et al. 1983)

Clinical diagnosis	No. Classified as BPH with probability p		
	$p > 0.9$	$0.9 > p > 0.1$	$p < 0.1$
BPH	107	2	0
Normal	1	7	79

Figs. 5 and 6 share common properties of urination which do align them with each other and segregate them from normal patients and those with other diseases. In a series of 109 patients with benign prostatic hypertrophy and 87 individuals who are clearly normal, it was possible to score 96% of the normal voidings correctly and 80% of the BPH voidings correctly based upon a one-parameter analysis (Fig. 10). Of course, such a result means that 20% of the patients with BPH would have been missed. However when the same subjects' voidings were submitted to multiparameter analysis, nearly every voiding was classified correctly (Fig. 11, Table 1) (Zinner et al. 1983). The results show the error factor to be one-half of one percent

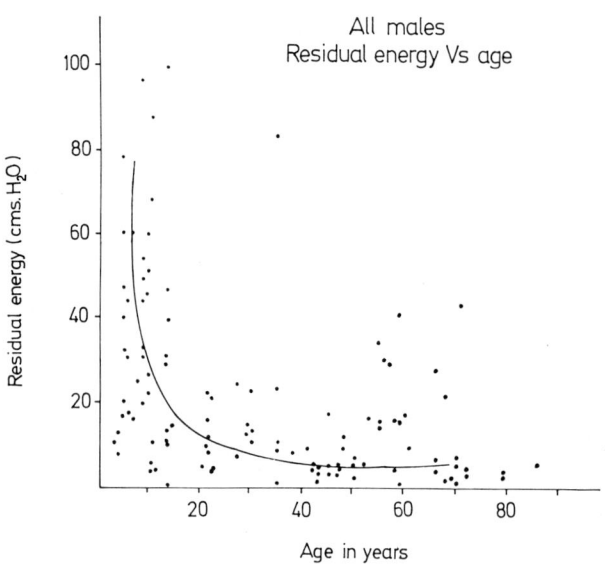

Fig. 12. Relationship between urinary stream energy and age. (From Bottaccini et al. 1973)

even though the determination is based on a single voiding performed on command and "in public". While it is nice to show these data, we must be fair. The patients studied here were known to have BPH. One is not helped by confirming a known clinical fact which requires no other study. What we need is to be able to make a diagnosis of BPH in the patient who is not suspected of having this disorder. The problem scientifically is – "How do we prove it?" In order to do this, I believe that we will need to perform longitudinal studies on subjects beginning in their middle years and continuing into older age. We could then evaluate the early progressive changes of obstruction associated with BPH.

So much for flow.

The study of flow alone as conducted was not sufficient to reveal the entire story concerning the impact of obstructive uropathy upon voiding dysfunction. Research turned to energy factors. Bottacini along with Gleason (1973) demonstrated that in the male, there is a relationship between energy loss and age (Fig. 12). Cass and Hinman also assessed this subject in an animal model in a rather elaborate and beautiful study in 1971. Prior to 1964, the anatomy books described the female urethra as if it were a tube 1 cm in diameter. In view of the belief that the urethra was a 1 cm diametral tube, urologists clinically were calibrating the urethra to 30 French using sounds or bougies. In 1961, Rogers Ritter, a young physics professor at the University of Virginia proved to me that if the urethra were to function as if it were even as large as a 0.75 cm diametral tube, it would empty a 280 cc bladder in about two seconds. Of course, this is absurd.

Using data I had obtained in volunteer student nurses and female prisoners in Virginia in 1960, Ritter calculated that the functional equivalent diameter of the urethra is about 2.7 mm (7 French). This work was published in 1964. The two graphs shown in Fig. 13, taken from our 1964 manuscript, permit an iterative determination of effective urethral diameter (resistance if you will) based upon the flow rate – bladder pressure combination.

In speaking of a 2.7 mm functional urethral diameter, we mean that the normal female urethra functions as if it were the equivalent of a 7 French rigid tube. Such a designation can be used as a "resistance factor". Use of such a resistance factor (which is probably as good as one can get) is subject to criticism however because it

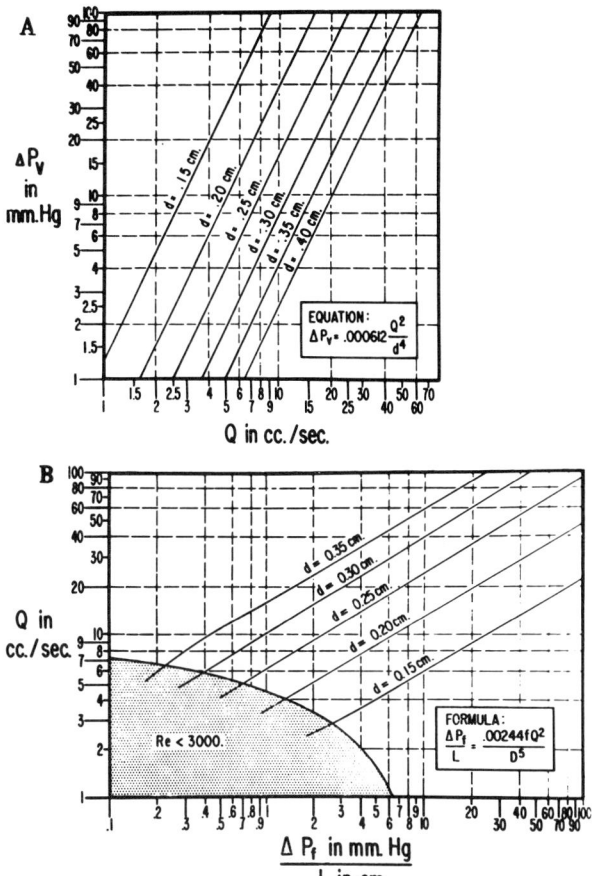

Fig. 13. Effective diameter is sought for round tube which is equivalent in function to urethra by trial and error solution if flow is turbulent. If flow is not turbulent, method is still valid but solution is direct. These graphs apply only to turbulent flow. Diameter (d) is assumed hypothetically when rate of flow (Q) and pressure drop (ΔP_{total}) have been measured. Graphs are entered for assumed value of Q, and values of ΔP_f and ΔP_v which correspond to assumed diameter are read off. (Note that ΔP_f is indicated in cm of urethral length. The value indicated must be multiplied by the estimated or measured urethral length in cm.) Interpolation between drawn parametric curves for d is usually necessary. Values of ΔP_v and ΔP_f are then added and if sum agrees (within 5 percent) with measured value for ΔP_{total}, trial result is sufficiently close. If these values do not equal ΔP_{total}, different value of d is assumed and process is repeated. Iterations are continued until agreement is obtained. Accuracy within 5 percent is sufficient because error of value d is very insensitive to error in ΔP

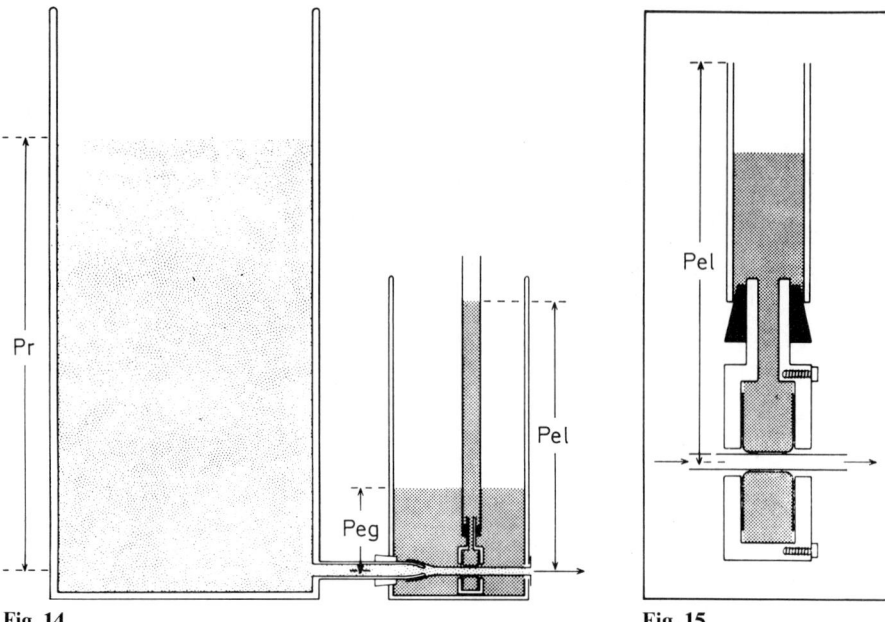

Fig. 14. Arrangement for studying flow through flexible models. (From J.E.S. Scott et al. 1971)

Fig. 15. Arrangement for producing localized extrinsic pressure. (From J.E.S. Scott et al. 1971)

presumes that the urethra is a static rigid system. Bottacini and Gleason (1971) held that it may be all right to view the urethra in this manner whereas those in our group do not share this view. J. E. S. Scott presented some outstanding research along these lines as long ago as 1968 (Scott et al. 1971). Scott used a reservoir with a constant pressure head to drive water through a Penrose drain system. The flexible Penrose drain was itself submerged inside a water-filled tank (Fig. 14). The pressure in the tank which could be adjusted independent of reservoir pressure imposed extrinsic compression upon the flexible Penrose drain. In addition, Scott's model allowed for a further local compression as shown in Fig. 15. If this system were to model the female urethra, the region of local compression would represent the external sphincter. Scott found that the flow rates in the flexible system were less than the flow rates expected if the system were to have been rigid (Fig. 16).

Griffiths, during this period (1969 and 1971) examined both pressure and flow and concluded that the urethra behaves as a flexible system – not a rigid one. Accordingly, we believe that it is incorrect to think of a resistance factor in terms of a single number and that *the clinician should consider the interaction* between the pressure and the flow as a continuum. This was studied by Abrams and Griffiths in 1979. These workers plotted pressure against simultaneous flow to demonstrate differences in pressure-flow patterns between patients with proximal obstruction, distal obstruction, and the normal state. In pursuing his studies, Griffiths (1973) finally proposed the concepts of the *Bladder Output Relation* and the urethral resistance relation (BOR and URR). He described the relationships among the force of bladder contraction, intravesical pressure, and urinary flow rate. He demonstrated that, for a given force of bladder contraction, the bladder pressure will vary inversely with the flow rate. Initially, as the bladder builds up pressure, there is no flow rate. The contraction is isometric. As flow begins, intravesical pressure is maximum. It drops during flow. These interactions are demonstrated by the BOR curve. In addition to the BOR, Griffiths describes the URR (Fig. 17). The crossing of the BOR and the URR defines the lower urinary system at the instant of that particular measurement. Since the system is flexible and changing continuously, the instantaneous BOR and URR interactions are also changing continuously. More recently, Schafer (1983) has come to clarify further Griffiths' work and to add to it. Schafer summarizes most of the material embraced by Griffiths and others regarding the functions of a flexible tube system and adds other dimensions he terms passive urethral resistance relationship (PURR) and dynamic urethral resistance relationship (DURR). Simply (and probably loosely) stated, Schafer's concept holds that before voiding, the bladder muscle contains a predetermined quantity of energy (strength). This energy is used to produce urination. The original bladder energy can be recharged during the micturitional cycle itself. In this sense, the bladder behaves as if it were a battery which contains a finite resource rather than if it were a motor driven by the electrical cur-

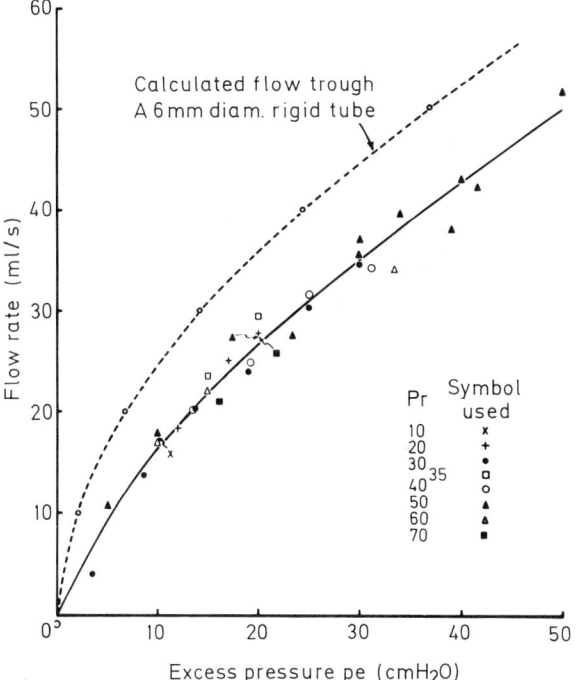

Fig. 16. Flow through 6 mm diameter latex tube. *Solid curve* shows how rate of flow of water through thin-walled collapsible tube 9 cm long with 0.6 cm diameter depends on excess pressure. Rates measured for wide range of reservoir pressures all lie close to same curve. *Dotted curve* shows how calculated flow rate through a rigid-walled tube having same dimensions would depend on total pressure head. (From J.E.S. Scott et al. 1971)

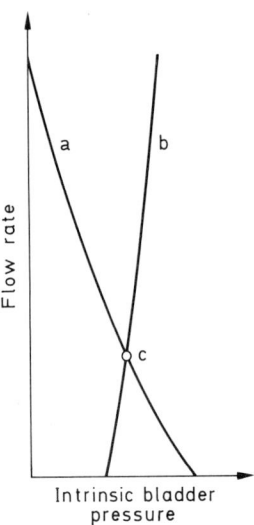

Fig. 17. Relationships among force of bladder contraction, intravesical pressure and urinary flow rate. See text for explanation. (From Griffiths 1973)

rent drawn from the wall outlet. It can wear down. If the bladder contains more urine than can be voided with the available initial power, it will stop the voiding before the bladder empties. However, initial bladder power increases with bladder volume. This, according to Schafer is why there is a relation between flow rate and bladder volume. Schafer goes on to say that while there is a finite amount of power within the bladder for a given volume, the *use* of that power depends upon the resistiveness of the urethra during the voiding. In other words, the urethra controls the *use* of the power whereas the bladder supplies the *source* of that power. As the bladder begins to contract, it forces the urethra open. In doing this, a certain portion of the total initial detrusor power is used to open the urethra to allow flow to begin. The power consumed in this phase creates the condition of urethral openness. The remaining initial bladder power is now available for flow. As voiding occurs, the bladder length shortens and the power decreases. That is, as the bladder volume decreases, the muscle length shortens. If the person is normal, the remaining power produces flow at appropriate rates and the bladder empties. If the person is abnormal, the parameters may change. Schafer describes two types of obstruction: *Compressive* and *Constrictive.* Compressive obstruction is found in benign prostatic hypertrophy (BPH). The bladder neck or proximal urethra opens poorly and causes a dissipation of power during the opening phase. Since more bladder power is spent in the opening phase, less remains for the flow. Since the bladder does not have limitless resources, it runs out of energy before all of the urine has been expelled. Having run out of detrusor power, the bladder neck shuts and leaves residual urine. There is simply a lack of remaining power to sustain the bladder neck opening. While still but a theory, Schafer's concepts tie in nicely with previous work in flexible systems. Discussion of constrictive obstruction is beyond the scope of this report. The interested reader is referred to Schafer's chapters in our recent book on *Benign Prostatic Hypertrophy* (1983).

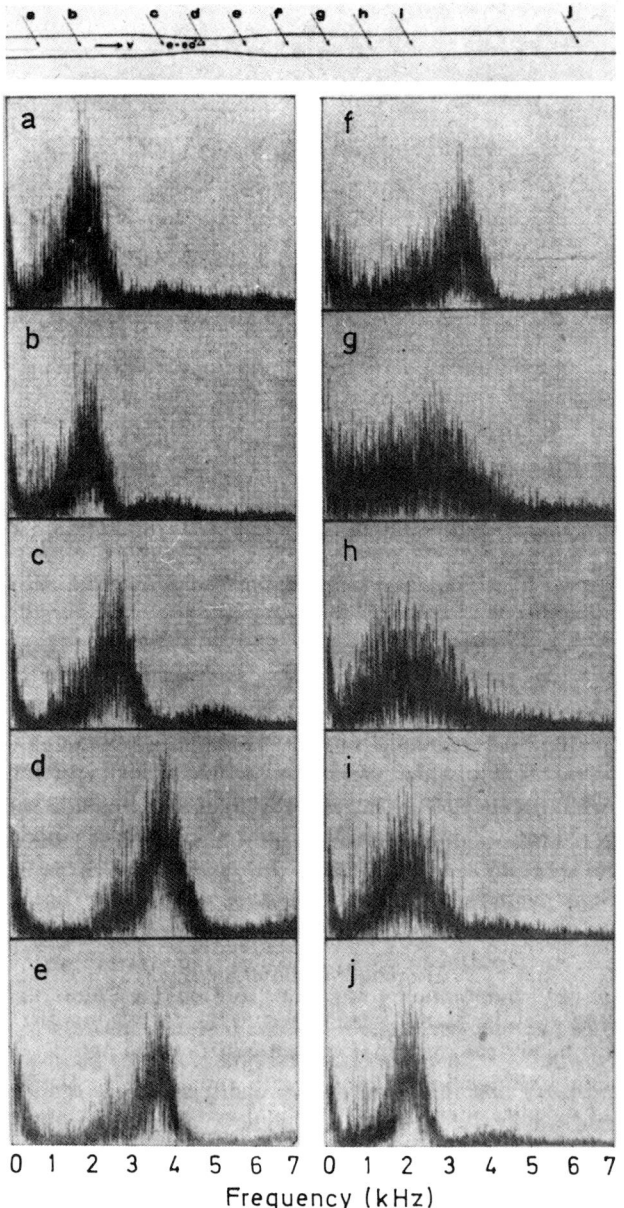

Fig. 18. Spectral analysis of signals from C-W doppler unit when used in model flow system shown at top of this illustration. Observe stricture at location *d*. Spectral analysis of measurements made at locations *a–j* are shown in correspondingly labelled tracings. Spectral peak indicates average axial flow velocity. Higher velocity produces proportionately higher frequency or return signals. Note that highest velocity is in region of strictured segment (location *c*) and that greatest spectral bandwidth (indicating greatest turbulence) is downstream of stricture. (From Zinner et al. 1973)

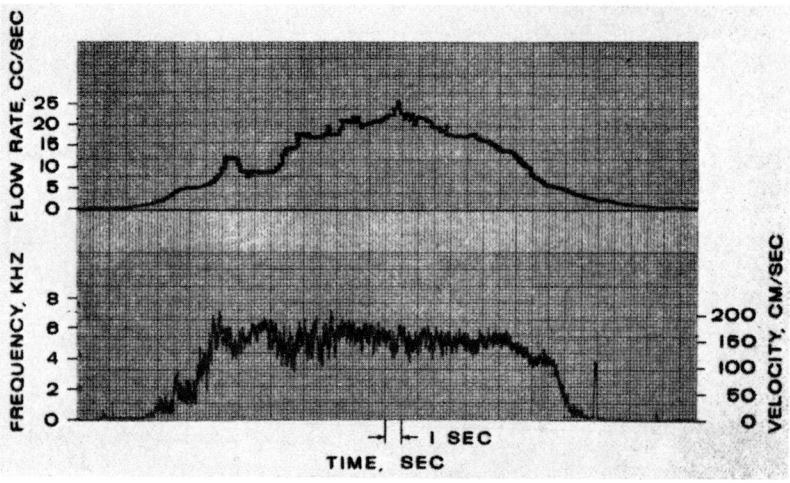

Fig. 19. Analysis of signals from C-W Doppler unit when used in normal human male subject. *Top* tracing represents voiding flow rate as measured with standard flow meter. *Bottom* tracing is simultaneous measurement of stream velocity within the mid-pendulous urethra using the C-W Doppler probe on the outside of the urethra. (From Zinner 1973)

I would like now to review some of the additional material my group presented at the 1971 meeting in Aachen. At that time, we were focused not only on bladder pressures, urinary flow rates and the urinary drop spectrometer, but also on the structure of turbulence within the urethral system. In 1971, we had the benefit of inventions by imaginative engineers which permitted study of local *urethral effects* (Albright, Harris and Zinner 1969, 1970; Gessner and Zinner 1970; Gessner, Nykvist and Zinner 1971; Zinner et al. 1971, 1973). Some techniques were external to the canal – some were not. One of these methods employed a Doppler probe set on the urethra (Albright et al. 1970). Using this probe, we were able to determine local fluid velocities and to understand some local effects without disturbing events inside the urethra. Figure 18 demonstrates the Doppler data obtained from flow within a system containing a local obstruction. From this analysis, it is evident that stream velocity increases as expected within the contricted area and that the spectrum of Doppler signals from stream turbulence broadens as one passes distally beyond the constriction. Figure 19 shows results of use of the Doppler probe when applied to

---

Fig. 20 A–G. Cross sections of normal human male penis in mid pendulous location during normal voiding. **A–C** represent different locations; **D–G** represent same location at different phases of that voiding. Corpora cavernosa appear as black spaces and corpora spongiosum appears as region of white fluffy spots. Ventral surface of penis represented by transverse white line. Rotating scan real-time Doppler used for measurement. **A** Mid shaft of penis prior to voiding. **D** Mid shaft with voiding just starting. **E** Mid shaft of penis with flow increasing. Note larger cross-section of urethra. **F** Mid shaft during maximum flow. Note urethral size now nearly fills space (*3–4*), (*b–c*). **G** Mid shaft at end of urination. Note, urethra again closed. **B** and **C** represent corona of *penis* and mid glans (not voiding) respectively. (From Zinner et al. 1973)

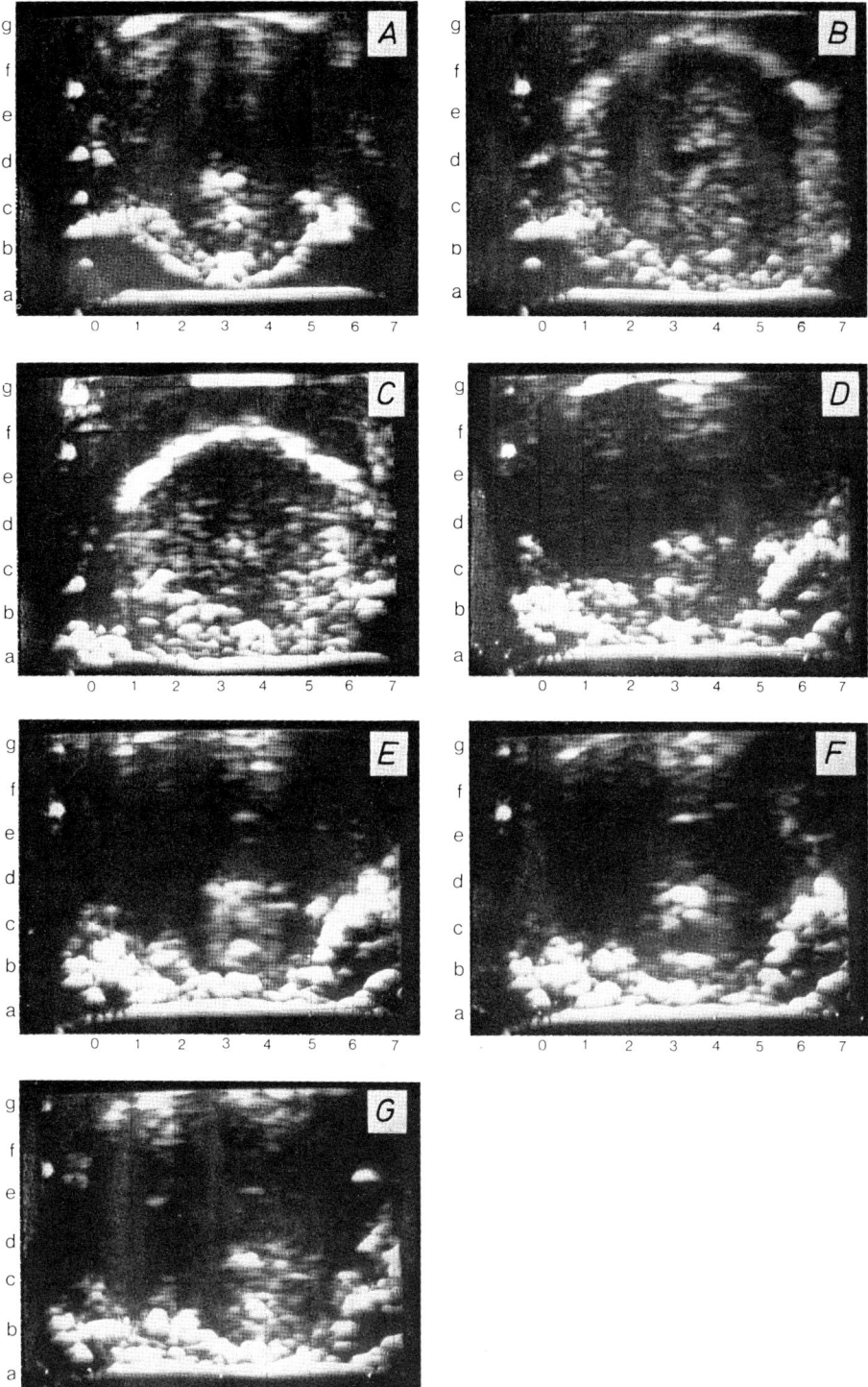

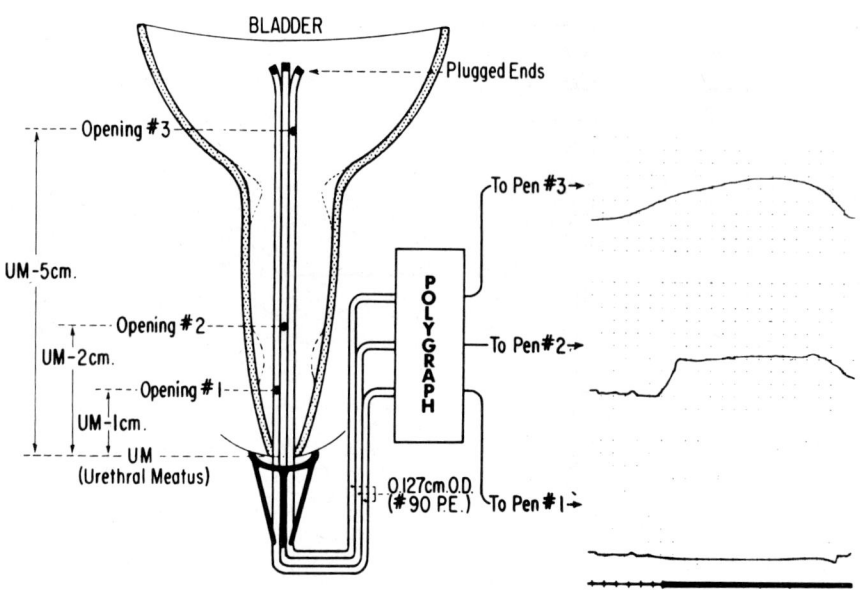

Fig. 21. Triple lumen catheter designed to measure static urethral pressure profiles during voiding. Catheter position held in place by specially designed device shown in illustration. Sample measurement shown on right of diagram. Timing marks indicate seconds. Solid line shows period of urination. Note curve from pen-3 corresponds to opening-3 and represents intravesical pressure. Sudden pressure rise in pen-2 indicates moment of opening of bladder neck. Note that pressure drop occurs accross distal urethra throughout urination. (From Zinner et al. 1963)

the human male urethra. To my knowledge, this is the only measurement of human male urethral urine flow velocity ever made without inserting a probe inside the urethra. Using this information, we were able to calculate that the velocity in this subject was 170 cm/s near the meatus but that within a few centimeters of this location, the flow velocity was only 20 cm/s. In short, we learn that there was more than an eightfold change in velocity along a 2 cm length of normal human male urethra. Another method employed a rotating scan Doppler (Zinner et al. 1973). Using this instrument, in 1965, we were able to demonstrate in real time on a video screen, the transverse lumen of the urethra during an actual urination (Fig. 20). More recently, this writer has used a small parts ultrasound to demonstrate longitudinal urethral geometric changes during flow.

Finally, a word about static pressure profiles. Figure 21 shows work conducted in 1959 together with Dr. Albert Paquin at the University of Virginia. Three small polyethyline tubes were secured to each other. Ends were plugged and side holes cut at preselected locations. The three locations were used to simultaneously measure static pressure at different sites within the bladder and along the urethra, both at rest and during urination. Figure 22 shows measurements both prior to and during urination. The voiding portion demonstrates that the energy loss of the female urethra occurs at the distal 2 centimeters of the urethra. We termed this location of loss, the "control zone". Later, it was to be determined by Rogers Ritter that this

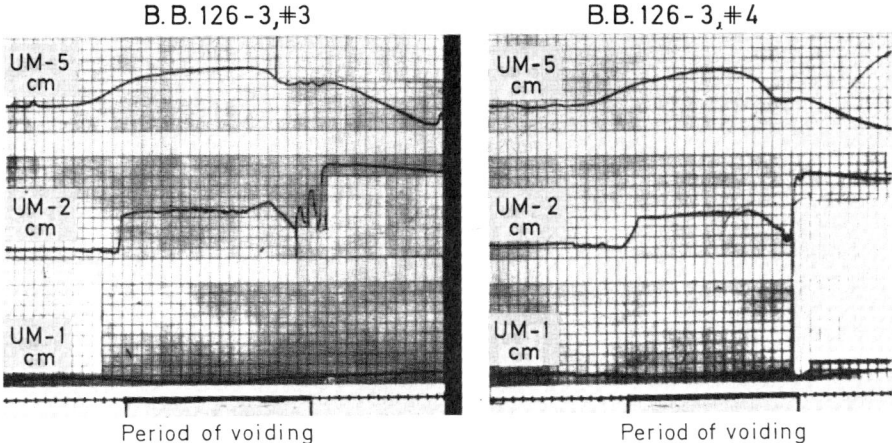

Fig. 22. Tracings from triple lumen catheter in normal adult female subject in two consecutive voidings. Catheter locations same as shown in figure 21. (From Zinner, Ritter, Arbuckle, and Paquin, unpublished data, 1961)

control zone functions as if it had an effective diameter of about 7 French (1964). In 1971, Melchior and Simhan, both of Aachen introduced a catheter-tip transducer. While their device was not intended for static pressure measurements, it could have served in this manner quite well. In this regard, we must again return attention to the work of J. E. S. Scott performed prior to 1968 and published in 1971. In his model, Scott demonstrated static pressure drops across local lengths of increased resistance (Fig. 15). Thus, even as far back as the 1960's, much was known about our subject. In the case of Scott (and others), the work has largely been undiscovered but is now again coming to light. Yalla (1980, 1981, 1983) more recently, has employed static profilometry in extensive studies of human urination. Yalla continues to contribute and has become the most active person in the field of micturitional static pressure profile measurement. The last figures show another type of pressure profile – the total urethral pressure profile (Fig. 23) (Gessner and Zinner 1970, 1983). Using this method, we have also been able to discover the extent and location of pressure loses within the intact urethra during flow.

Summary

This presentation represents an effort to demonstrate the breadth and scope of work which has been conducted in hydrodynamics of bladder and urethral function during the past fifteen or twenty years. It is not intended to be exhaustive nor is it intended as a teaching exercise. It is an overview. We see that in earlier days, much progress was made because of involvement among physicians, engineers and physical scientists. Over the years, the field has grown and now incorporates new com-

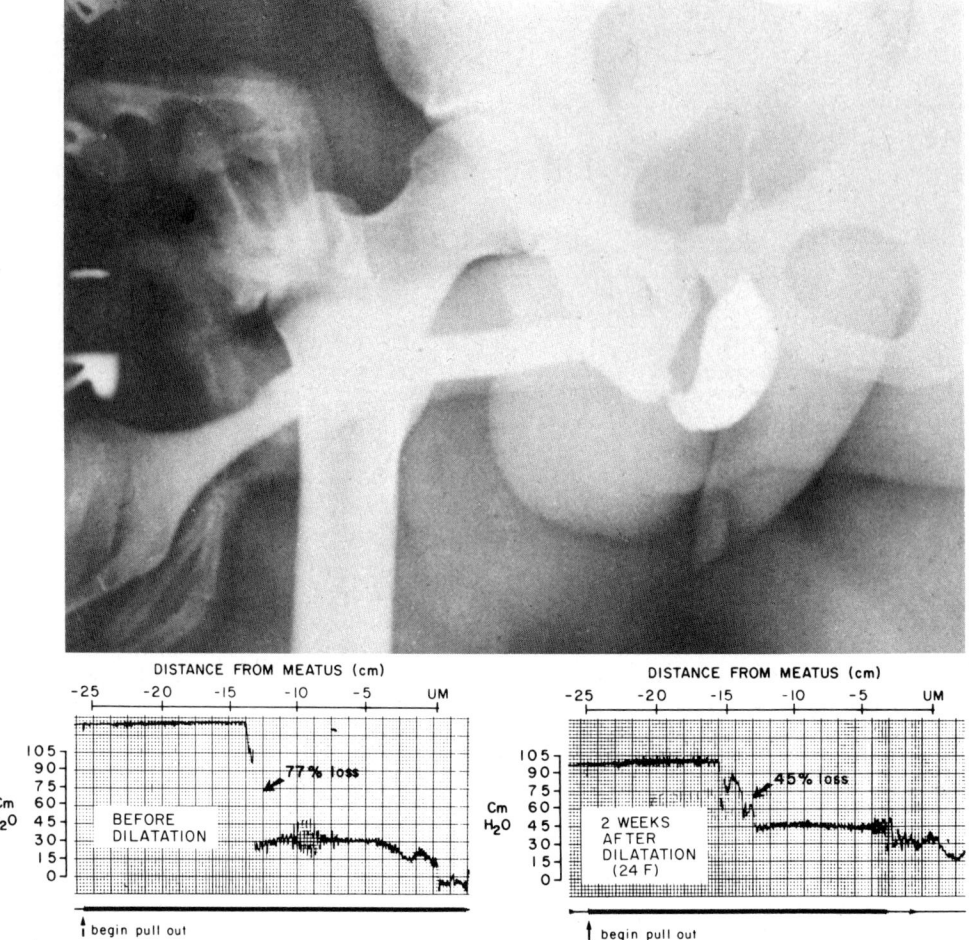

Fig. 23. Total urethral pressure profile measurement during urination in 19 year old male made before and after urethral dilatation. Note quantitiation and localization of urethral energy loss. (From Zinner and Gessner, unpublished data, 1967)

ponents including neurophysiology, anatomy, pharmacology, and the like. I think it is fair to say that we have developed a good understanding of much of what happens during micturition. More importantly, perhaps, I believe that we have developed a healthy basis for communication. Many problem areas remain and new information must be developed. There are many unexplored scientific leads concerning benign prostatic hypertrophy and urinary incontinence and research in hydromechanics should continue on. We need to begin longitudinal studies of BPH starting with subjects at relatively young ages and moving through their later years. This sort of investigation is being performed in cardiovascular centers and should be conducted for urological disease as well. We need to be able to measure bladder pressure from outside. We must learn to better assess the impact of being measured upon the measurement and to understand how voiding performance is or may be altered. Despite the continuing needs which help to keep us all young and invigorated, it has been a pleasure to look back and review just how far we have come and how much we owe to all those people who have helped pave the way for those of us who are here today.

References

Abrams PH, Griffiths DJ (1979) The assessment of prostatic obstruction from urodynamic measurements and from residual urine. Br J Urol 51:129
Albright RJ, Harris JH, Zinner NR (1969) Ultrasonic diagnosis of micturition. 8th Intern Conf on Med and Bio Eng Proc Chicago, 3th of July 1969
Albright JR, Harris JH, Zinner NR (1970) Transcutaneous measurement of the urethral lumen. Invest Urol 8:340
Backman KA (1965) Urinary flow during micturition in normal women. Acta Chir Scand 130:357
Bottacini MR, Gleason DM, Byrne JC (1973) Resistance measurements in the human urethra. In: Lutzeyer W, Melchior H (eds) Urodynamics. Springer, Berlin Heidelberg New York pp 301–316
Cass AS, Hinman F Jr (1971) Constant urethral flow in female dog model. In: Hinman F Jr (ed) Hydrodynamics of micturition. Thomas, Springfield, pp 136–145
Denny-Brown D, Robertson EG (1933) On the physiology of micturition. Brain 56:149
Gessner FB, Zinner NR (1970) On the measurement of local urethral resistance. I. Analytical Considerations. Inv Urol 8:331
Gessner FB, Zinner NR (1983) Urethral pressure profiles. In: Hinman F Jr (ed) Benign prostatic hypertrophy. Springer, Berlin Heidelberg New York, pp 566–576
Gessner FB, Nykvist WE, Zinner NR (1971) Pressure pulse reflection as a means of diagnosing obstructions in the lower urinary tract. J Biomechanics 4:391
Gleason DM, Lattimer JK (1962) A miniature radio transmitter which is inserted into the bladder and which records voiding pressures. J Urol 85:507
Griffiths DJ (1969) Urethral elasticity and micturition hydrodynamics in females. Med Biol Eng 7:201
Griffiths DJ (1971) Hydrodynamics of male micturition. I. Theory of steady state flow through elastic-walled tubes. Med Biol Eng 9:581
Griffiths DJ (1971) Hydrodynamics of male micturition. II. Measurements of stream parameters and urethral elasticity. Med Biol Eng 9:589
Griffiths DJ (1973) The mechanics of the urethra and of micturition. Br J Urol 45:497
Langworthy OR, Kolb LC, Lewis LG (1940) Physiology of micturition. Williams & Wilkins, Baltimore
Melchior H, Simhan KK (1973) A new uro-rheomanometer. In: Lutzeyer W, Melchior H (eds) Urodynamics. Springer, Berlin Heidelberg New York, pp 30–34
Miller ER (1967) Techniques for simultaneous display of X-ray and physiologic data. In: Boyarsky S (ed) The neurogenic bladder. Williams & Wilkins, Baltimore, pp 79–85
Miller ER (1973) Studies of mechanisms of continence, incontinence and voiding. In: Lutzeyer W, Melchior H (eds) Urodynamics. Springer, Berlin Heidelberg New York, pp 204–214
Mosso A, Pellacani P (1882) Sur les fonctions de la vessie. Arch Ital Biol 1:97
Platenkamp GJJM, Kramer C, Hermans J, Sterling A, Van Ness J, Ouverkerk Th, Bout C (1976) Voiding Characteristics of normal man. Proceedings Int Cont Soc VI Annual Mtg, Antwerp
Reyfish E (1897) Über den Mechanismus des Harnblasenverschlusses und der Harnentleerung. Virchow Arch Pathol Anat 150:111
Ritter RC, Zinner NR, Paquin AJ Jr (1964) Clinical urodynamics II: Analysis of pressure flow relations in normal female urethra. J Urol 91:161

Ritter RC, Zinner NR, Sterling AM (1974) Analysis of drop intervals in jet modelling obstruction of the urinary tract. Physics Med Biol 19:161

Rose DK (1927) Cystometric bladder pressure determinations: Their clinical importance. J Urol 17:487

Schafer W (1983) Detrusor as the energy source of micturition. In: Hinman F Jr (ed) Benign prostatic hypertrophy. Springer, Berlin Heidelberg New York, pp 450–469

Schafer W (1983) The contribution of the bladder outlet to the relation between pressure and flow rate during micturition. In: Hinman F Jr (ed) Benign prostatic hypertrophy. Springer, Berlin Heidelberg New York, pp 470–496

Scott FB (1973) Correlation of flow rate profile with diseases of the urethra in man. In: Lutzeyer W, Melchior H (eds) Urodynamics. Springer, Berlin Heidelberg New York, pp 292–300

Scott JES, Clayton CB, Dee PM, Simpson W (1971) Dynamic and flexible models of the urethra. In: Hinman F Jr (ed) Hydrodynamics of micturition. Thomas, Springfield, pp 124–135

Siroky MB, Krane RJ (1983) Hydrodynamic significance of flow rate determination. In: Hinman F Jr (ed) Benign prostatic hypertrophy. Springer, Berlin Heidelberg New York, pp 507–522

Sterling AM, van Ness J, Zinner NR, Ritter RC (1979) Consistency of human urination. In: de Voogt, Miranda (eds) Current and future trends in urology. Bunge Scientific Publishers, Utrecht

Straub LR, Ripley HS, Wolf S (1950) Res Publ Assoc Res Nerv Ment Dis 29:1019

Tammen H (1973) The mictiograph – A new principle in the measurement and recording of urinary flow. In: Lutzeyer W, Melchior H (eds) Urodynamics. Springer, Berlin Heidelberg New York, pp 40–41

von Garrelts B (1956) Analysis of micturition, a new method of recording the voiding of the bladder. Acta Chir Scand 112:326

von Garrelts B (1957) Intravesical pressure and urinary flow during micturition in normal subjects. Acta Chir Scand 114:49

von Garrelts B (1957) Micturition in the normal male. Acta Chir Scand 114:197

von Garrelts B (1958) Micturition and urethral stricture. Acta Chir Scand 114:466

von Garrelts B (1958) Micturition in disorders of the prostate and posterior urethra. Acta Chir Scand 115:227

Yalla SV (1983) Urethral static pressure profiles. In: Hinman F Jr (ed) Benign prostatic hypertrophy. Springer, Berlin Heidelberg New York, pp 577–588

Yalla SV, Sharman GVRK, Barsamian EM (1980) Micturitional static urethral pressure profile: A method of recording urethral pressure profile during voiding and the implications. J Urol 124:649

Yalla SV, Blute R, Waters WB, Snyder H, Fraser L (1981) Urodynamic evaluation of prostatic enlargements with micturitional vesicourethral static pressure profiles. J Urol 125:685

Zinner NR (1971) The need for accurate non-destructive measurements of voiding flow properties. In: Hinman F Jr (ed) Hydrodynamics of micturition. Thomas, Springfield, pp 269–279

Zinner NR, Harding DC (1971) Velocity of the urinary stream, its significance and a method for its measurement. In: Hinman F Jr (ed) Hydrodynamics of micturition. Thomas, Springfield, pp 186–203

Zinner NR, Paquin AJ Jr (1963) Clinical urodynamics. I. Studies of intravesical pressure in normal female subjects. J Urol 90:719

Zinner NR, Ritter, RC, Arbuckle CD Jr, Paquin AJ Jr (1963) Clinical urodynamics. III. Pressure profiles of the female urethra. Surg Forum 14:481

Zinner NR, Ritter RC, Sterling AM, Harding DC (1969) Drop spectrometer: A non-obstructive non-interfering instrument for analysing hydrodynamic properties of human urination. J Urol 100:915

Zinner NR, Ritter RC, Sterling AM, Harding DC (1969) High speed cinematography of human urination. Invest Urol 6:605

Zinner NR, Harding DC, Sterling AM, Ritter RC (1971) Detection and location of obstruction in the human male by analysis of the urinary stream. J Urol 106:115

Zinner NR, Sterling AM, Ritter RC, Harris JH, Gessner FB, Reid JM, Hedges J, Chow D, Barber FE (1973) The velocity profile of the human urethra: Measurement and significance. In: Lutzeyer W, Melchior H (eds) Urodynamics. Springer, Heidelberg Berlin New York, pp 274–291

Zinner NR, Sterling AM, Ritter RC (1983) The urinary drop spectrometer in diagnosis. In: Hinman F Jr (ed) Benign prostatic hypertrophy. Springer, Berlin Heidelberg New York

Ureteric Ultrastructure – 12 Years on

R. G. Notley[1]

In 1971 I was privileged to present to the meeting in Aachen my paper entitled "Electron Microscopic Observations on Human Ureteric Structure". I was greatly honoured to be invited back to take part in the Special Anniversary Meeting 12 years later.

12 years of modern scientific observation is a long time. Many areas of Urological Science have been revolutionised in such a time span. Some observations have been shown to be entirely spurious, some forms of urological management have changed radically, but a few facts have stood the test of time and remain more or less unchanged.

The observations which I presented to the Aachen meeting in 1971 are one of those which have remained unchallenged. That is not to say that none of my conclusions have been challenged – indeed they have – and considerable doubt has been cast upon some of the deductions which I took from fact into the theory of function where the ureter was concerned.

The intention of this paper is to review my original presentation in the light of work which has followed. I must stress that none of this work is my own because when I was appointed as Consultant Urological Surgeon in Guildford my research into ureteric structure ceased within a year as the pressures of creating a Department of Urology in a District General Hospital in Great Britain grew. I have, however, maintained an interest in the ultrastructure of the human ureter. Two separate groups, one in the United States of America in the mid-70's (Hanna et al. 1976) and one in Great Britain have continued to study the ureter with the electron microscope. Claude Schulman, of course, has made great contributions in this field. Hanna and his colleagues did little more than repeat my original observations on a wider scale with more sophisticated micrographs, but probably John Gosling and his co-workers in Manchester have made the greatest contribution to the ultrastructural study of the human ureter in the late 70's and 80's.

I would remind you that the ureter has but one function, to transport urine from the kidney to the bladder. It does not absorb, secrete or in any way modify its contents. The co-ordinated muscular contraction propagated along its length is the mechanism by which this function is discharged. The nature of ureteric peristalsis has been the subject of much speculation and study, but until my observations in the late 1960's no satisfactory anatomical basis had been provided to support any such hypothesis.

The first hurdle was the word "peristalsis", a word truly applicable only to the intestine and defined as a muscular contraction coordinated by a ganglionated in-

---

1 Royal Surrey County Hospital, GB-Guildford

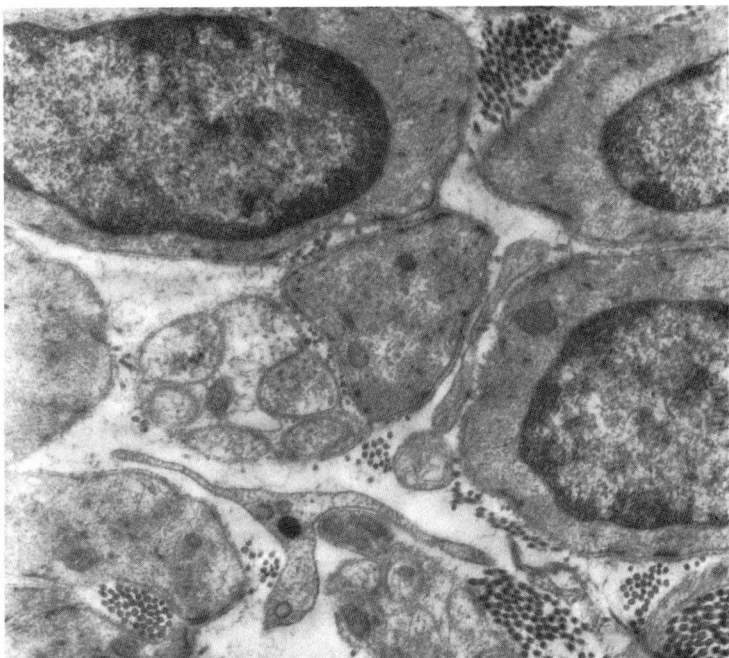

Fig. 1. Unmyelinated nerve fibres within the muscular wall of the human ureter

tramural nerve plexus. The ureter had been thought to be similarly arranged, but the improved resolution of the electron microscope exposed the flaw in this theory. There are many unmyelinated nerve fibres in the wall of the ureter (Notley 1968, 1969, 1970) and many nerve terminals can be found in association with the ureteric smooth muscle cells and its blood vessels, but the number and distribution of terminal axons in the muscular layer are simply not adequate to organise the co-ordinated muscular contraction which we observe. Similarly the nature of the action potentials associated with ureteric peristalsis and their rate of propagation is not compatible with nerve fibre conduction (Prosser et al. 1955) and finally normal ureteric peristalsis can be observed in the isolated ureter. These facts, together with the observation that autonomic ganglia are not a feature of ureteric anatomy (except in Waldeyer's sheath), make it apparent that the innervation of the ureter does not control its normal propulsive activity.

Having cast aside autonomic innervation as the controlling mechanism of ureteric contraction it was necessary to explain how the ureter behaves as a "single unit" visceral smooth muscle (Bozler 1938, 1942). Action potentials passing along the ureter travel at a rate compatible with transmission along muscle fibres (Prosser et al. 1955) and it was here that the electron microscope provided the answer.

Examination of smooth muscle from other organs with the electron microscope has shown points of fusion between the walls of adjacent muscle fibres (Dewey and Barr 1964) which could be shown to offer areas of low electrical resistance which would permit the spread of electrical excitation from cell to cell (Barr et al. 1968).

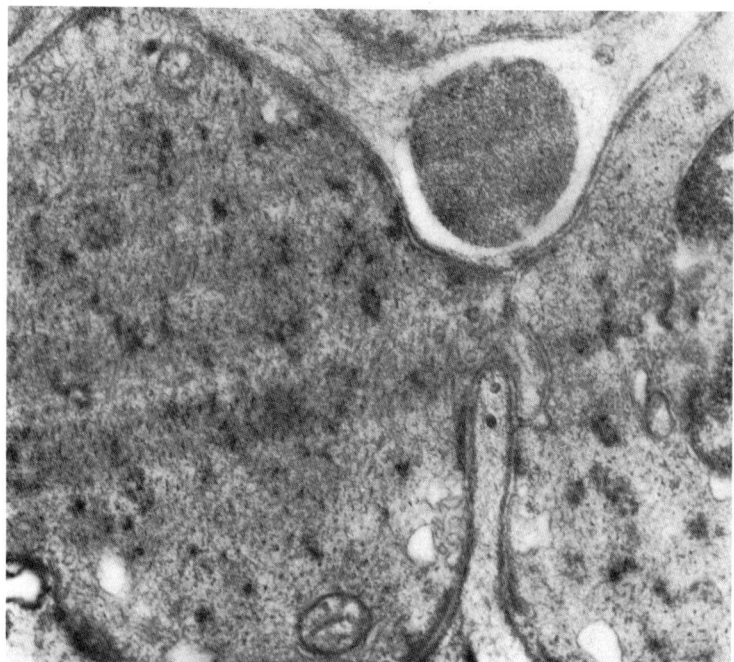

Fig. 2. A nexus, or "close approach", between two smooth muscle cells of the human ureter

That such areas of intimate cell wall apposition or "close approach", exist in the human ureter was demonstrated in my observations (1968). Gosling and Dixon (1978) confirmed these observations nearly 10 years later.

The electron microscope thus provided evidence for an anatomical pathway by which the electrical excitation necessary to produce muscular contraction may be propagated along the ureter without involvement of nerve fibres. Claude Schulman (1974) has shown how innervation may modify peristalsis, but the general agreement is that it is a phenomenon of ureteric smooth muscle itself. Peristalsis normally proceeds from the renal end of the ureter to the bladder, although its direction may be reversed by stimulation of the lower end of the ureter, which is to be expected if this concept of conduction of electrical activity from cell to cell is correct as the cells have no directional conductivity.

Following naturally from these observations comes a consideration of ureteric pacemaker activity. This is an old concept (Bozler 1942), but one which is still very much alive. The most enthusiastic contemporary advocate is probably Constantinou (1974) who has made a number of compelling and convincing observations and studies in this field. Similarly Hannappel and Lutzeyer (1978) provide strong physiological evidence to support the concept of an ureteric pacemaker. The necessary ultrastructural evidence for the ureteric pacemaker is not, however, quite so compelling. Dixon and Gosling (1982) have shown two morphologically and histochemically distinct types of smooth muscle cell which can be identified within the walls of the renal calyces and pelvis. They suggest that a group of cells devoid of non-specific cholinesterase and exhibiting characteristic ultrastructural features are capable of spontaneous contractility and can perform a pacemaker function which is responsible for the initiation of ureteric peristalsis. These cells are unusually elongated and irregular, often with many lateral protrusions or branches. The myofilaments tend to be arranged in elongated bundles and are separated by clusters of granular reticulum, small mitochondria and glycogen granules. A layer of these "atypical" cells is continuous across the minor calyces of the human ureter and it may be that this layer of cells is responsible for the almost synchronous activity of the minor calyces observed by Constantinou and Djurhuus (1981). Positive evidence that these "atypical" ureteric muscle cells act as centres of spontaneous muscular contraction is still lacking, although their enzyme content suggests that they could well do so.

In Aachen in 1971 I put forward evidence of increased amounts of collagen fibres between muscle cells and bundles and in the subepithelial layers of the ureter in the pelviureteric region in cases of idiopathic hydronephrosis and in the juxta-

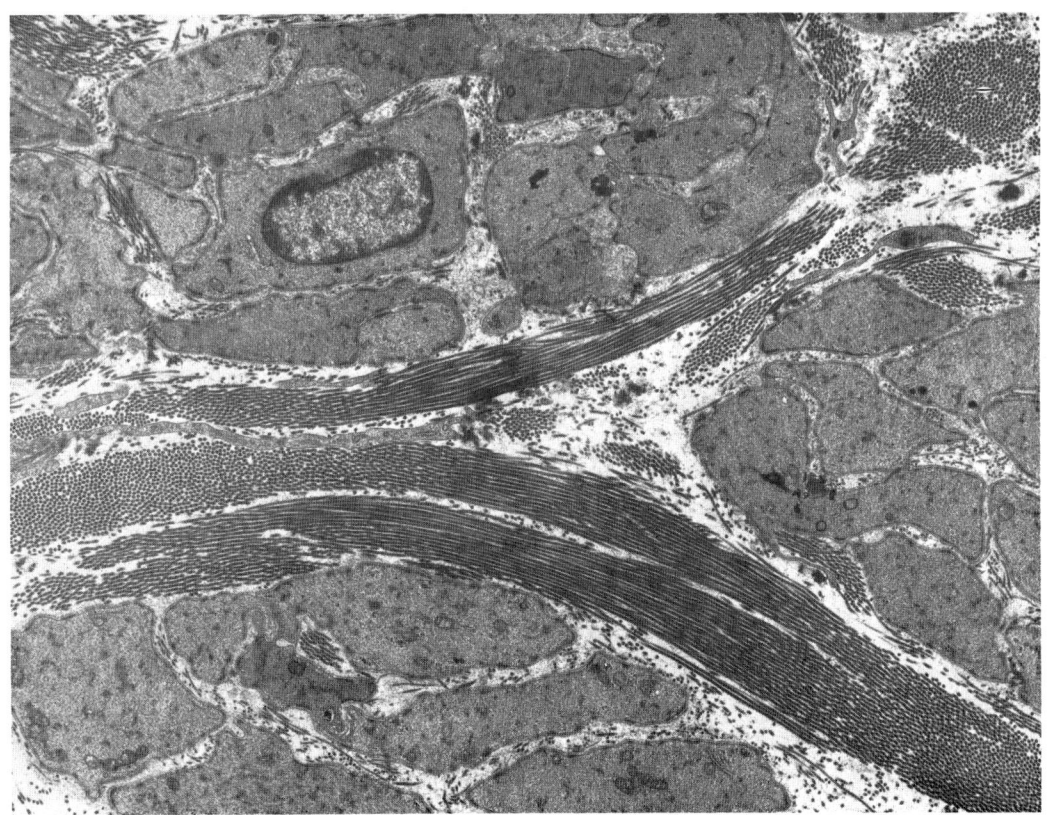

Fig. 3. Smooth muscle cells of the human ureter, in primary obstructive megaureter showing increased bundles of collagen fibres between the muscle cell groups

vesical segment of the primary obstructive megaureter (Notley 1968, 1972). I concluded that these excessive amounts of collagen could act as inelastic segments to produce a functional obstruction of the ureter at these points. Hanna et al. (1976) took the observations further and showed disruption or attenuation of nexuses in the narrow segments as well as excessive accumulation of collagen fibres between the cells, the changes being more obvious immediately above the narrowed segments. Gosling and Dixon (1978) disagreed with Hanna and found, as I did, that the arrangement and fine structure of the nexuses were not different from the rest of the ureter and that the innervation was normal. Thus, on morphological grounds, confirming that it was unlikely that the basic aetiology of these conditions is caused either by failure of electrotonic coupling between smooth muscle cells or by abnormalities in the autonomic innervation.

Gosling and Dixon, however, went much further than I had done in the 1960's and extended their study to include samples throughout the obstructed ureter and renal pelvis above these two forms of functional obstruction. They found that in primary obstructed megaureter and in idiopathic hydronephrosis structural and histochemical changes extend throughout the distended segment of ureter and renal pelvis. On this basis it seems unlikely that the pathological conditions are caused by a discrete, inelastic segment confined to the distal end of the dilated portion. Two alternative hypotheses can be provided – either a primary anomaly of ureteric and renal pelvic smooth muscle is present in both conditions so that an intrinsic malfunction of muscle cells is the cause of these condition or, in contrast, the morphological features seen arise as secondary changes in response to distension, the latter being due to an as yet undetermined cause. We await further information.

To turn for a moment from the musculature of the ureter to the epithelium few new facts have emerged since my observations of the epithelial ultrastructure with its layers, asymmetrical luminal cell wall structure and typical epithelial junctional complexes (Notley 1978).

My title is "Ureteric Ultrastructure – 12 years on". Many of the observations put before the meeting in Aachen in 1971 remain as our modern view of ureteric ultrastructure. We have refined the concept of autonomic innervation – and agree on ganglia in Waldeyer's sheath. The nexus remains, although we may now call it an area of "close approach". The increase in collagen deposition in the obstructed ureter is confirmed, but has a wider distribution than originally noted. Specialised cells which may exhibit pacemaker activity can now be defined ultrastructurally.

The 12 years before 1971 took ureteric ultrastructure from darkness to positive morphological information. In the 12 years from 1971 to 1983 these morphological features have been clarified and extended, but still much in the field of correlation between morphology and function awaits new research. What will the next 12 years bring?

Summary

The original descriptions of ureteric ultrastructure made in the 1960's remain unchanged, the nature of the muscle cells, their distribution in the ureteric wall as a single layer and their intimate relationships being confirmed in later works. The arrangement of the autonomic innervation which was described then, without autonomic ganglia and with insufficient nerve endings to control ureteric pacemaker was developed in the 1970's and 80's by many physiological observations and recently specialised cells in the calyces which may be the pacemaker cells have been demonstrated. It has also been shown that obstruction of the ureter produces specific ultrastructural changes in the proximal ureter and pelvi-calyceal system.

References

Barr L, Berger W, Dewey MM (1968) Electrical transmission at the nexus between smooth muscle cells. J Gen Physiol 51:347–368
Bozler E (1938) Electrical stimulation and conduction of excitation in smooth muscle. Am J Physiol 122:614–623
Bozler E (1942) The action potentials accompanying conducted responses in visceral smooth muscles. J Physiol 136:553–560
Constantinou CE (1974) Renal pelvic pacemaker control of ureteral peristaltic rate. Am J Physiol 226:1413–1416
Constantinou CE, Djurhuus JC (1981) Urodynamics of the multicaliceal upper urinary tract. In: O'Reilly PH, Gosling JA (eds) Idiopathic hydronephrosis. Springer, Berlin Heidelberg New York, pp 16–43
Dewey MM, Barr L (1964) a study of the structure and distribution of the nexus. J Cell Biol 23:553–585
Dixon JS, Gosling JA (1982) The musculature of the human renal calices, pelvis and upper ureter. J Anat (Lond) 135:129–137
Gosling JA, Dixon JS (1978) Functional obstruction of the ureter and renal pelvis. A histological and electron microscopic study. Br J Urol 50:145–152
Hanna MK, Jeffs RD, Sturgess JM, Barkin M (1976) Ureteral structure and ultrastructure. Part II. Congenital ureteropelvic junction obstruction and primary obstructive megaureter. J Urol 116:725–730
Hannappel J, Lutzeyer W (1978) Pacemaker localisation in the renal pelvis of the unicaliceal kidney. In vitro study in the rabbit. Eur Urol 4:192–194
Notley RG (1968) Electron microscopy of the upper ureter and the pelvi-ureteric junction. Br J Urol 40:37–52
Notley RG (1969) The innervation of the upper ureter in man and in the rat: an ultrastructural study. J Anat (Lond) 105:393–402
Notley RG (1970) Electron microscopy of the lower ureter in man. Br J Urol 42:439–445
Notley RG (1972) Electron microscopy of the primary obstructive megaureter. Br J Urol 44:229–234
Notley RG (1978) Ureteral morphology. Urology 12:8–14
Prosser CL, Smith CE, Melton CE (1955) Conduction of action potentials in the ureter of the rat. Am J Physiol 181:651–660
Schulman CC (1974) Electron microscopy of the human ureteric innervation. Br J Urol 42:609

Innervation of the Ureter: A Histochemical and Ultrastructural Study

C. C. Schulman[1]

Summary

The role of the autonomic nervous system in the physiology of the ureter remains controversial.

Histochemical studies using catecholamine fluorescence and actetylcholinesterase have revealed a rich network of adrenergic and cholinergic nerve fibers in the human and animal ureter. Terminal fibers and mixed ganglia (adrenergic and cholinergic), which are located in the end of the ureter, represent this innervation.

Ultrastructural studies of the ureter's nerve supply confirm the presence of both adrenergic and cholinergic fibers. Both types of nerve form terminal and preterminal vegetations throughout the length of their axons. The existence of adrenergic nerve fibers is further confirmed by the use of 5-hydroxydopamine, a false transmitter, which permits selective identification of such fibers. Both types of fiber are to be found side by side in a single nerve bundle, suggesting a functional interaction between them in the ureter. The cholinergic endings are thought to be sensory. 'Purinergic' terminals possibly releasing cyclic nucleotides as transmitters are also found in the ureteral muscle and submucosa.

A model of the ureteral nerve supply is proposed in the light of these ultrastructural studies; it takes particular account of the numerous fine intramuscular connections and the rarity of direct neuromuscular contact.

This model regards ureteral peristalsis as an essentially myogenic phenomenon, the influence of the autonomic nerve supply being secondary and likely to play an important role in modulating peristalsis and influencing ureteral tone.

The ureterovesical ganglia represent "short adrenergic neurones", so-called because they arise from sympathetic ganglia situated in the innervated organ in contrast to the classical arrangement of the autonomic nervous system.

Electron microscope studies cast further light on the nature of these ureterovesical ganglia. They emphasize the presence of adrenergic structures such as adrenergic nerve endings and tiny cells rich in cathecholamines. These components of the system probably modulate ganglionic function in order to integrate the activities of bladder and ureter.

The nerve supply to the ureter comprises the superior, middle and inferior ureteral nerves derived respectively from the renal and aortic plexuses, from the superior hypogastric nerve and from the pelvic plexus (Mitchell 1938; Kuntz 1953; Pick 1970).

---

[1] Department of Urology, University Clinics of Brussels, Erasme Hospital, B-1070 Brussels

While there is agreement about the extrinsic innervation of the ureter among most authors, the distribution and structure of the intramural nerve fibres remains controversial.

The control of the ureteral function is in fact far from resolved. Despite a large number of morphological and physiological studies, some very different and frequently opposing views on the role of the autonomic nervous system have been expressed.

Various physiological and pharmacological studies lend support to the notions that ureteral peristalsis is either purely myogenic in its control, or purely neurogenic.

The myogenic theory derives from the fundamental studies of Engelmann (1869). Later pharmacological and electrophysiological studies by Bozler (1938), Lapides (1948) and Kiil (1957) all tend to confirm the myogenic hypothesis. The theory is further supported by the continuing normal peristaltic function of the transplanted ureter (O'Connor and Dawson-Edwards 1959), by the persistence of the normal antegrade peristalsis even after in situ inversion of a segment of ureter (Melick et al. 1961) and the failure of certain authors to modify peristaltic activity with sympathetic and parasympathetic drugs (Bozler 1938; Lapides 1948; Kiil 1957).

Others believe that the response of the ureter to different pharmacological agents could be due to a direct effect of such drugs on the muscle cells rather than the modification of autonomic reflex activity (Kaplan et al. 1968). However subsequent physiological and pharmacological studies reached to the contrary conclusion that the autonomic nervous system *does* influence ureteral activity (see review by Boyarsky and Labay 1972). Thus eventual proof of autonomic influence in ureteral peristalsis must depend on the demonstration of α and β adrenergic receptors (McLeod et al. 1973; Rose and Gillenwater 1974; Weiss 1975) and a high concentration of catecholamines in the ureter (Boyarsky et al. 1966).

It should also be noted that much of the impetus towards the development of the myogenic theory arose out of the past failure to demonstrate nerve endings in the ureteral muscle histologically (Engelmann 1869; Disselhorst 1894; Satani 1919; Pieper 1953; Gosling 1970).

One of the major difficulties in assessing the role of the autonomic nervous system in the control of peristalsis stems is due to the lack of any defined structure or distribution of nerve endings in the musculature of this organ. Indeed, for decades morphological studies have been limited to classical histological techniques such as methylene blue uptake and silver impregnation, which as they failed to distinguish sympathetic from parasympathetic fibres have always been inconclusive.

Specific histochemical techniques with the ability to distinguish between adrenergic (catecholamine fluorescence) and cholinergic (acetylcholinesterase) structures, have provided a new approach to this controversial subject. By using the electron microscope it was possible to examine the ultrastructure of the nerve supply to the smooth muscle of the ureter and therefore to propose a model of the ureteral innervation at cellular level.

Our own ultrastructural studies have similarly been able to establish the distribution of the various components of the autonomic nervous system, giving some idea of the motor and sensory roles played by these nerves in the ureter.

Material and Methods

Material included the human ureters removed during surgical operations and specimens from different animal species (rabbits, dogs, guinea-pigs).

The histochemical studies were directed towards the cholinergic fibers, identified by their acetylcholinesterase (AchE) content according to the technique of Karnovsky and Roots (1964) as modified by El-Badawi and Schenk (1967).

Adrenergic structures were located by the method of catecholamine fluorescence described by Falck et al. (1962) and modified for frozen section study according to the method described by Spriggs et al. (1966).

Ultrastructural studies were made on specimens fixed by 4% glutaraldehyde in cacodylate buffer and stained with osmium tetroxide.

Medium sections were stained with toluidine blue and finer cuts with uranyl acetate and lead citrate. Certain specimens were further stained with 1–3% potassium permanganate in veronal acetate buffer at pH 7.4, after incubation for 2 h in Krebs-Ringer solution at 37 °C (Dewey and Barr 1962; Richardson 1966).

The greater part of the electron microscopic studies were carried out on human ureters.

In addition, one series of animals received an intravenous injection of 5-hydroxydopamine (5-OH-DA) 10 mg/kg preceded by an intraperitoneal injection of α-methylmetatyrosine (α-MMT) 200 mg/kg 20 h and 4 h before the experiment. Some of the human ureters were incubated for 30 min in a Krebs-Ringer solution containing 1 mg/ml of 5-OH-DA (Tranzer and Thoenen 1967) at 37 °C before being submitted to electron microscopy as described above.

Results and Discussion

This article is limited to the principal results obtained and a discussion of their implications. For the sake of clarity the innervation of the ureter itself is described first, followed by a study of the ureterovesical ganglia.

Innervation of the Ureter

Our own work has shown that the nerve supply to the ureter includes both sympathetic and parasympathetic elements (Schulman 1973; Schulman et al. 1972, 1973).

Generally speaking the nerve fibres enter the ureter alongside the vessels. They ramify throughout the different layers of the ureter where, according to the model described by Hillarp (1946) they form an autonomic ground plexus.

The intrinsic innervation is characterized by perivascular plexuses situated in the adventitia, smooth muscle and submucosa. An independent network of fibers traverses the different layers of the ureter. This system is particularly well represented in the ureteral submucosa where the nerve-endings are predominantly cholinergic. The intrinsic nerve supply also includes a series of perivascular adrenergic and

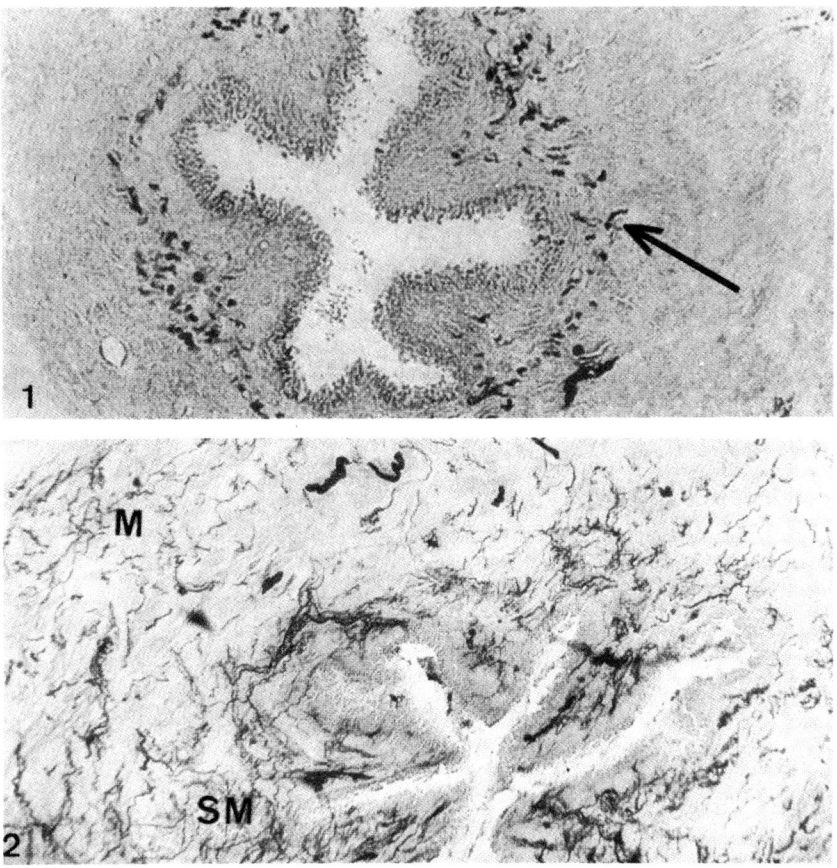

Fig. 1. Upper ureter (dog) – acetylcholinesterase (AChE) staining: only a few fibres are to be seen in the ureteral submucosa (x50)

Fig. 2. Terminal ureter (dog) – AChE: rich innervation of a submucosa (*SM*); less dense cholinergic supply to the muscle layer (*M*) (x50)

cholinergic plexuses distributed throughout the different layers of ureteral tissue (Figs. 1–4).

The density of the nerve supply increases progressively from the top end of the ureter towards the bladder, the pelvic segment being more richly innervated than the lumbar. This variation in density of innervation might eventually explain the different responses of different segments of ureter to certain drugs, tested under standard conditions (Kiil 1957; Hannappel and Golenhofen 1974).

Ultrastructural examination confirms the presence of adrenergic and cholinergic fibres.

In fact two types of terminal fiber can be recognized in the ureteral smooth muscle depending on the type of synaptic vesicle contained in the terminal swellings (Richardson 1966). The first type, representing the cholinergic endings, contains mostly small, pale vesicles (25–60 nm) and a few which are large and granular

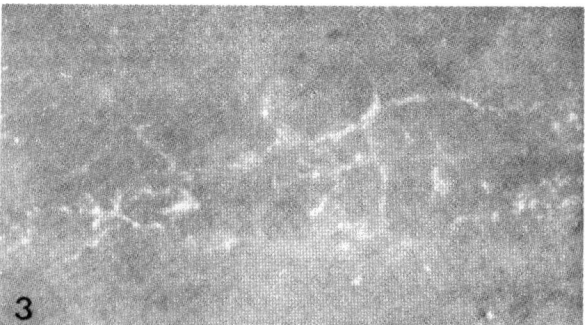

Fig. 3. Lower ureter (dog) – catecholamine fluorescence: network of fluorescing adrenergic fibres in the muscle coat (x80)

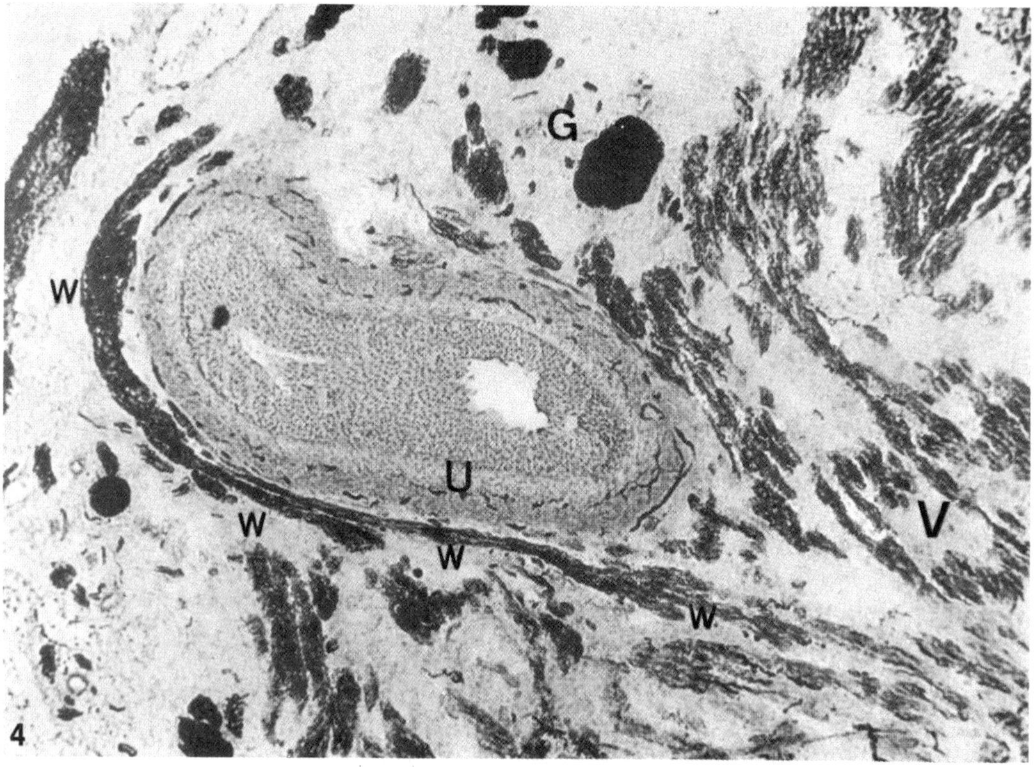

Fig. 4. Ureterovesical junction (rabbit) – AChE: major difference in the richness of nerve supply between the ureteral (*U*) and vesical (*V*) muscle. The innervation of the peri-ureteral sheath of Waldeyer (*W*) is identical to that of the bladder musculature. Ganglia (*G*) are to be seen at the ureterovesical junction (x60)

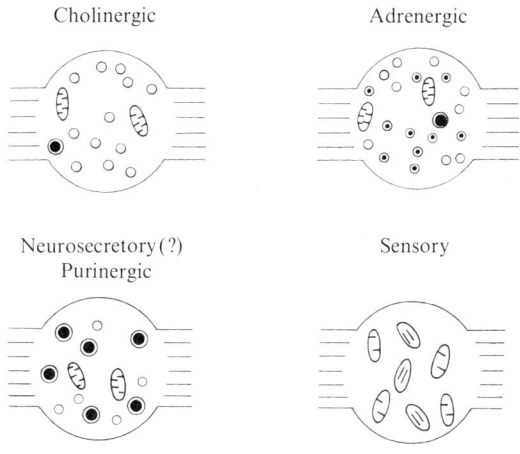

- ○ Agranular synaptic vesicle (30–50 nm)
- ⊙ Vesicle with small dense grain (30–50 nm)
- ● Vesicle with large dense grain (60–200 nm)
- 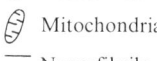 Mitochondria
- ≡ Neurofibrils

Fig. 5. Diagram of the different types of synapse-like swellings

(70–160 nm) (Fig. 5). The other group contains mainly large granular vesicles and a few smaller granular vesicles (25–60 nm) corresponding to the electron-dense vesicles which contain noradrenaline (Taxi and Droz 1966; Wolfe et al. 1967; Hokfelt 1969).

Most physiological and pharmacological studies of the ureter have demonstrated the presence of α-stimulant and β-inhibitory receptors. Knowing that the ureter is able to contract without any nervous stimulation these studies suggest that the adrenergic fibres in the ureteral wall are likely to function as modulators of ureteral tone and force of contraction.

The current electron microscopic study confirms the presence of adrenergic nerve terminals in the different layers of both animal and human ureters (Fig. 6).

Their existence is further confirmed by the use of false chemical transmitters such as 5-hydroxydopamine. It has recently been demonstrated that these substances can act as selective markers for adrenergic nerve endings in the peripheral autonomic nervous system (Tranzer and Thoenen 1967).

False transmitters displace the endogenous noradrenaline contained in the terminal vesicles, and because of their affinity to osmic acid, permit a localization of terminal fibres which are capable of taking up and storing biogenic amines (Tranzer et al. 1969).

Thus, after treatment with 5-OH-DA, in numerous axons in the muscle coat and submucosa vesicles can be found which contain very dense particles. Cholinergic fibres, on the other hand, are unchanged by such a treatment (Tranzer et al. 1969).

Cholinergic and adrenergic fibres are commonly found in the same nerve bundle running parallel to each other suggesting a possible functional interaction between

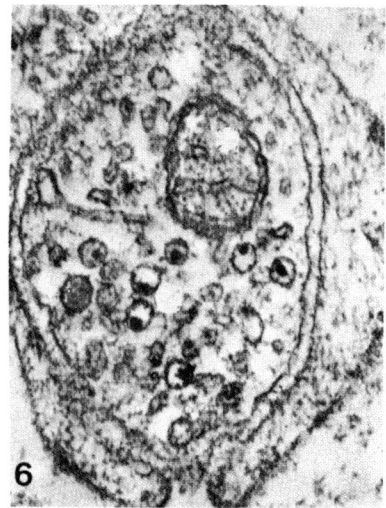

Fig. 6. Enlargement of adrenergic axon characterized by numerous small vesicles containing dense granules, a few large granular vesicles and some mitochondria (incubation in a solution of noradrenaline) (x120,000)

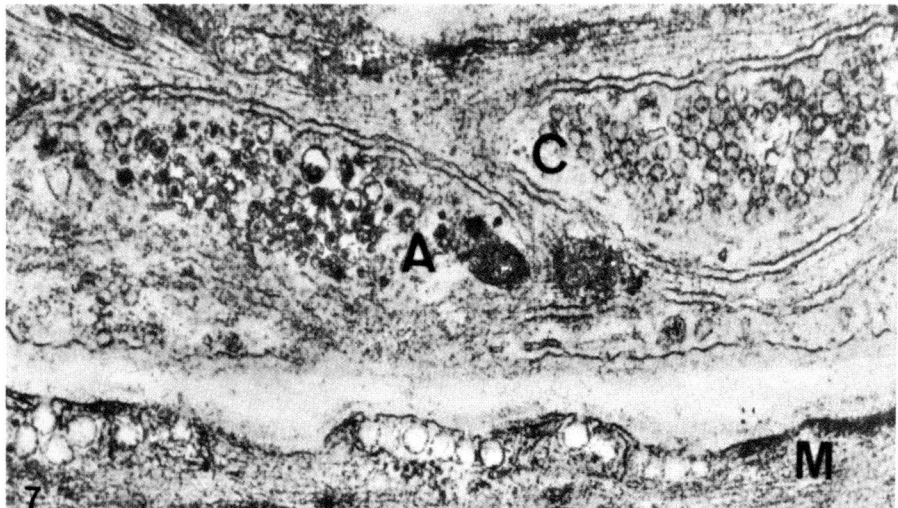

Fig. 7. Treatment with 5-hydroxydopamine: an adrenergic axon (*A*) contains numerous small vesicles with a dense granule while the cholinergic axon remains clear (*C*). The two types of axon run parallel to each other in the same nerve close to a muscle cell (x48,000)

the two. Our observations provide the anatomical basis which is necessary for the interpretation and localization of action of the sympathomimetic agents that are liable to influence the mobility of the ureter (Fig. 7).

There is also a third type of nerve fibre to be found in the ureter. They are neither cholinergic nor adrenergic, are characterized by their large granular vesicles, and have been identified as "purinergic". According to Burnstock (1971, 1972) the neuro-transmitters in these nerves are cyclic nucleotides. Purinergic nerve endings

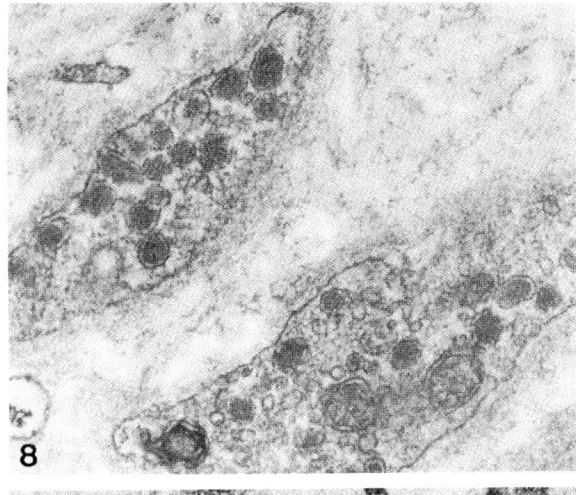

Fig. 8. "Purinergic" axon characterized by a predominance of large granular vesicles; some of these vesicles are fusiform (x60,000)

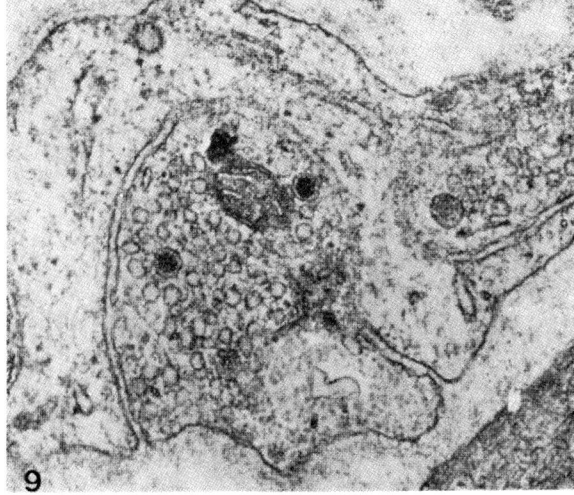

Fig. 9. Enlargement of a cholinergic axon characterized by numerous small clear vesicles, some large granular vesicles and some mitochondria (x60,000)

appear in the muscle and submucosa of the ureter. Little is known about their role as a result of the scant information available on the action of cyclic nucleotides on ureteral tissue. Again, our observations may explain the influence of various drugs such as theophylline, caffeine and certain sympathomimetics which modify ureteral function by changes in the production of cyclic AMP (Fig. 8).

The cholinergic nerve supply to the ureter is particularly rich in the submucosa where, taking an analogy from other organs (Cauna et al. 1969; Nadol et al. 1970), the fibres might well have a sensory function.

There are bundles of nerve fibres in the different layers of the ureter (Fig. 10). Occasional axons denuded of Schwann cells can be seen among the smooth muscle fibres and sometimes narrow neuromuscular contacts, of the order of 15–50 nm, between an axon and smooth muscle cell (Fig. 11) can be observed.

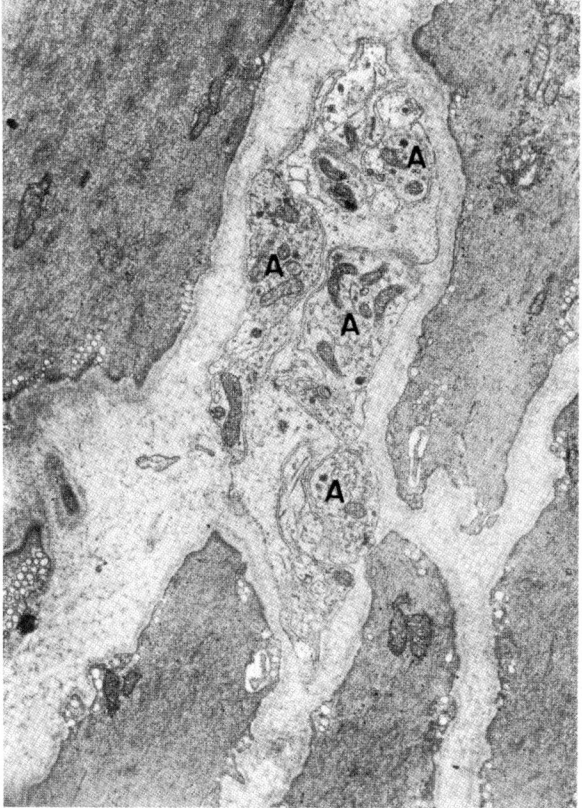

Fig. 10. A nerve bundle comprising 4 axons (*A*) running between smooth muscle cells (x18,400)

Model for the Innervation of the Ureteral Musculature

Ever since the basic studies of Bozler (1941, 1948) smooth muscle has been classified into two types: individualized units such as those of the intestine which are autonomous, with spontaneous fibre-to-fibre activity, and multiple units such as found in the iris, bladder and vascular wall. Activity in the latter is dependent on stimulation by the nervous system and is never spontaneous. In the past this division into myogenic and neurogenic smooth muscle fibres served a useful purpose but is now considered rigid and outmoded. Studies using electrophysiology, neurohistochemistry and electron microscopy have shown that several smooth muscles such as those of the bladder, the digestive tract and the vas deferens for example have characteristics common to both types (reviewed by Burnstock 1970; Bennett 1972). Burnstock (1970), furthermore, has proposed a new classification which takes these new findings into account. It is mostly based on the nature of the relationship between peripheral autonomic nervous system and smooth muscle cell.

The outcome of our own study is to suggest a model of the autonomic innervation of the ureter (inspired by the general model of smooth muscle innervation pro-

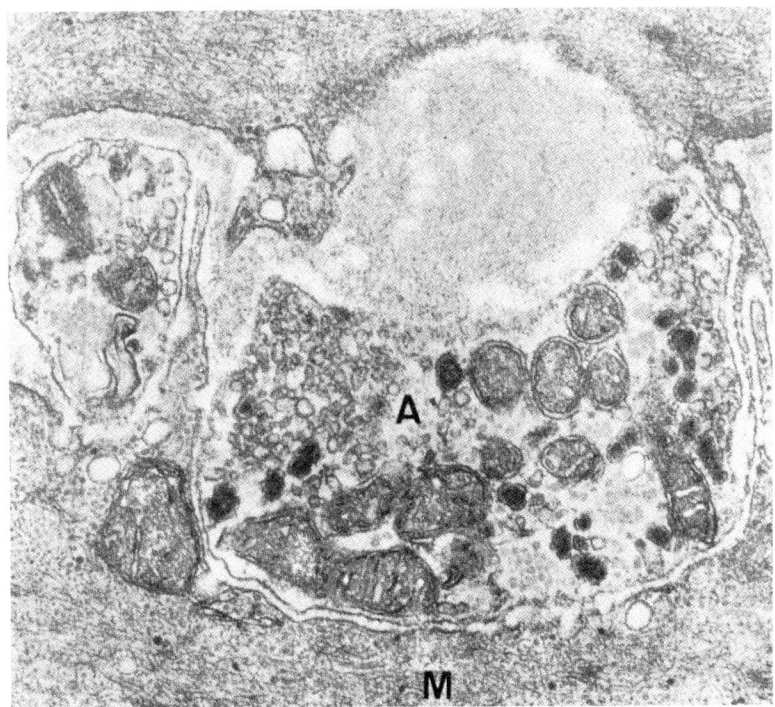

Fig. 11. Another view of a narrow neuromuscular junction; the axon (*A*) is situated in a depression in the muscle cell's membrane (*M*) (x46,000)

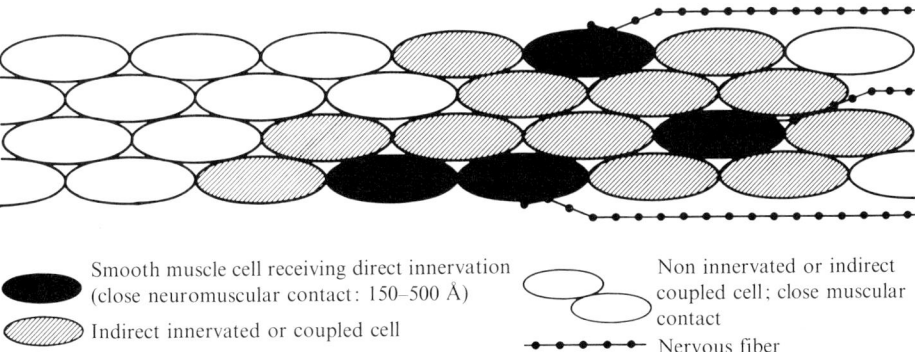

Fig. 12. Diagram of a model for the innervation of smooth muscle. (Modified after Burnstock 1970)

posed by Burnstock et al. 1971), the principle tenets of which are the following (Fig. 12):

1. *The direct innervation* of muscle cells is rare. When present, it is seen as a swelling of the axon which is in direct contact with the muscle cell, separated only by a space of some 20 nm (Fig. 11). At the level of contact the axon is without Schwann cells and generally sits in a small depression in the muscle cell's surface.

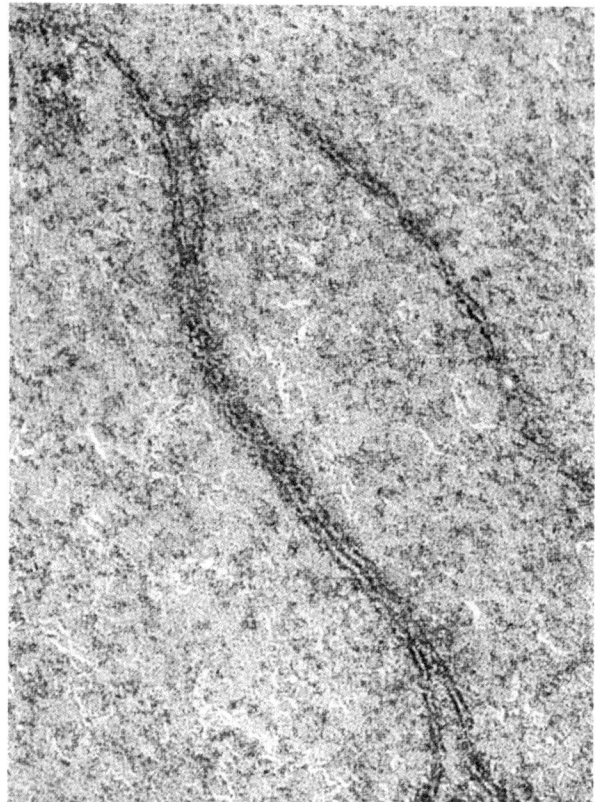

Fig. 13. Narrow contact between smooth muscle cells: contact between plasma membranes after fixation in potassium permanganate (x120,000)

There is no specialized area of membrane like the interneural synapses or motor end-plate of striated fibres. The few who have previously studied he ultrastructure of the ureter's nerve supply have not been able to demonstrate these neuromuscular contact points (Notley 1969; Dixon and Gosling 1971) and our findings provide the first evidence of such structures in the human and animal ureter.

Those few muscle cells receiving direct innervation are electrically coupled to their neighbours by contact zones of low electrical resistance.

2. The majority of ureteral cells are of the non-innervated type, in which *muscle-to-muscle connections,* represented by further zones of less electrical resistance, play a vital role in the integration of muscle cell activity (Barr et al. 1968; Loewenstein 1970; Staehelin and Hull 1978).

3. The detailed structure of these connections merits further discussion insofar as they represent one of the factors fundamental to any explanation of ureteral muscle function.

The areas of contact between the membranes of adjacent muscle cells were originally termed 'nexus' by Dewey and Barr (1962). At first it was thought that the plasma membranes were partially fused together like the narrow junction between

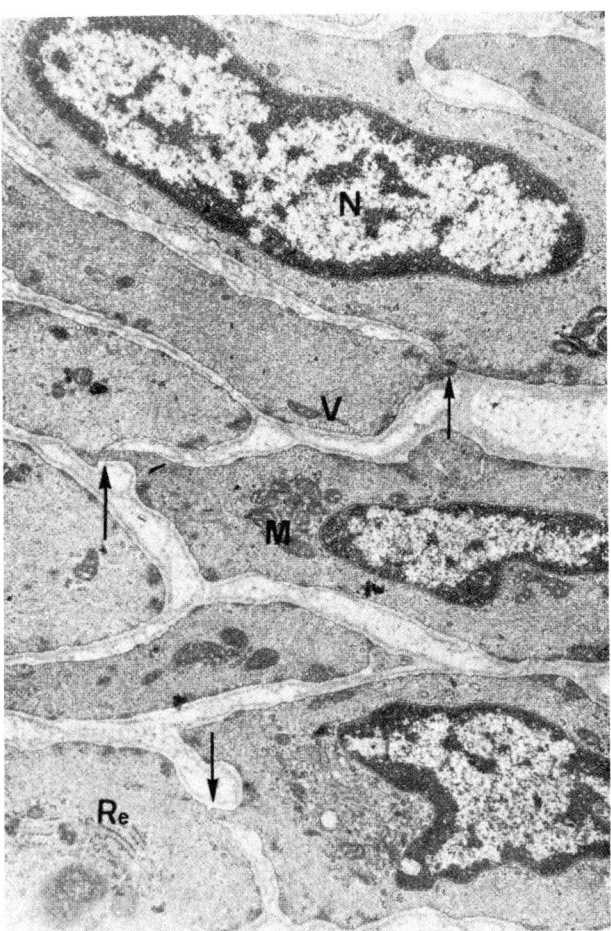

Fig. 14. Characteristic appearance of muscle cells from the human ureter on electron microscopy. The cells have established narrow zones of contact with each other (↑) (x24,000). *N* nucleus; *M* mitochondria; *Re* endoplasmic reticulum; *V* micropinocytotic vesicle

epithelial cells. Subsequent studies, however, have shown that there is a distinct space of some 2–3 nm between the membranes for which the term "junction gap" has been adopted (Revel et al. 1967; Nehara and Burnstock 1970). These junctions permit the passage of molecules and of electrical activity from one cell to another, without the intervention of a neurotransmitter as mediator (Bennett and Merrillées 1966; Loewenstein 1970; Staehelin and Hull 1978). The area of contact and size of the junction gap depend on the methods of preparation and fixation used (Gabella 1973), but the former are particularly well demonstrated after fixation in potassium permanganate (Dewey and Barr 1964). Their apparent number increases after preincubation of the tissue in physiological saline at 37 °C for 2 h, which allows the muscle fibres to relax somewhat from the trauma of surgical removal. Such technical details are probably of fundamental importance and explain why other authors

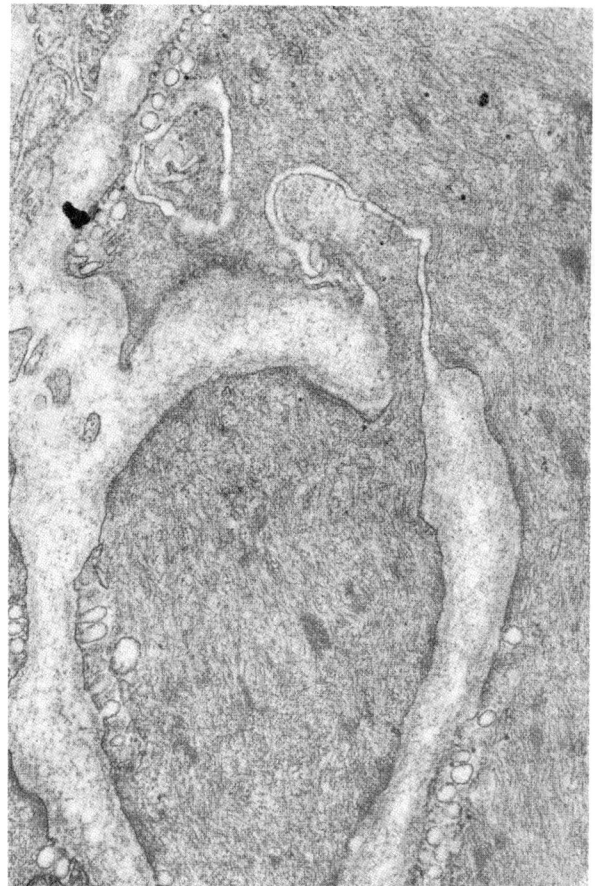

Fig. 15. Prolongation of one cell into another; the clubbed extension invaginates the neighbouring cell (x60,000)

have been unable to demonstrate the same structures. Thus Notley (1970), Dixon and Gosling (1971), Libertino and Weiss (1972) and Hanna et al. (1976) used conventional staining methods without prior incubation. Our study is the first to show these narrow zones of intercellular contact (Fig. 13).

There are also other forms of connection between the smooth muscle cells of the ureter, such as the numerous protrusions which give the impression of intercellular cytoplasmic bridges (Bergmann 1958), the interdigitations between neighbouring cells being particularly evident on cellular contraction. Finally, there are frequent and deep diverticular-like invaginations between adjacent cells (Figs. 14, 15).

4. Neurotransmitters can be released by axons "en passage" through the smooth muscle coat of the ureter, influencing cellular activity at distances of 80 to 1,000 nm (Burnstock 1970). As Burnstock (1970) has very properly emphasized, the three varieties of smooth muscle differ neither in structure nor in properties. On the contrary,

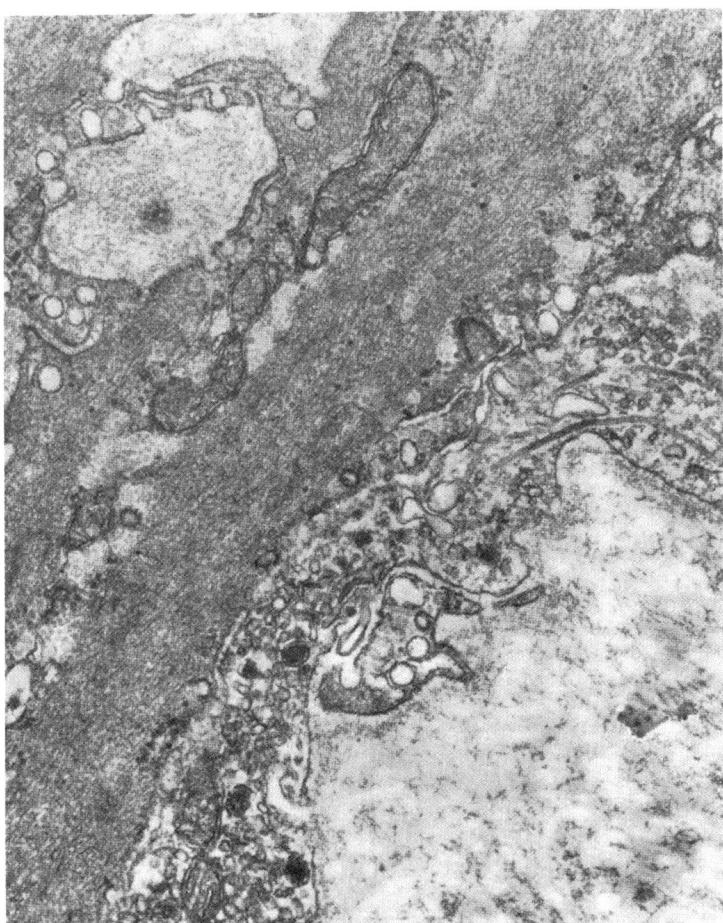

Fig. 16. Axon establishing contact "en passage" with a muscle cell (x46,000)

many cells may pose as "direct innervated", "coupled" or "indirectly coupled" at different phases of physiological activity of the same organ (Fig. 16).

Ureteral peristalsis is an essentially myogenic phenomenon in which the contraction is passed from one cell to another by means of numerous narrow intercellular connections. Nevertheless, the presence of nerves, albeit few, among the muscle cells, is sufficient to explain the effects of certain drugs on ureteral activity (Malin et al. 1970; Vereecken et al. 1971, 1973; Boyarsky and Labay 1972; Raz et al. 1972; McLeod et al. 1973; Weiss et al. 1974; Hannappel and Golenhofen 1974; Weiss 1975, 1978).

Therefore our model regards ureteral peristalsis as essentially myogenic, the influence of the autonomic nervous system playing a secondary role in the modulation of activity and maintenance of muscle tone.

Ganglionic Structures

Whether or not ganglia are present in the ureter is a matter of controversy. However, we have regularly found ganglion-like structures at the lower end of the ureter, although they appear to be rare or even absent more cranially. These structures are part of a ureterovesical ganglionic plexus situated mostly around the orifices of the ureters and in the floor of the bladder as far down as the neck (Figs. 4–17). This complex is in turn part of the pelvic plexus which derives branches from the pelvic (sacral parasympathetic component) and hypogastric nerves (lumbar sympathetic component) (Kuntz and Moseley 1936; Bradley and Teague 1968; Foroglou and Winckler 1973; Gabella 1976). They are largely composed of cholinergic cells the cytoplasm of which exhibits strong cholinesterase activity (Fig. 18). Nevertheless, in the heart of this predominantly parasympathetic milieu adrenergic cells are to be found whose cytoplasm shows a fluorescence of variable intensity (Fig. 19). In the same setting, catecholamine fluorescence picks out yet other adrenergic structures.

These are represented by numerous fluorescing swellings corresponding to the terminal adrenergic fibres which sometimes completely surround certain cholinergic and adrenergic neurones (Hamberger et al. 1965) (Fig. 19).

These nerve terminals represent the branches of post-ganglionic axons – collections of small intensity fluorescent (SIF) cells (Eränkö and Härkönen 1965) which are analogous to the extra-adrenal chromaffin tissue (Coupland 1972) and are to be found dispersed throughout these ganglia (Fig. 19).

Electron microscopic studies have detailed the ultrastructure of the ureterovesical ganglia and shown them to be composed of neurones (Figs. 20, 21). These studies further emphasize the presence of intraganglionic adrenergic structures represented by nerve endings and SIF cells distributed throughout these mixed ganglia.

The adrenergic nerve endings are characterized by small, densely granular axonal swellings. The axons lie close to the ganglion cells and synapse with their corresponding dendrites (Fig. 22), as far as can be ascertained. These terminals correspond to the ganglionic fibres which fluoresce under catecholamine staining.

The SIF cells are typically smaller (5–15 µm) than the ganglion neurones (200 µm approx.) and are relatively much more granular (Elfvin 1968) (Fig. 23).

The granules in many of the cells tend to be located towards the periphery of the cytoplasm (Fig. 23).

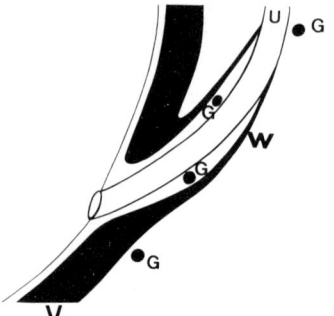

Fig. 17. Diagram to show the distribution of the mixed cholinergic/adrenergic ganglionic structures of the ureterovesicle group. *G* ganglion; *U* ureter; *V* bladder; *W* periureteral sheath of Waldeyer

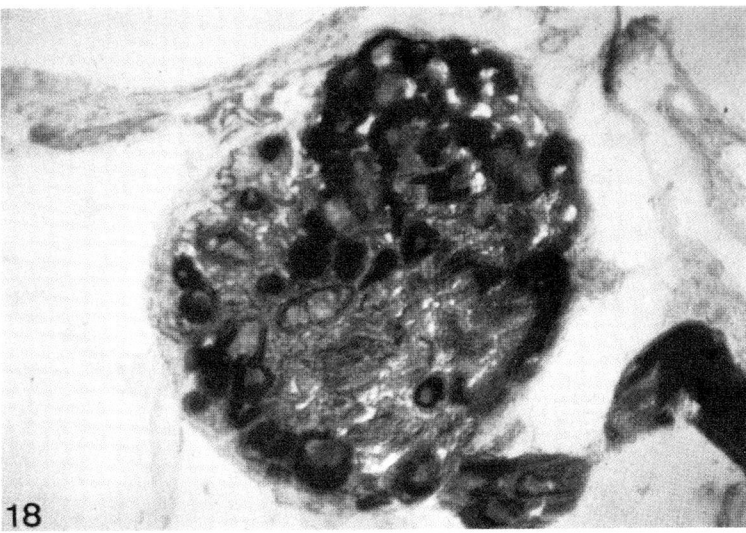

Fig. 18. Ureteral ganglion (man) AChE. Characteristic appearance of a ganglion composed of cholinergic cells (x100)

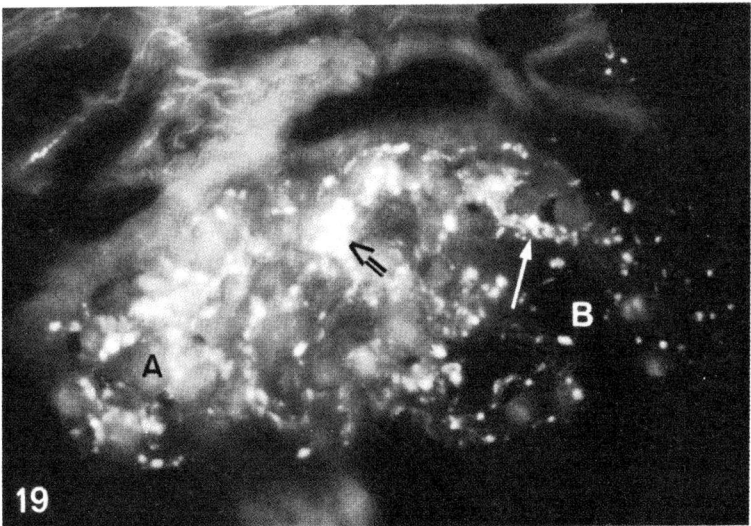

Fig. 19. Ureteral ganglion (dog) catecholamine fluorescence: mixed ganglion composed of cells whose cytoplasm is fluorescent (*A*) and others where it is not (*B*). Fluorescing adrenergic nerve fibres are present in the ganglion and surround numerous fluorescing and non-fluorescing ganglionic cells (↑). Small intensely fluorescent (SIF) cells are dispersed throughout the ganglion (↟) (x125)

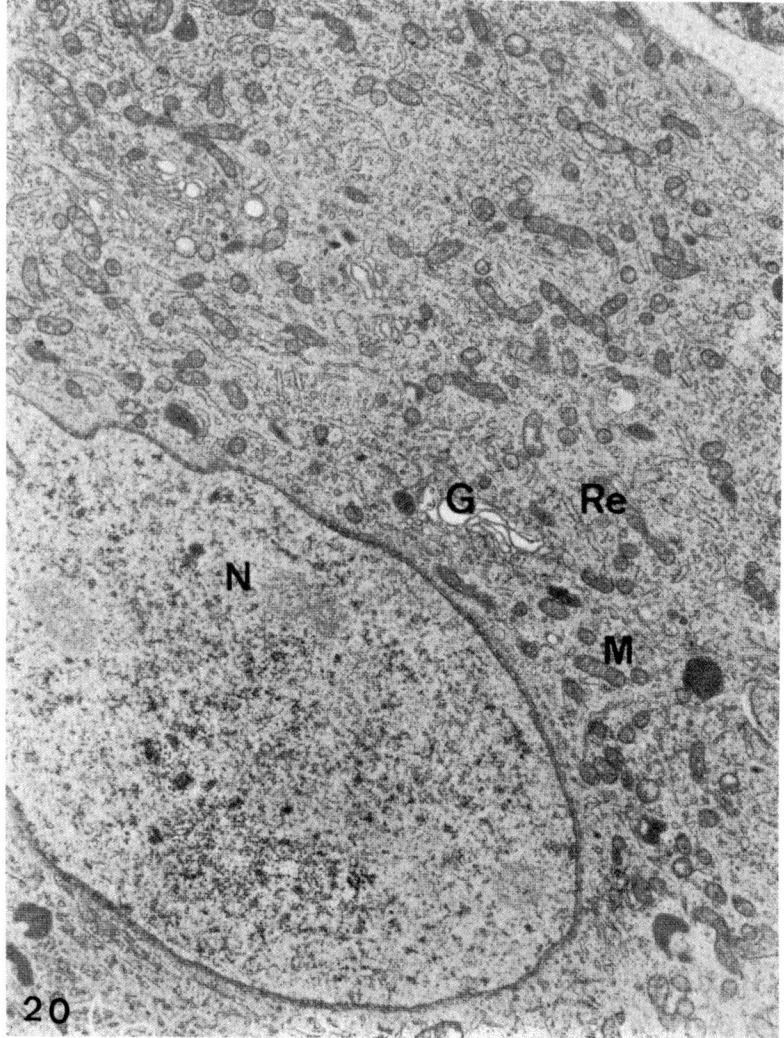

Fig. 20. Ganglionic cells: *N* nucleus; *M* mitochondria; *Re* endoplasmic reticulum; *G* Golgi apparatus (x9,600)

These granular cells possess extensions containing characteristic granules as well as mitochondria, filaments and microtubules (Fig. 24). The presence of numerous large granules in the extensions provide a simple means of distinguishing these axons from ordinary neurons (Fig. 25).

Capillaries are often close to the granular cells and their extensions. The cells themselves are frequently surrounded by cholinergic axons containing small nongranular vesicles.

Physiological and pharmacological studies have shown that the catecholamines may modulate the activity of the sympathetic ganglia (Marrazzi 1939; Bulbring

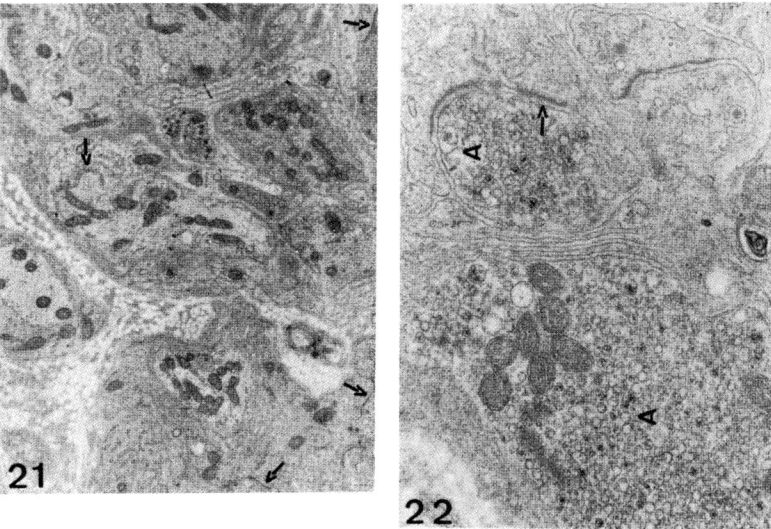

Fig. 21. Examples of some ganglionic neurones with axodendritic synapses (↑) (x6,000)

Fig. 22. Ureteral ganglion: adrenergic axons (*A*) one of which (↑) has synapsed with a dendrite (x15,000)

1944, Pasternak and Larrabée 1948; Lundberg 1952; Costa et al. 1961; Trendelenburg 1961; Curtis 1963; Giller and Baker 1963; Reinert 1963; Weir and McLennan 1963; Norberg and Sjoqvist 1966; Libet 1970; Libet and Tosaka 1970; Kebabian and Greengard 1971; Libet and Owman 1974; Bloom 1975).

Further studies, though few in number, have been carried out which indicate the presence of adrenergic inhibitory mechanisms in certain parasympathetic ganglia (Tum Suden et al. 1951; McDougal and West 1954; Kosterlitz and Robinson 1957; Kewenter 1965; de Groat and Saum 1971; Cantino and Mugnaini 1974), in particular the pelvic ganglia. From observations of diverse ganglia, in particular from our own studies in man, it has been possible to identify two types of adrenergic structure likely to play an inhibitory role. The first are the terminal adrenergic fibres considered to be the branches of postganglionic neurones synapsing with ganglionic neurones (Elfvin 1961; Eranko and Eranko 1971; Hamberger et al. 1964; Jacobowitz 1970). The second group are the SIF cells whose ultrastructure is that of granular catecholaminergic cells (Elfvin 1968; Siegrist et al. 1968; Matthews and Raisman 1969; Williams 1967; Williams and Palay 1969; Taxi et al. 1969; Watanabe 1971; Kanerva 1972; Gabella 1976) which some authors regard as autonomic interneurones (Williams 1967; Matthews and Raisman 1969; Kebabian and Greengard 1971; Benitez et al. 1974; Williams et al. 1975; Taxi and Mikulajova 1976). These cells, whose extensions are short and infrequent, run close to the intraganglionic vessels and probably release *dopamine*, which is capable of acting on large numbers of receptors (Eranko and Eranko 1971; Libet and Owman 1974) and in particular of inhibiting the release of acetylcholine from preganglionic nerve terminals (Dun and Nishi 1974).

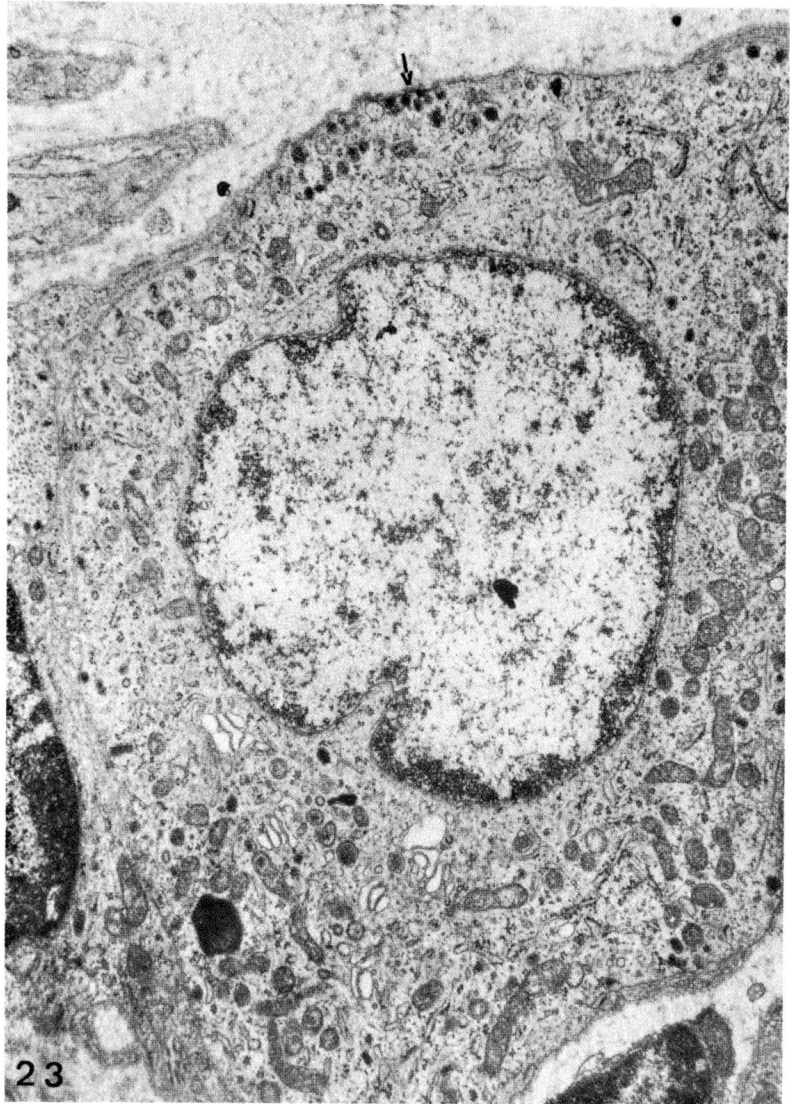

Fig. 23. Another example of a small catecholaminergic cell containing numerous dense vesicles of varying size. Towards the periphery of the cell there are some smaller vesicles (↑) (×12,000)

The results of fluorescence and electron microscopy together suggest that the function of the ureterovesical ganglia of the pelvic plexus may be modulated by two separate adrenergic systems: on one hand granular cells rich in catecholamines and capable of influencing the ganglionic cells or of acting as neurosecretory elements by releasing amines into the blood capillaries, and on the other hand the postganglionic adrenergic axons which synapse with certain neurones (Fig. 26).

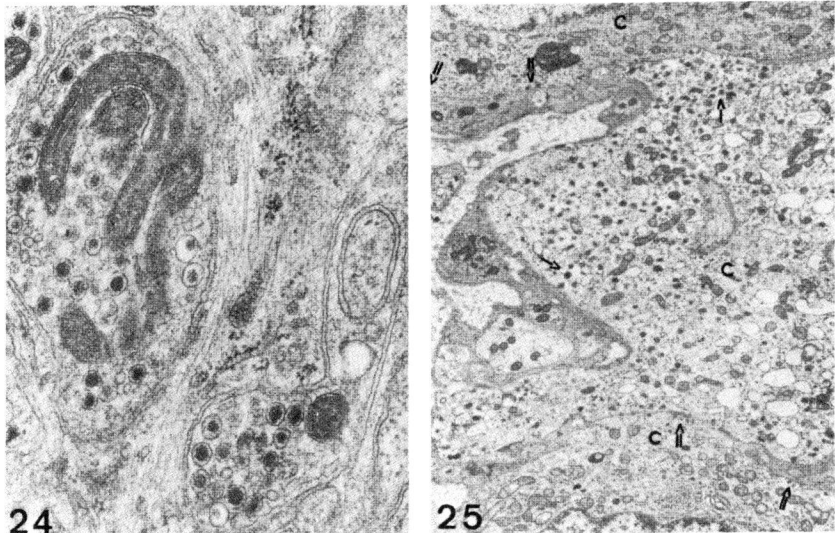

Fig. 24. Ureteral ganglion. Some of the cellular extensions contain a predominance of large granular vesicles whose granule is variably situated. These structures probably represent extensions of the small catecholaminergic cells (x15,000)

Fig. 25. Example of small catecholaminergic cells (SIF cells) (*C*). These small cells are characterized by the presence of numerous large dense vesicles (↑); in certain cells the vesicles, sometimes of smaller size, are located peripherally (↟) (x6,900)

The adrenergic neurones of the pelvic plexus belong to a category different from that of other sympathetic ganglia. They are termed "short adrenergic neurones", being situated in the immediate vicinity of their effector organ. Their axons run only a very short distance to reach their organs, in contrast to the classical arrangement whereby the nerve cells are situated in the pre- or para-vertebral ganglia and their axons run a considerable distance to reach the tissue they innervate (Sjostrand 1965; Owman and Sjostrand 1965). The possibility of sympathetic ganglionic cells being close to the pelvic organs was suggested by Langley and Anderson as long ago as 1895 and since then confirmed for a large number of different pelvic tissues, principally the vas deferens (Sjostrand 1962 a,b; Ferry 1963; Merrilees et al. 1963; Birmingham and Wilson 1963; Owman and Sjostrand 1965; El-Badawi and Schenck 1968; Birmingham 1970; Owman et al. 1971; Dail and Evan 1974).

This unusual arrangement of short adrenergic neurones is roughly similar to the layout of the peripheral parasympathetic nervous system (Fig. 26). Furthermore, the differences between the short and the ordinary fibres are not only topographical but pharmacological and functional as well (see review by Swedin 1971). The short axon is currently regarded as a separate entity representing a specific peripheral neuroendocrine mechanism (Owman et al. 1974).

The ureterovesical ganglion complex innervates the terminal ureter, the ureterovesical junction, the trigone, and the base and neck of the bladder. These structures are thus neurologically interdependent and their function is most prob-

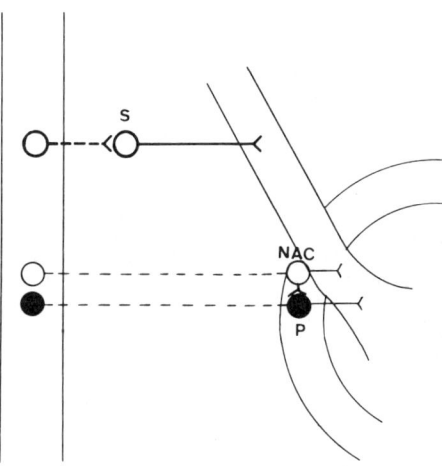

Fig. 26. Diagram of the "short adrenergic system". The adrenergic neurons of the pelvic plexus are called "short adrenergic neurons" (*NAC*) because they originate close to their effector organ and have a relatively short distance to run. This is in contrast to the classical adrenergic nerve which arises in the pre- or para-vertebral ganglia (*S*) and has a much longer distance to reach the organ it innervates. This unusual lay-out of the NAC is roughly similar to that of the peripheral parasympathetic system (*P*)

ably co-ordinated by the different components of the autonomic nervous system. The existence of a "short neurone system" introduces a new concept of the innervation of the urinary tract, that of a peripheral mechanism responsible for the integration and modulation of the terminal ureter and bladder.

References

Barr L, Berger W, Demey MM (1968) Electrical transmission at the nexus between smooth muscle cells. J Gen Physiol 51:346–368
Benitez HH, Masurovsky EB, Murray MR (1974) Interneurons of the sympathetic ganglia, in organotypic culture. A suggestion as to their function, based on three types of study. J Neurocytol 3:363–384
Bennett MR (1972) Autonomic neuromuscular transmission. Cambridge University Press, Cambridge
Bennett MR, Merrillées MCR (1966) An analysis of the transmission of excitation from autonomic nerves to smooth muscles. J Physiol (Lond) 185:520
Bergman RA (1958) Intercellular bridges in ureteral smooth muscle. Bull Johns Hopkins Hosp 102:195–202
Birmingham AT (1970) Sympathetic denervation of the smooth muscle of the vas deferens. J Physiol (Lond) 206:645–661
Birmingham AT, Wilson AB (1963) Preganglionic and postganglionic stimulation of the guinea-pig isolated vas deferens prepation. Br J Pharmacol Chemother 21:569–580
Bloom FE (1975) The role of cyclic nucleotides in central synaptic function. Rev Physiol Biochem Pharmacol 74:1
Boyarsky S, Labay P (1972) Ureteral dynamics. Williams & Wilkins, Baltimore
Boyarsky S, Kirshner N, Labay P (1966) Catecholamine content of the normal dog ureter. Invest Urol 4:97
Bozler E (1938) Electrical stimulation and conduction of excitation in smooth muscle. Am J Physiol 122:614
Bozler E (1941) Action potentials and conduction of excitation in muscle. Biol Symp 3:95–110
Bozler E (1948) Conduction automaticity and tonus of visceral smooth muscle. Experientia 4:213–218

Bradley WE, Teague C (1968) The pelvic ganglia. J Urol 100:649–652
Bulbring E (1944) The action of adrenaline on transmission in the superior cervical ganglion. J Physiol 103:55–67
Burnstock G (1970) Structure of smooth muscle and its innervation. In: Bulbring, Brading, Jones and Tomita (eds) Smooth muscle. Arnold, London, pp 1–69
Burnstock G (1971) Neural nomenclature. Nature 229:282–283
Burnstock G (1972) Purinergic nerves. Pharmacol Rev 24:509–581
Burnstock G, Iwayama T (1971) Fine structural identification of autonomic nerves and their relation to smooth muscle. Prog Brain Res 34:389–404
Cantino D, Mugnaini E (1974) Adrenergic innervation of the parasympathetic ciliary ganglion in the chick. Science 185:279–281
Cauna N, Hinderer KH, Wentges RT (1969) Sensory receptor organs of the human nasal respiratory mucosa. Am J Anat 124:187–209
Costa E, Revzin AM, Kuntzman R, Spector S, Brodie BB (1961) Role of ganglionic norepinephrine in sympathetic synaptic transmission. Science 133:1822–1823
Coupland RE (1972) The chromaffin system. In: Blaschko H, Muscholl E (eds) Catecholamines. Springer, Berlin Heidelberg New York, pp 16–39
Curtis DR (1963) The pharmacology of central and peripheral inhibition. Pharmacol Rev 15:333–364
Dail WG, Evan AP Jr (1974) Experimental evidence indicating that the penis of the rat is innervated by short adrenergic neurones. Am J Anat 141:203–218
De Groat WC, Saum WR (1971) Adrenergic inhibition in mammalian parasympathetic ganglia. Nature (London) New Biol 231:188–189
Dewey MM, Barr L (1962) Intercellular connection between smooth muscle cells: the nexus. Science 137:670–672
Dewey MM, Barr L (1964) A study of the structure and distribution of the nexus. J Cell Biol 23:553–585
Disselhorst R (1894) Der Harnleiter der Wibeltiere. Anat Hefte 4:129–191
Dixon JS, Gosling JA (1971) Histochemical and electron microscopic observations on the innervation of the upper segment of the mammalian ureter. J Anat 110:57–66
Dun N, Nishi S (1974) Effects of dopamine on the superior cervical ganglion of the rabbit. J Physiol (Lond) 239:155–164
Eccles RM, Libet B (1961) Origin and blockade of the synaptic responses of curarized sympathetic ganglia. J Physiol 157:484–503
El-Badawi A, Schenck EA (1967) Histochemical methods for separate consecutive and simultaneous demonstration of acetylcholinesterase and norepinephrine in cryostat sections. J Histochem Cytochem 15:580–588
El-Badawi A, Schenck EA (1968) A new theory of the innervation of bladder musculature. Part I. Morphology of the intrinsic vesical apparatus. J Urol 99:585–587
Elfvin LG (1961) The electron-microscopy investigation of filaments structures in unmyelinated fibres of cat splenic nerve. J Ultrastruct Res 5:51
Elfvin LG (1968) A new granule-containing nerve cell in the inferior mesenteric ganglion of the rabbit. J Ultrastruct Res 22:37–44
Engelmann TW (1869) Zur Physiologie der Ureter. Pflügers Arch Ges Physiol 2:243
Eranko O, Eranko L (1971) Small intensely fluorescent, granule-containing cells in the sympathetic ganglion of the rat. Prog Brain Res 34:39–51
Eranko O, Harkonen M (1965) Monoamine containing small cells in the superior cervical ganglion of the rat and an organ composed of them. Acta Physiol Scand 63:511–512
Falck B, Hillarp NA, Thieme G, Torp A (1962) Fluorescence of catecholamines and related compounds condensed with formaldehyde. J Histochem Cytochem 10:348–454
Ferry CB (1963) The post-ganglionic fibres of the vas deferens in the guinea-pig. J Physiol (Lond) 169:72
Foroglou Ch, Winckler G (1973) Characteristiques du plexus hypogastrique inférieur (pelvien) chez le rat. Bull Assoc Anat 57:853–866
Gabella G (1973) Fine structure of smooth muscle. Philos Trans R Soc Lond Biol 265:7–16
Gabella G (1976) Structure of the autonomic nervous system. Chapman & Hall, London
Giller FB, Baker WW (1963) Adrenergic mechanisms in ganglionic transmission. Am J Pharmacol 135:334–350

Gosling JA (1970) The innervation of the upper urinary tract. J Anat 106:51–61

Hamberger B, Norberg KA (1965) Studies on some systems of adrenergic synaptic terminals in the abdominal ganglia of the cat. Acta Physiol Scand 65:235–242

Hamberger B, Norberg KA, Sjoqvist F (1964) Evidence for adrenergic nerve terminals and synapses in sympathetic ganglia. Int J Neuropharmacol 2:279–282

Hanna MK, Jeffs RD, Sturgess JM, Barkin M (1976) Ureteral structure and ultrastructure. Part I. The normal human ureter. J Urol 116:718–724

Hannappel J, Golenhofen K (1974) The effect of catecholamines on ureteral peristalsis in different species (dog, guinea-pig and rat). Pflügers Arch 350:55–68

Hillarp NA (1976) Structure of the synapse and the peripheral innervation apparatus of the autonomic nervous system. Acta Anat [Suppl. IV] 1–153

Hokfelt T (1969) Distribution of noradrenaline storing particles in peripheral adrenergic neurons as revealed by electron microscope. Acta Physiol Scand 76:427–440

Jacobowitz D (1970) Catecholamine fluorescence studies of adrenergic neurons and chromaffin cells in sympathetic ganglia. Fed Proc 29:1929–1944

Kanerva L (1972) Ultrastructure of sympathetic ganglion cells and granule-containing cells in the paracervical ganglion of the newborn rat. Z Zellforsch 126:25–40

Kaplan N, Elkin M, Sharkey J (1968) Ureteral peristalsis and the autonomic nervous system. Invest Urol 5:468

Karnovsky MJ, Roots L (1964) A-direct-coloring-thiocholine technique for cholinesterase. J Histochem Cytochem 12:219–221

Kebabian JW, Greengard P (1971) Dopamine-sensitive adenyl cyclase as a possible role in synaptic transmission. Science 174:1346–1349

Kewenter J (1965) The vagal control of the jejunal and ileal motility and blood flows. Acta Physiol Scand [Suppl] 65:251

Kiil F (1957) The function of the ureter and renal pelvis. Saunders, Philadelphia

Kosterlitz MV, Robinson JA (1957) Inhibition of the peristaltic reflux of the isolated guinea-pig ileum. J Physiol 136:249–262

Kuntz A (1953) The autonomic nervous system. Lea & Febiger, Philadelphia

Kuntz A, Moseley RL (1936) An experimental analysis of the pelvic autonomic ganglia in the cat. J Comp Neurol 64:63–75

Lapides J (1948) The physiology of the human intact ureter. J Urol 59:501

Libertino JA, Weiss RM (1972) Ultrastructure of human ureter. J Urol 108:71–76

Libet B (1970) Generation of slow inhibitory and excitatory postsynaptic potentials. Fed Proc 29:1945–1956

Libet B, Owman Ch (1974) Concomitant changes in formaldehyde induced fluorescence of dopamine interneurons and in slow inhibitory post-synaptic potentials of the rabbit inferior cervical ganglion, induced by stimulation of the preganglionic nerve or by a muscarinic agent. J Physiol (Lond) 237:635–662

Libet B, Tosaka T (1970) Dopamine as a synaptic transmitter and modulator in sympathetic ganglia: A different mode of synaptic action. Proc Natl Acad Sci USA 67:667–673

Loewenstein WR (1970) Intercellular communication. Scientific Am 222:78

Lundberg A (1952) Adrenaline and transmission of the sympathetic ganglion in the cat. Acta Physiol Scand 26:252–262

Malin JM Jr, Deane RF, Soyarsky S (1970) Characterization of adrenergic receptors in human ureter. Br J Urol 42:171

Marrazzi AS (1939) Electrical studies on the pharmacology of autonomic synapses. II. The action of a sympathomimetic drug (epinephrine) on sympathetic ganglia. J Pharmacol 67:395–404

Marrazzi AS (1939) Adrenergic inhibition at sympathetic synapses. Am Physiol 127:738–744

Matthews MR, Raisman G (1969) The ultrastructure and somatic efferent synapses of small granule-containing cells in the superior cervical ganglion. J Anat 105:255–282

McDougal MD, West GB (1954) The inhibition of the peristaltic reflux by sympathomimetic amines. Br J Pharmacol 9:131–137

McLeod DG, Reynolds DG, Swan KG (1973) Adrenergic mechanisms in the amine ureter. Am J Physiol 224:1054

Melick WF, Naryka JJ, Schmidt JH (1961) Experimental studies of ureteral peristaltic patterns in the pig. II. Myogenic activity of the pig ureter. J Urol 86:46

Merrilles NCR, Burnstock G, Holman ME (1963) Correlation of fine structure and physiology of the innervation of smooth muscle in the guinea-pig vas deferens. J Cell Biol 19:529

Mitchell GAG (1938) The innervation of the kidney, ureter, testicule and epididymis. J Anat 72:508

Nadol JB Jr, Brzin M, de Lorenzo AJD (1970) Fine structural localization of acetylcholinesterase in sensory and motor neurons of the muscle receptor organ in Homarus. J Comp Neurol 140:399–420

Norberg KA, Sjoqvist F (1966) New possibilities for adrenergic modulation of ganglionic transmission. Pharmacol Rev 18:743–751

Notley RG (1969) The innervation of the upper ureter in man and in the rat: an ultrastructural study. J Anat 105:393–402

Notley RG (1970) The musculature of the human ureter. Br J Urol 42:724–727

O'Connor VJ Jr, Dawson-Edwards P (1959) Role of the ureter in renal transplantation. I. Studies of denervated ureter with particular reference to uretero-ureteral anastomosis. J Urol 82:566

Owman C, Sjostrand NO (1965) Short adrenergic neurons and catecholamine-containing cells in vas deferens and accessory male genital glands of different mammals. Z Zellforsch 66:300–320

Owman Ch, Owman T, Sjoberg NO (1971) Short adrenergic nerves innervating the female urethra in the cat. Experientia 27:313–315

Owman Ch, Sjoberg NO, Sjostrand NO (1974) Short adrenergic neurons, a peripheral neuroendocrine mechanism. In: Fujiwara M, Tanaka C (eds) Amine fluorescence histochemistry. Igaku Shoin, Tokyo, 47–66

Pasternak JM, Larrabée MG (1948) Dépression de la transmission synaptique dans les ganglions sympathiques par l'adrénaline. Helv Physiol Acta 6:62c–63c

Pick J (1970) The autonomic nervous system. Lippincott, Philadelphia

Pieper A (1953) Neurovegetative Gebilde in der Wand des menschlichen Nierenbeckens und Ureters sowie ein Beitrag zur neurogenen Theorie der Nierensteinbildung. Z Urol 46:375

Raz S, Zeigler M, Caine M (1972) Hormonal influence on the adrenergic receptors of the ureter. Br J Urol 44:405–410

Reinert H (1963) Role and origin of noradrenaline in the superior cervical ganglion. J Physiol 167:18–29

Revel JP, Olson W, Karnovsky MJ (1967) A twenty-Angström gap junction with a hexagonal array of subunits in smooth muscle. J Cell Biol 35:112A

Richardson KA (1966) Electron microscopic identification of autonomic nerve endings. Nature (Lond) 210:756

Rose JG, Gillenwater JY (1974) The effects of adrenergic and cholinergic agents and their blockers upon ureteral activity. Invest Urol 11:439

Satani Y (1919a) Histological study of the ureter. J Urol 3:247

Satani Y (1919b) Experimental studies of the ureter. Am J Physiol 49:474

Schulman CC (1973) L'innervation autonome de l'uretère et de la vessie. J Urol Nephrol 79:12 bis, 534–542

Schulman CC (1974a) Ultrastructure de l'uretère. J Urol Nephrol 80:12bis, 559–571

Schulman CC (1974b) Electron microscopy of the human ureteral innervation. Br J Urol 46:609–623

Schulman CC (1975) Ultrastructural evidence for adrenergic and cholinergic innervation of the human ureter. J Urol (Baltimore) 113:765–771

Schulman CC, Duarte-Escalante O, Boyarsky S (1972) The ureterovesical innervation. Br J Urol 44:698–712

Schulman CC, Duarte-Escalante O, Boyarsky S, Gregoir W (1973) New concepts of ureterovesical innervation. J Urol (Baltimore) 109:381–384

Sjostrand NO (1962a) Inhibition by ganglionic blocking agents of the motor response of the isolated guinea-pig vas deferens to hypogastric nerve stimulation. Acta Physiol Scand 54:306–315

Sjostrand NO (1962b) Effect of reserpine and hypogastric denervation on the noradrenaline content of the vas deferens of the guinea-pig. Acta Physiol Scand 56:376–380

Sjostrand NO (1965) The adrenergic innervation of the vas deferens and accessory male genital glands. Acta Physiol Scand [Suppl. 257] 63:1:82

Spriggs TLB, Lever JD, Rees PM, Graham JDP (1966) Controlled formaldehydecatecholamine condensation in cryostat sections to show adrenergic nerves by fluorescence. Stain Techn 41:323–327
Staehelin LA, Hull BE (1978) Junctions between living cells. Scientific Am 238:140–152
Swedin G (1971) Studies on neurotransmission mechanisms in the rat and guinea-pig vas deferens. Acta Physiol Scand [Suppl. 369] 83
Taxi J, Droz B (1966) Etude de l'incorporation de noradrénaline-^{3}H(Na-^{3}H) et de 5-hydroxytryptophene-^{3}H(5-HTP-^{3}H) dnas les fibres nerveuses du canal déférent et de l'intestin. CR Acad Sci Paris 263:1237–1240
Taxi J, Mikulajova M (1976) Some cytochemical and cytological features of the so-called SIF cells of the superior cervical ganglion of the rat. J Neurocytol 5:283–295
Taxi J, Gautron J, L'Hermitte P (1969) Données ultrastructurales sur une éventuelle modulation adrénergique de l'activité du ganglion cervical supérieur du rat. CR Acad Sci Paris 269:1281–1284
Thoa NG, Axelrod J, Eccleston D (1967) Uptake and release of C^{14} serotonin in the noradrenergic neurons of the guinea-pig vas deferens. Pharmacol 9:251
Tranzer JP, Thoenen H (1967) Electromicroscopic localization of 5-hydroxytryptamine (3,4,5-trihydroxyphenyl-ethylamine) a new "false" sympathetic transmitter. Experientia 23:743–745
Tranzer JP, Thoenen H, Snipes RL, Richards JG (1969) Recent developments on the ultrastructural aspect of adrenergic nerve endings in various experimental conditions. Prog Brain Res 31:33 46
Trendelenburg U (1961) Pharmacology of autonomic ganglia. Annu Rev Pharmacol 1:219–438
Tum Suden C, Hart ER, Lindenberg R, Marrazzi AS (1951) Pharmacologic and anatomic indications of adrenergic neurons participating in synapses at parasympathetic ganglia. J Pharmacol Chemother 103:364–365
Uehara Y, Burnstock (1970) Demonstration of "gap junctions" between smooth muscle cells. J Cell Biol 44:215–217
Vereecken RL (1973) Dynamical aspects of urine transport in the ureter. Thesis, Katholieke Universiteit van Leuven, Belgium
Vereecken RL, Hendrickx H, Casteels R (1971) Modification of the action potential of the guinea-pig's ureter by catecholamines. Arch Inter Pharmacodyn 192:208
Watanabe H (1970) Adrenergic nerve endings in the peripheral autonomic ganglion. Experientia (Basel) 26:69–70
Weir MCL, McLennan (1963) The action of catecholamines in sympathetic ganglia. Can J Biochem 41:2672–2636
Weiss RM (1975) Autonomic mediators of ureteral function. Fed Proc 34:362
Weiss RM (1978) Ureteral function. Urol 12:114–133
Weiss RM, Biancani P, Zabinski MP (1974) Adrenergic control of ureteral tonus. Invest Urol 12:30
Williams TH (1967) Electron microscope evidence for an autonomic interneuron. Nature (Lond) 214:309–310
Williams TH, Palay SL (1969) Ultrastructure of the small neurons in the superior cervical ganglion. Brain Res 15:17–34
Williams TH, Balck AC Jr, Chiba T, Bhalla RC (1975) Morphology and biochemistry of small, intensely fluorescent cells of sympathetic ganglia. Nature 256:315–317
Wolfe DE, Potter LT, Richardson KC, Axelrod J (1962) Localizing tritiated norepinephrine in sympathetic axons by electron microscopic autoradiography. Science 138:440–441

Progress in Diagnosis of Ureteral Urodynamics

H. MELCHIOR[1]

At the 1971 meeting we presented the uro-rheomanometry, the method of simultaneous measurement of pressure and flow in the ureter (Melchior 1971). The intraureteral flow measurement, the uro-rheography, was based on the principle of heat conduction. Heat conduction is – with some limitations – a function of the flow velocity of the surrounding medium. Combined with electromanometry, uro-rheography formed the basis of our program for urodynamic investigations of the upper urinary tract (Fig. 1).

In collaboration with the Institute of Aerodynamics Aachen, in 1971 we developed a probe which combined the measuring systems for endoluminal pressure and flow measurements in a single unit. The flow measuring system was located in the probe tip, and the pressure system in the stem. This new uro-rheomanometer was distinguished by better dynamical qualities, but it had an inconstant shift of the zero reference (Melchior and Simhan 1973).

The clinical value of uro-rheomanometry is in diagnostics of ureteral dilatation.

Example 1 (Fig. 2)

48 year old female with megaureters on both sides, on the right the condition after surgical correction by psoas bladder hitch procedure, X-ray pictures of which showed a positive result (Fig. 2a). However, urodynamic examination shows that the ureteral peristaltic activity is nearly the same on both sides. In the dilated left ureter as well as in the operated right ureter, we can see only minimal peristaltic contractions without any effective urine transport. In addition, the basic pressure in the operated right ureter is higher than that in the dilated left ureter (Fig. 2b).

Example 2 (Fig. 3)

22 year old male with colics in the right flank. The IVP shows a megaureter with ureterocele on the right (Fig. 3a). By means of uro-rheomanometry, a high intraureteral pressure and a peristaltic, but irregular urine transport are shown as criteria of dilatation by obstruction (Fig. 3b). Therefore, a transvesical resection of the ureterocele and a ureteroneocystomy were performed. The IVP shows the result of the operation (Fig. 3c).

In spite of all its advantages, the uro-rheomanometry has not been completely satisfactory. It is an invasive procedure with all the hazards of infection and/or misinterpretation.

---

1 Klinik für Urologie, Städtische Kliniken Kassel, Mönchebergstr. 41/43, D-3500 Kassel

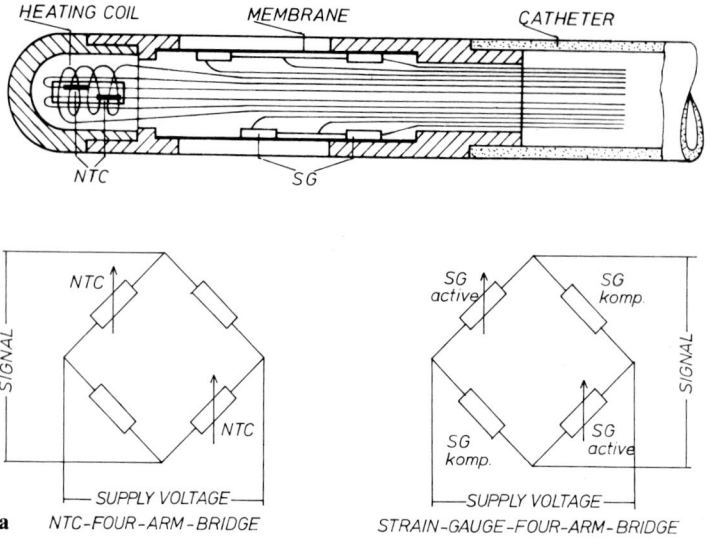
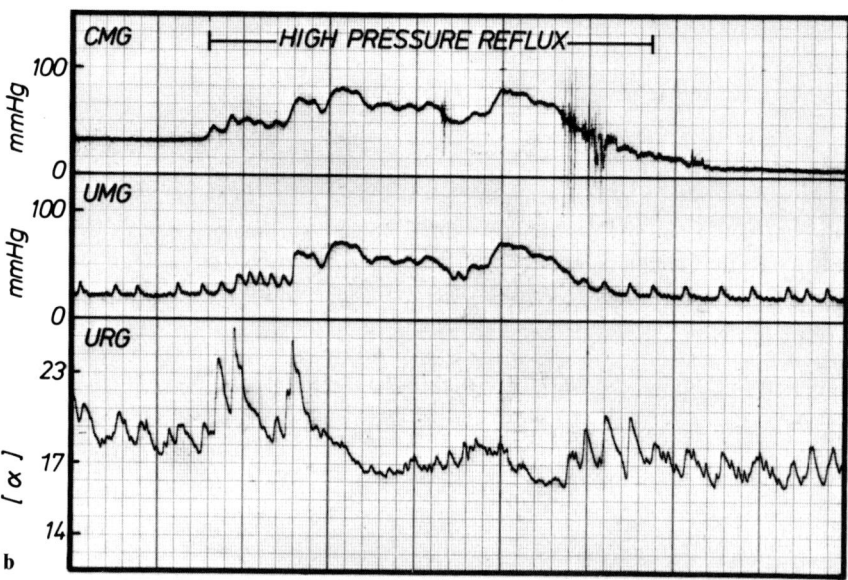

Fig. 1a,b. Uro-Rheomanometry. **a** Schematic drawing and circuit diagram of the uro-rheomanometer. **b** Simultaneous cystometry and uro-rheomanometry in a 22 year old female with vesico-ureteral reflux. The diagram shows the intraureteral pressure increase and the intraureteral urine stasis during micturition because of vesico-ureteral reflux. *CMG* intravesical pressure, *UMG* intraureteral pressure, *URG* intraureteral flow velocity

Progress in Diagnosis of Ureteral Urodynamics

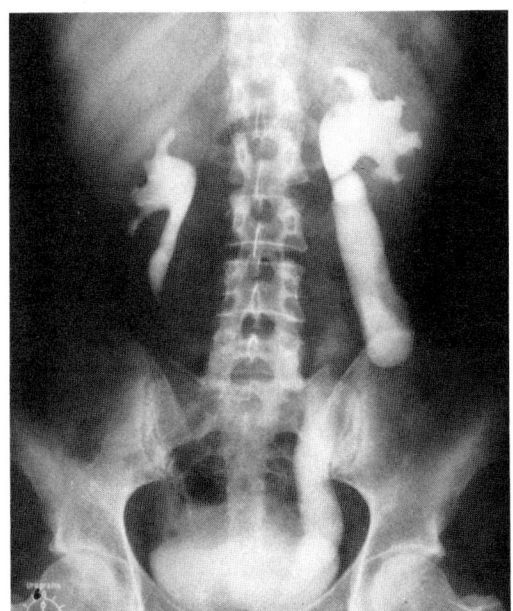

Fig. 2a, b. 48 year old female with megaureters on both sides, on the right side the condition after ureter tailoring and uretero-cystoneostomy by psoas bladder hitch procedure (Example 1). **a** Excretion urography. **b** Simultaneous cystometry and urorheomanometry. The diagram shows the peristaltic insufficiency of the megaureters on both sides. *CMG* intravesical pressure, *UMG* intraureteral pressure, *URG* intraureteral flow velocity

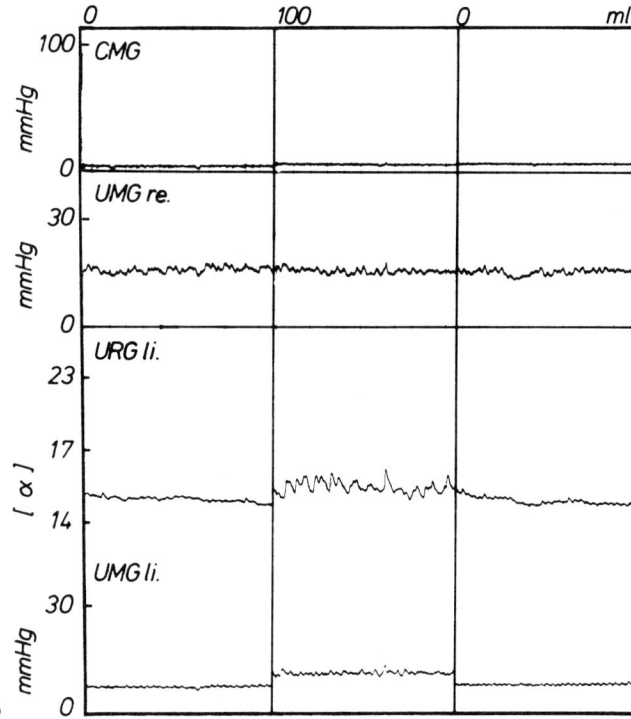

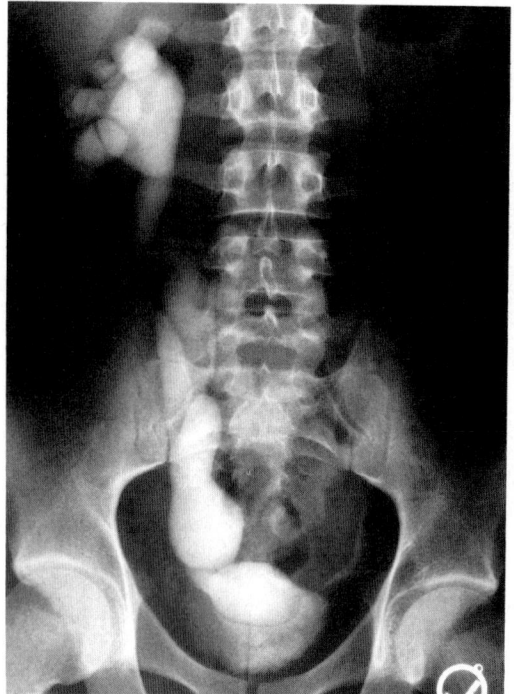
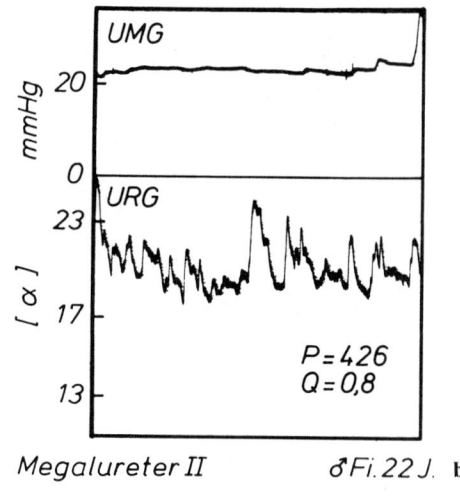
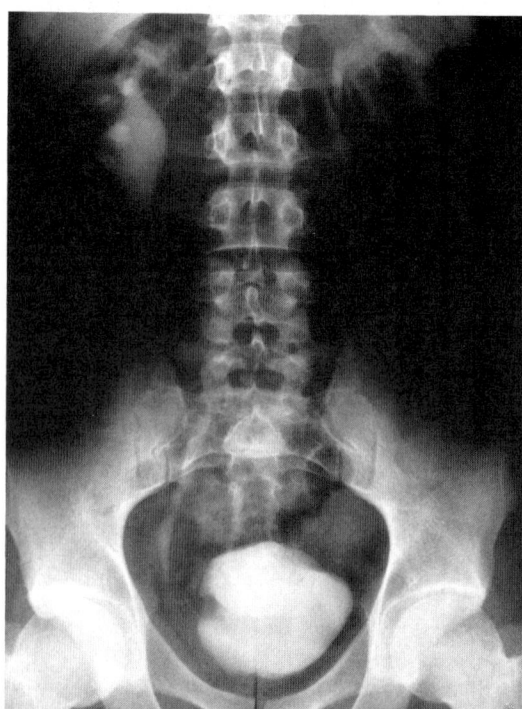

Fig. 3a–c. 22 year old male with a megaureter and ureterocele on the right side (Example 2). **a** Excretion urography. **b** The preoperative urorheomanometry shows the obstruction by a high intraureteral pressure (*UMG*) and an irregular urine transport (*URG*). **c** The excretion urography after uretero-cystomeostomy on the right side

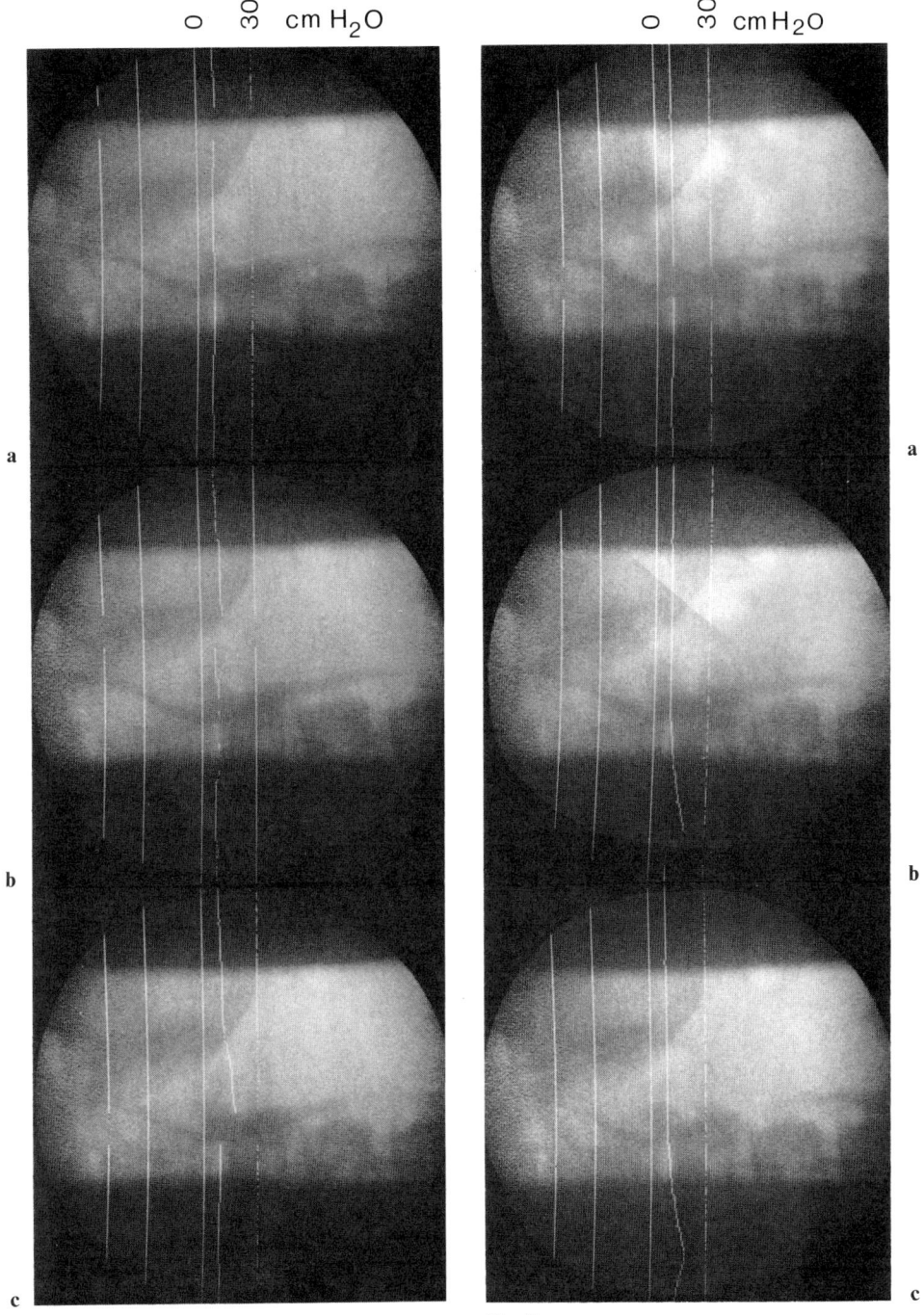

Fig. 4a–c. Intraureteral video-pressure measurements of a normal ureter with bolus urine transport (Example 3)

Fig. 5a–c. Intraureteral video-pressure measurements of a dilated ureter (Example 4)

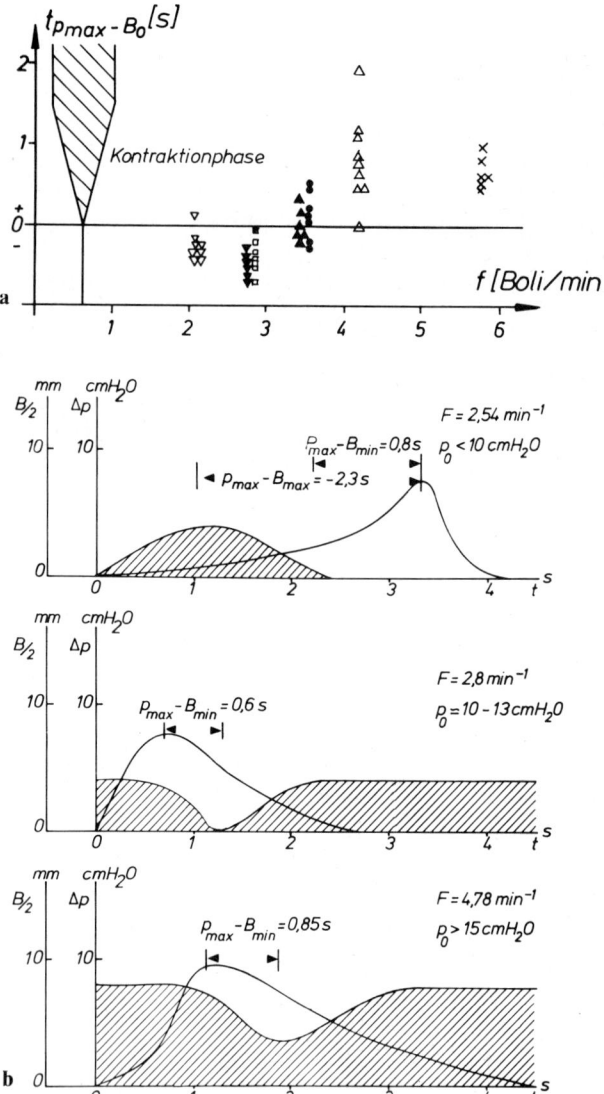

Fig. 6a, b. Intraureteral video-pressure measurements: The relationship between the maximum intraureteral pressure and the end of the urine bolus. **a** The time from the intraureteral pressure maximum to the end of urine bolus depends on the peristaltic frequency. **b** In case of normal peristaltic bolus transport the maximum intraureteral pressure is after the urine bolus. In case of obstruction with increased ureter dilatation the maximum pressure is shifting into the end of the radiologically visible urine bolus

Fig. 7a–f. Panurography in a 7 year old girl (Example 5). **a** Excretion urography 5 min p.i. (14″ image intensifier). **b** Excretion urography 5 min p.i. (9″ zoom). **c** Excretion urography 90 min p.i. (14″ image intensifier). **d–f** Flow triggered micturition urography 90 min p.i. (14″ image intensifier)

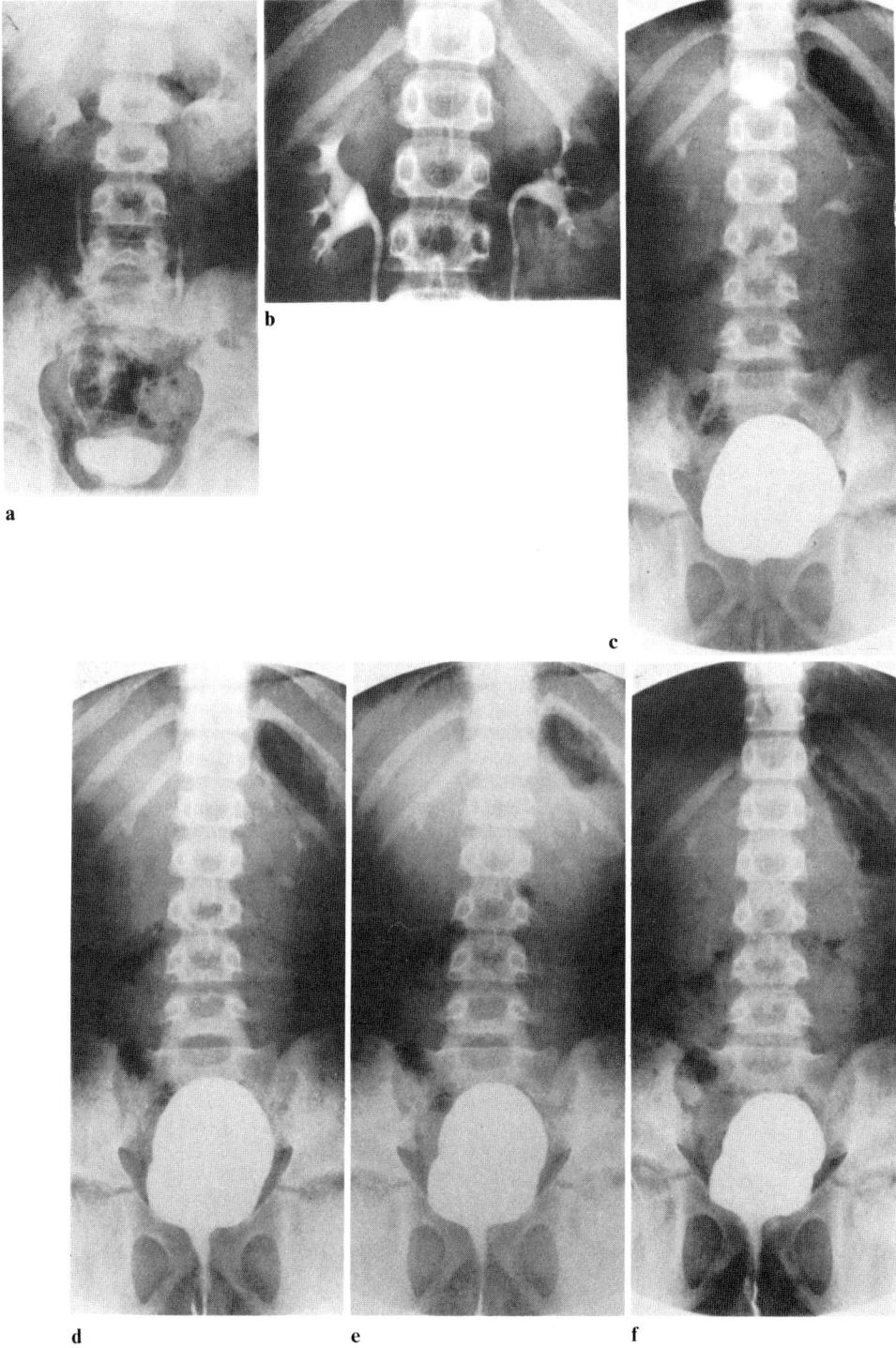

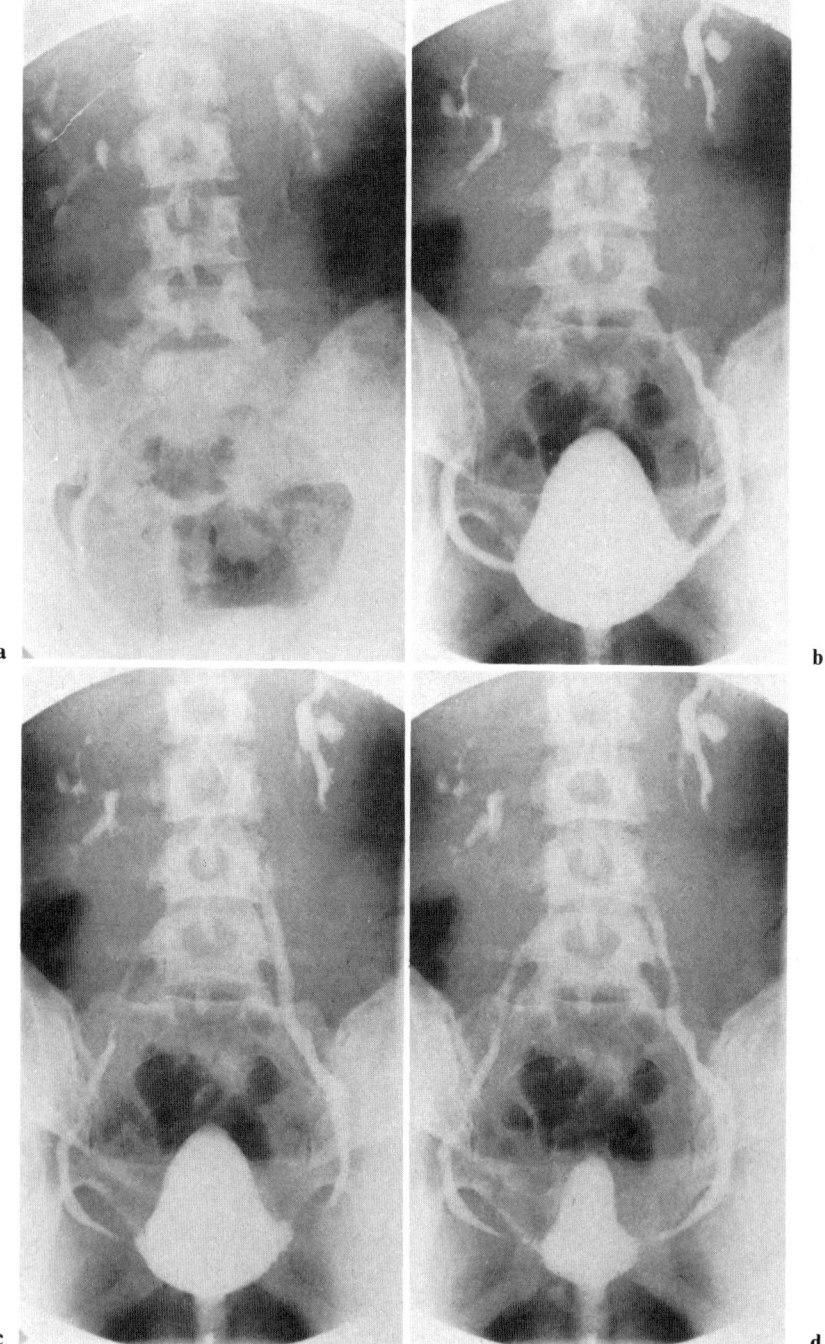

Fig. 8a–f. Panurography in a 22 year old female with bilateral vesicorenal reflux (Example 6). **a** Excretion urography 4 min p.i. (14″ image intensifier). **b–d** Flow triggered micturition urography 120 min p.i. (14″ image intensifier). **e,f** Conventional retrograde micturition cystography (9″ image intensifier)

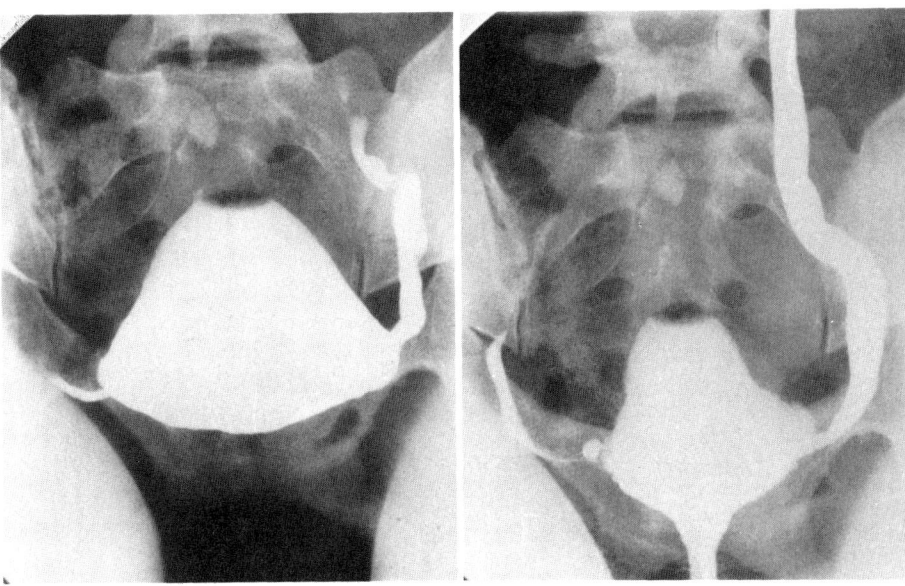

The Whitaker-procedure (Whitaker 1973) is an invasive procedure, too. Therefore, we have been looking for a non-invasive technique of functional ureter diagnostics. Thus, a large number of biotechnical studies have been performed by Shapiro et al. (1969), Simhan (1971), Fung (1971) and Gerlach (1976) with regard to analysing the relationship between the peristaltic contractions of the ureter and the intraureteral pressure and flow distribution.

Simhan (1971) demonstrated the flow profile depending on the relation between the maximum and the minimum diameter of the ureter lumen during the peristaltic contraction.

Durben et al. (1978) created the uro-dynamogram, the variation of the urine bolus passing the ureter, as a method of examining the function of the upper urinary tract.

Schumann (1983) investigated the pressure profile of the urine bolus by video manometry.

Example 3 (Fig. 4)

Normally configurated ureter filled with contrast urine (Fig. 4a). When the peristaltic wave starts in the upper ureter, the intraureteral pressure in the middle segment rises (Fig. 4b). But the maximum pressure is reached before the visible contraction wave passes the probe (Fig. 4c).

Example 4 (Fig. 5)

A dilated ureter (Fig. 5a). The peristaltic wave starts in the upper ureter, while the pressure is increasing in the middle ureter (Fig. 5b). Then the pressure decreases in the middle segment before the contraction wave reaches the probe (Fig. 5c).

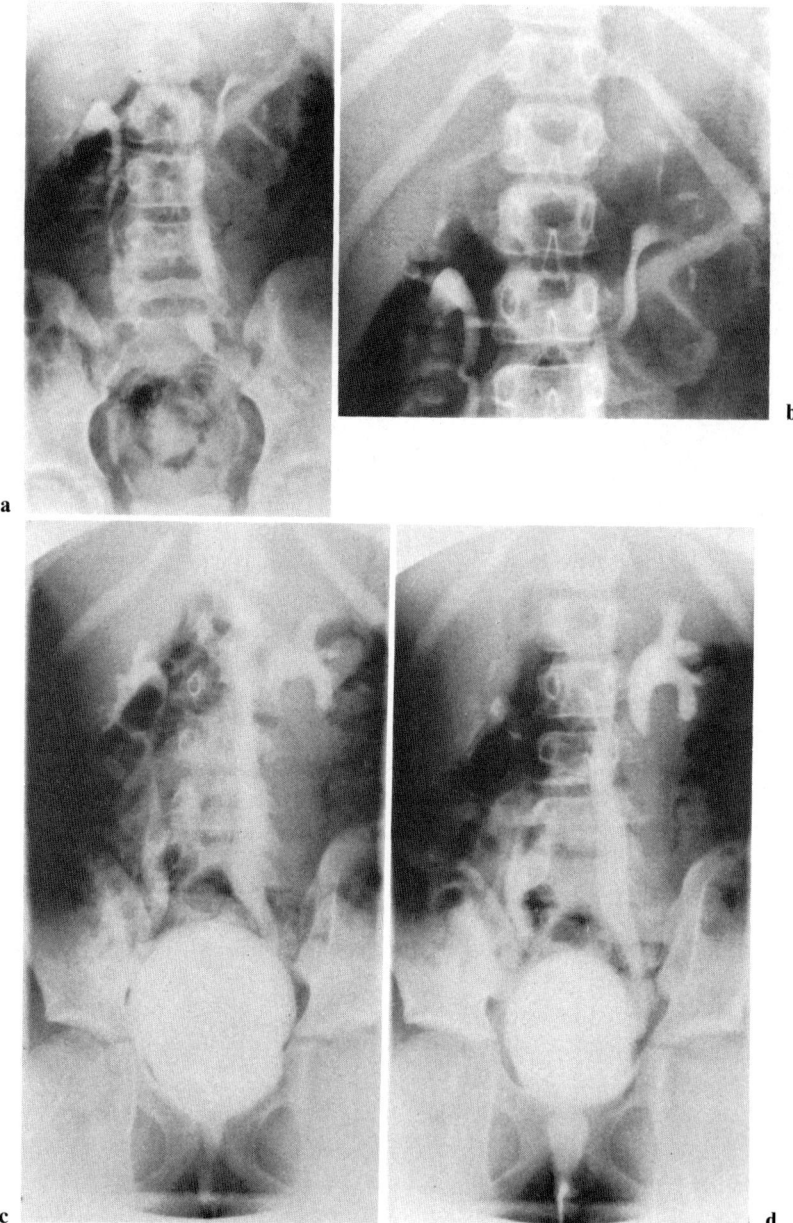

Fig. 9a–f. Panurography in an 8 year old girl with bilateral vesicorenal reflux (Example 7). **a** Excretion urography 5 min p.i. (14″ image intensifier). **b** Excretion urography 5 min p.i. (9″ zoom) **c–f** Flow triggered micturition urography 70 min p.i. (14″ image intensifier)

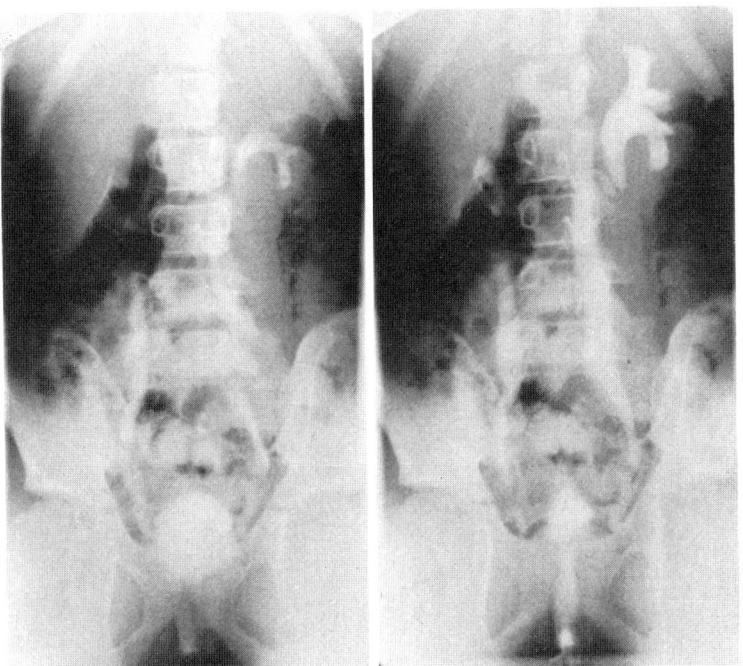
f

Schumann (1983) analysed about 1,500 peristaltic waves. He showed that the relation of the maximum contraction pressure to the end of the urine bolus depends on the frequency of peristaltic and the transport capacity. In low-frequency ureter peristalsis, the maximum contraction pressure lies behind the urine bolus at the site of the visible contraction wave (Fig. 6). With rising frequency, the maximum contraction pressure is shifting into the end of the urine spindle.

The time between the maximum pressure and the end of the urine bolus depends not only on the frequency but also on the degree of peristaltic occlusion. If the peristaltic wave is non-occlusive the maximum contraction pressure shifts into the end of the urine bolus.

Although we do not have sufficient hydrodynamic explanations for these phenomena, the results will stimulate our efforts in non-invasive ureterdynamics.

It may be possible that the 'Panurography' is the first step on this path. 'Panurography' is how we describe the one-stage procedure of intravenous excretion and micturition urography (Melchior et al. 1984).

Example 5 (Fig. 7)

7 year old girl with recurrent urinary tract infections. The IVP by 14″ image intensifier shows 5 min p.i. normal kidneys and ureters on both sides. The magnification photograph by 9″ zoom does not show any pyelonephritic destructions. 90 min p.i., at the time the girl desired to void, the bladder was optimally filled with contrast urine and only a trace of opaque urine remained in both kidneys. During micturition, the x-ray exposures automatically flow-triggered at 5 s intervals demon-

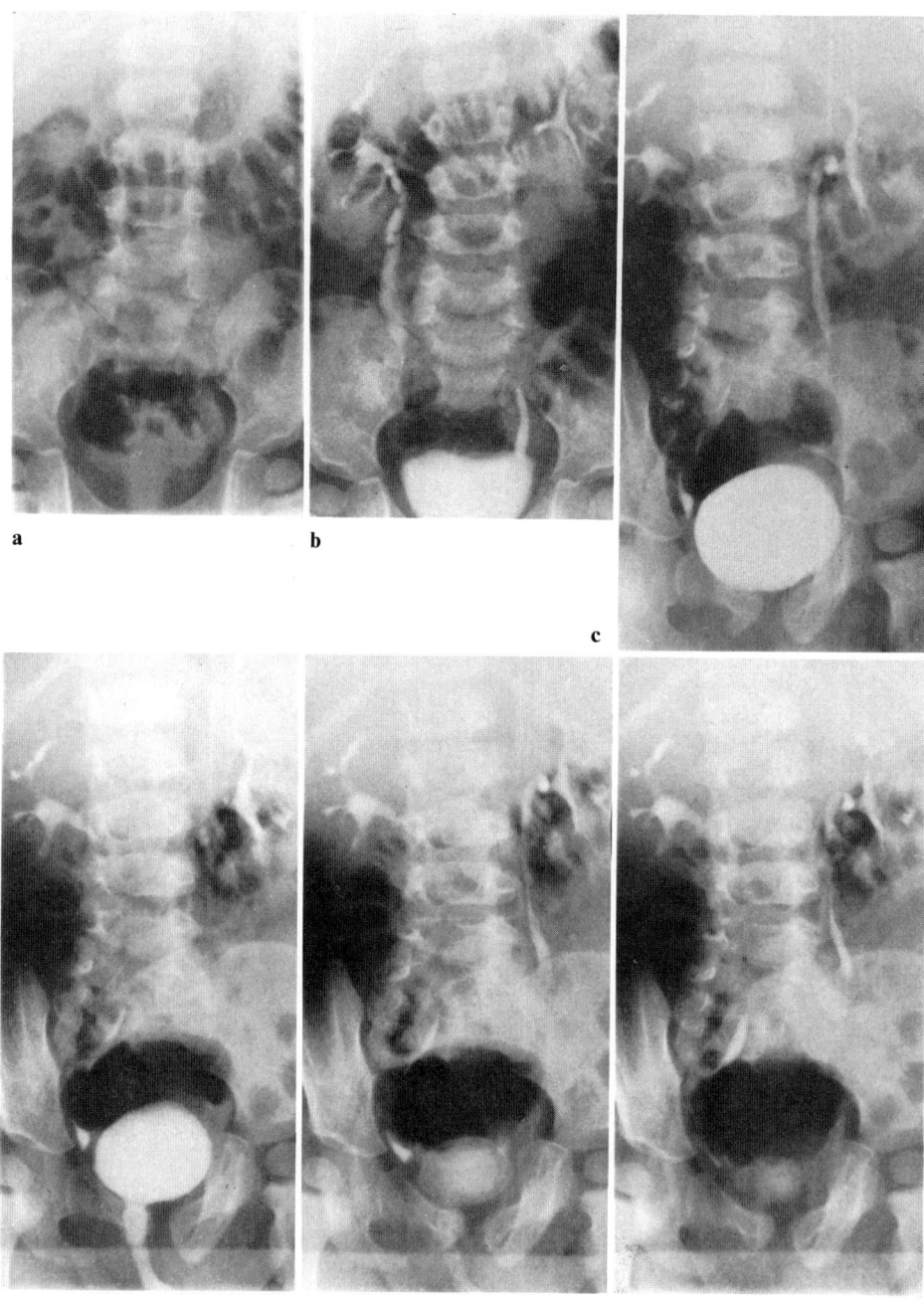

Fig. 10a–f. Panurography in a 20 months old boy with grade I reflux on the right side (Example 8). **a** Abdominal radiography (9″ zoom). **b** Excretion urography 5 min p.i. (9″ zoom). **c** Excretion urography 45 min p.i. (9″ zoom). **d–f** Flow triggered micturition urography 45 min p.i. (9″ zoom)

Progress in Diagnosis of Ureteral Urodynamics

strate the funnelling of the bladder neck and the urethra as well as the bladder emptying without any indication of reflux or bladder outlet obstruction.

Example 6 (Fig. 8)

22 year old female with a history of recurrent urinary infections and chronical pyelonephritis. The IVP by 14" image intensifier shows pyelonephritic destruction of both kidneys with significant scarring of the left one 4 min p.i. When the patient returned 2 h p.i. with a strong desire to void, the flow-triggered 10 cm exposures demonstrate the reflux of opaque urine from the bladder into both ureters and kidneys indicating a grade-II-reflux on the right and a grade-III-to -IV-reflux on the left side as well as a paraureteral diverticle on the right side.

The voiding cystourethrogram performed conventionally by bladder catheterisation confirms the diagnosis of bilateral reflux.

Example 7 (Fig. 9)

8 year old girl with a history of recurrent urinary infections and episodes of pyelonephritis. The IVP by 14" image intensifier shows dilated ureters on both sides 5 min p.i. The magnification exposure by 9" zoom demonstrates the pyelonephritic destructions and scarrings of both kidneys. After 70 min urgency occurred. On the X-ray exposure, the filled bladder with an open bladder neck indicates the attempt to suppress bladder emptying. The dilated ureters and the persistent contrast urine in both kidneys are suggestive of obstruction and of reflux on both sides. During spontaneous voiding, the flow-triggered exposures at 5 s intervals show the bolus reflux of bladder urine into both ureters and kidneys confirming a reflux on both sides. Moreover, these exposures suggest a distal urethral obstruction and secondary bladder neck disease.

Example 8 (Fig. 10)

20 months old boy with a history of two episodes of urinary infection. The IVP by 9" image intensifier does not show vertebral disorders or pyelonephritic destructions of the kidneys. However, the right ureter seems to be dilated in its abdominal segment. 45 min p.i. we find persistent contrast urine in both kidneys while the bladder is filled. The flow-triggered exposures during spontaneous micturition demonstrate the reflux of bladder urine into the right ureter indicating a grade-I-reflux as well as a suspicion of stenosis of the urethral bulb.

Example 9 (Fig. 11)

8 year old boy with a history of recurrent urinary infections and pyelonephritic episodes. The IVP does not show any sign of vertebral disorders, but demonstrates discrete pyelonephritic scarring and significant intrarenal reflux in the right kidney. About 2 h p.i. the bladder is completely filled with contrast urine. The opaque urine persistent in both kidneys and the pelvic ureters suggests bilateral reflux. The series of flow-triggered exposures during micturition confirms the bilateral grade-II-reflux.

The technical requirements for the procedure of flow-triggered micturition urography are a large format image intensifier, a 14" image intensifier and a mictur-

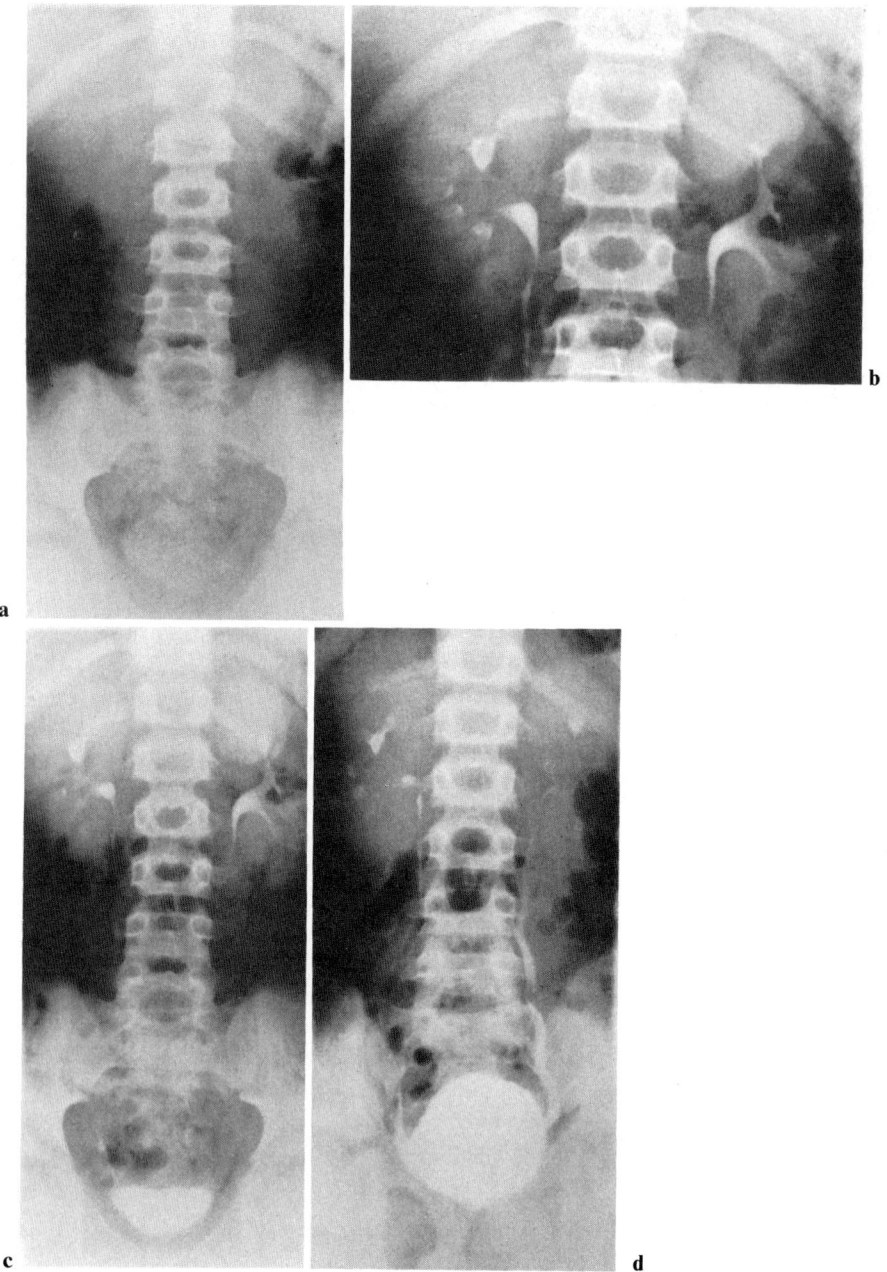

Fig. 11 a–f. Panurography in an 8 year old boy with bilateral vesicorenal reflux (Example 9). **a** Abdominal radiography (14″ image intensifier). **b** Excretion urography 5 min p.i. (9″ zoom). **c** Excretion urography 5 min p.i. (14″ image intensifier). **d–f** Flow triggered micturition urography 120 min p.i. (14″ image intensifier)

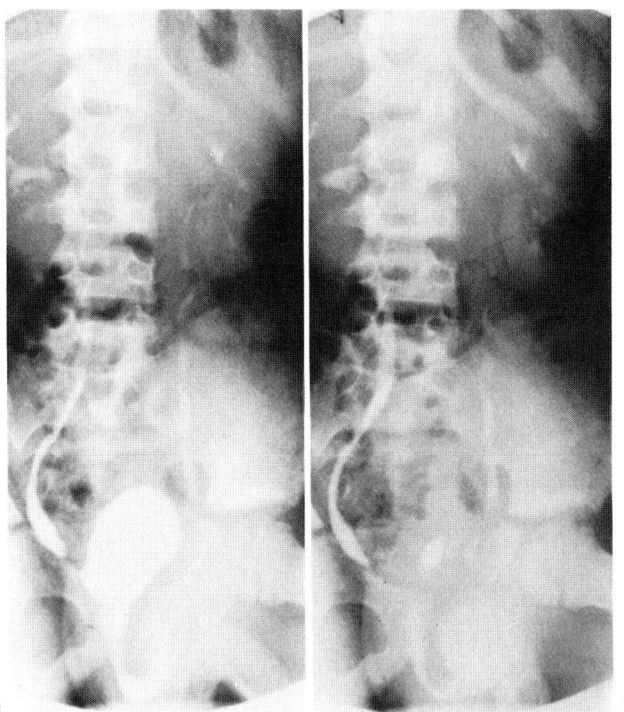

e   f

ition seat coupled with a uroflowmeter which automatically triggers exposures by a 10-cm-camera at preselected intervals as long as a measurable urine flow exists.

The present experiences with about 100 patients show that clinically relevant vesicorenal reflux – grade II and higher – as well as urethral obstructions could be diagnosed by the procedure of one-stage excretion and micturition urography. Only in less than 10 percent of the patients were additional investigations necessary to verify or exclude reflux.

Thus we can say that the flow-triggered intravenous MCU is a valuable screening procedure with a high diagnostic yield. Only in few cases, bladder catheterisation is not required for a complete diagnostic check-up.

References

Durben G, Gerlach R, Hannappel J (1978) Graphisch-radiologische Erfassung der unterschiedlichen Imbolis-Konfiguration beim peristaltischen Harntransport. 4. Symp Exp Urol, Kassel

Fung YC (1971) Peristaltic pumping; a bioengineering model. In: Boyarsky S et al. (eds) Urodynamics of the renal pelvis and ureter. Academic Press, New York

Gerlach R (1976) Untersuchungen zum peristaltischen Harntransport am zweidimensionalen hydrodynamischen Uretermodell. (Persönliche Mitteilung)

Melchior H (1971) Uro-Rheomanometrie (Simultane Uro-Reographie und Elektromanometrie). In: Lutzeyer W, Melchior H (eds) Ureterdynamik. Thieme, Stuttgart

Melchior H, Simhan KK (1973) A new uro-rheomanometer. In: Lutzeyer W, Melchior H (eds) Urodynamics. Springer, Berlin Heidelberg New York

Melchior H, Degeeter P, Borbe G (1984) Panurographie – eine neue Methode der kombinierten Ausscheidungs- und Miktionsurographie. Urologe A 23:55–60

Schumann W (1983) Das Ureterdruckprofil im Urinbolus. Inaug.-Dissertation, Marburg

Shapiro AH, Jaffrin MY, Weinberg SL (1969) Peristaltic pumping with long wavelengths at low Reynold's number. J Fluid Mech 37:799–825

Simhan KK (1971) Über ein theoretisches Modell zur Erfassung des peristaltischen Harntransportvorgangs. In: Lutzeyer W, Melchior H (eds) Ureterdynamik. Thieme, Stuttgart

Whitaker RH (1973) Diagnosis of obstruction in dilated ureters. Ann R Coll Surg Engl 53:153

Ureteral Urodynamics: Past and Future

S. BOYARSKY[1]

One of history's purposes is to teach us lessons in how to avoid the errors of the past. I feel that urodynamics seems to have "gone clinical" too eagerly and has devoted itself too much to problems of the lower urinary tract, commendably, but to the neglect of the ureter and renal pelvis. Homeostasis of the chemical composition of the bodily fluids, the very medium for life itself, depends upon renal function and thus upon urodynamics. There is a vast uncharted area between homeostasis and the retention or expulsion of urine.

The need for research is just as great in the upper urinary tract as it is in the lower urinary tract. If we define research challenges in terms of ignorance rather than opportunity, as all the great scientists have chosen to do, then it is very clear that the upper tract offers ten times as many possibilities for ultimate scientific reward as the lower tract does today. One must choose for himself.

Next, I will present some data that were presented ten years ago but may not be familiar to many here today. Then, I will discuss Narath's theory of calyceal function published in 1951, recent progress in renal neurology, and present some evidence from renal micropuncture work which will give these data a focus covered by the title of "integrative urodynamics."

The renal pelvis, calyces, ureter, ureterovesical junction and bladder are one unique dynamic system amongst the several systems which constitute the human organism. It is not valid to consider the ureter to be an isolated, autonomous, contractile muscle, even though its peristalsis may be under endocrine, vascular or neurologic control. The ureter and pelvis form an adaptive subsystem of the urinary tract which control and integrate its conduit and peristaltic functions.

To completely describe ureteral function will require that the following mechanisms be taken into consideration:
1) Renal secretory volume.
2) Neuro-endocrine demands and controls.
3) Circulatory.
4) Metabolic.
5) Probably respiratory.
6) Possibly urinary molecules.

The ureter truly does pump the urine out of the renal pelvis and calyx, but it may be possible that the peristaltic pattern may respond to more remote stimuli than renal pelvic content alone.

---

[1] Washington University School of Medicine, Division of Urology, Barnes Hospital, St. Louis, MO 63110, USA

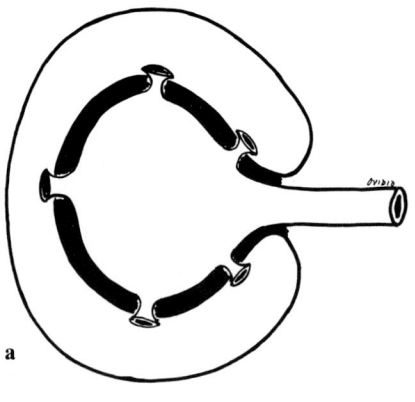
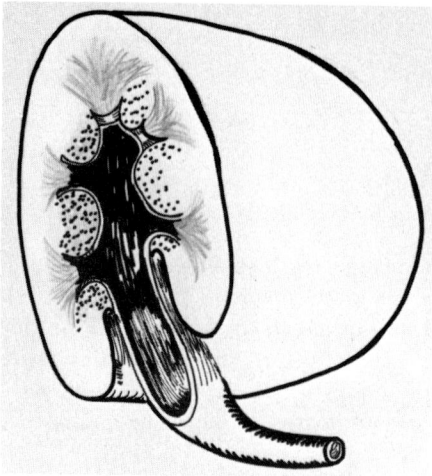
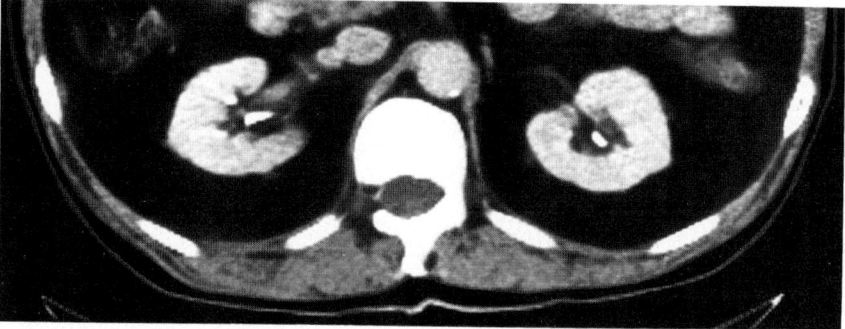

Fig. 1. a,b Artist's rendition and **c** modern computerized tomography scan of human kidney showing the encapsulated parenchymal mass to surround the renal pelvis as an acetabulum or ball-and-socket formation for maximal surface to surface contact. Physiologically, this would allow: 1. Transmission of mechanical pressure, and/or, 2. Neurological transduction facilitation or amplification of pressure events

In 1972, Labay and I proposed that the kidney and renal pelvis formed a morphologic ball and socket joint, or acetabulum, which had physiologic significance as well as physical reality. The diagrams in Fig. 1 show our artist's conception of the anatomy that the renal pelvis and upper ureter are surrounded almost completely by parenchyma to provide a maximum surface-to-surface contact which could allow for the transmission of mechanical pressure and the neurological transduction, facilitation or amplification of such pressures.

The circumstantial evidence for this hypothesis included 1) the well-accepted profound influence of urine flow upon peristalsis, 2) the initiation of peristalsis at the upper end of the system where a pacemaker has been proposed to reside, 3) the evidence that renal denervation is associated with diuresis, 4) the sensitive trigger areas in the peri-calyceal tissues which we have demonstrated to accelerate or decelerate peristaltic rate upon appropriate stimulation, and 5) the commonality of the renal and ureteral nerves in the same trunks (which can accelerate and decelerate peristalsis).

Circumstantial evidence suggested that a physiologic coupling of the kidney to the ureter could exist. It is the biologic pattern of the mammalian organism to back up its structural systems with functional systems, and to facilitate the responses of these systems with regulatory systems, such as neural and endocrine controls.

The method used in the laboratory to search for this possibility was simple. An anterior midline incision exposed the kidney, upper ureter and renal vessels in anesthetized dogs with minimum manipulation. The urine flow was monitored, maintained at a low level by a six-drop per minute infusion of glucose and water, and monitored. The ureteral peristaltic rate was observed and counted by two or three observers simultaneously. As soon as the rate became stable, the experiment was performed and the observations of peristalsis recorded every minute (Fig. 1).

The first maneuver was to compress the kidney, continuously or intermittently, for three minutes to raise the parenchymal pressure within the renal capsule surrounding the pelvic pressure so as to squeeze the pelvis.

Observations were continued for each of fifteen or more minutes until peristalsis returned to the baseline level.

In the second set of experiments, a fine silk ligature was passed and tightened around the renal vein for three minutes to raise the intrarenal pressure, with adequate controls.

In the third set of experiments, fine zero silk was passed around the renal artery to occlude it for three minutes; and observations made before, during, and after constriction. This dropped the intraparenchymal pressure immediately and, of course, slowed and stopped urine formation, but renal pelvic pressure would be less rapidly affected by sudden anuria than intraparenchymal pressure would be by sudden ischemia if the two could be separated, because secretion might continue but the blood pressure would fall immediately.

The chief factors being manipulated in these experiments were the intrarenal volume, intrarenal or parenchymal interstitial pressure and renal size, primarily for their possible impaction on renal pelvic pressure and volume. Data were analyzed at the start and at the finish, on the upswing and on the downswing on each of the 3 maneuvers, to give us 6 sets of observations where renal pressure may have departed from or diverged quickly in direction from pelvic pressure.

Over 50 studies were performed in 20 pairs of kidneys in 20 dogs.

When the renal artery was occluded by the ligature, shrinkage of the renal substance and volume, and lowering of the intrarenal pressure could be expected to result. In all but one study, the peristaltic rate fell from 10 to 40 per cent of the control rate in the first minute (Fig. 2).

The renal compression experiments showed over 90 per cent success in producing an accelerated ureteral peristaltic rate up to a nine-fold increase and as low as two-fold. After cessation, the peristaltic rate fell (Fig. 3).

When the renal vein was occluded, ureteral peristaltic rate was again seen to rise as high as six-fold. The boluses appeared to be longer and fuller. The kidney became tense after such occlusion. When the renal vein occlusion was terminated by release of the ligature, the peristalsis slowed to zero or one per minute (Fig. 4).

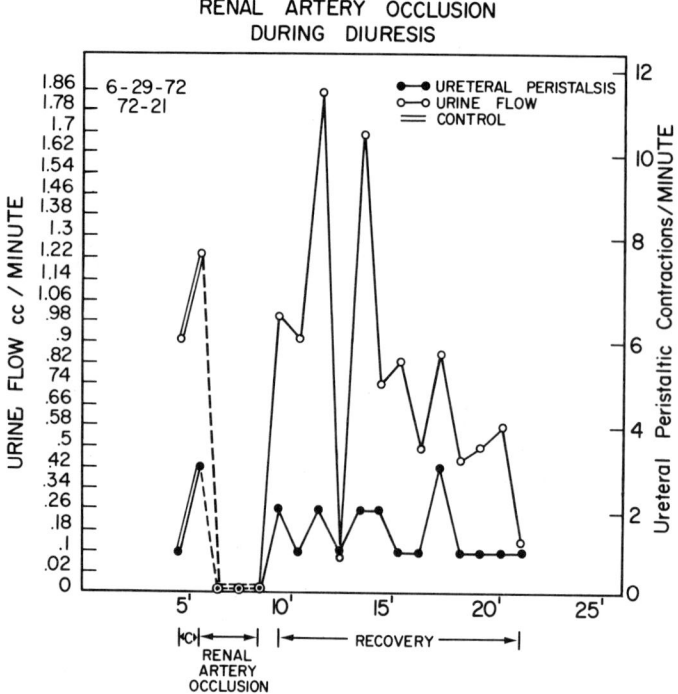

Fig. 2. Renal artery occlusion. Note drop in peristaltic rate, and recovery on release

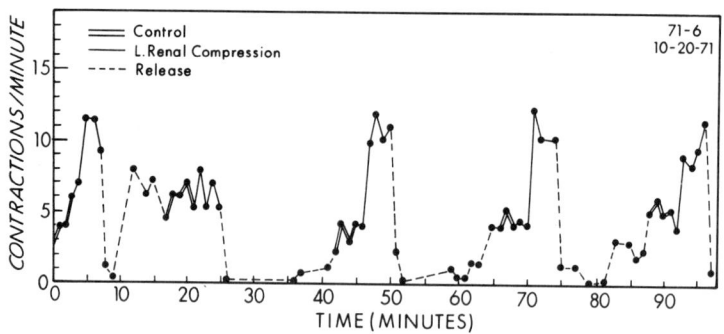

Fig. 3. Effect of renal compression was to raise the peristaltic rate; release slowed it

Re-analyzing the data, we found no correlation of peristaltic rate with changes in urine flow.

To *summarize* the observations:
1) Compression of the kidney accelerated the rate of the ureteral peristalsis.
2) Occlusion of the renal vein produced the same effect.
3) Occlusion of the renal artery lowered the peristaltic rate.

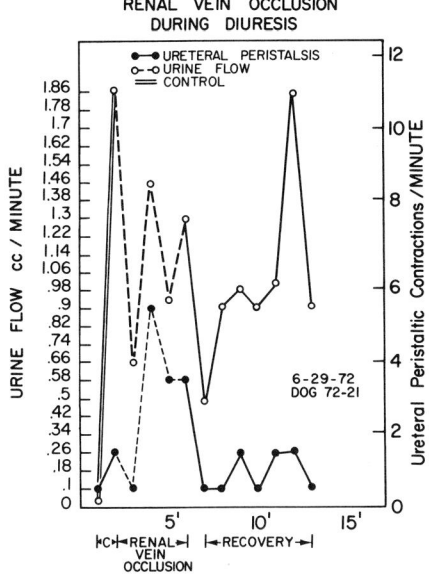

Fig. 4. Renal vein occlusion accelerated the peristaltic rate

4) In each case, the effect produced by the initial maneuver was opposite of its cessation.
5) These changes were unrelated to alterations in urine flow and to a moderate diuresis.

We concluded that renal mass and parenchymal pressure in relation to pelvic volume were manipulated in six ways. These exploratory experiments suggested that the anatomic juncture of the renal parenchyma and pelvis form an acetabular type structure, wherein sudden relative renal swelling accelerated peristalsis and sudden pelvic distension decelerated peristalsis. Clearly, they raised as many questions as they answered.

These, or similar experiments, need to be repeated by those who have the facilities, more than they need to be debated or defended, for the questions they raise.

Calyceal Milking Theory

The early literature contains some interesting speculations upon anatomic and physiologic evidence based on serial pyelograms of calyceal function which can no longer be disregarded. Narath in 1951 reasoned from the pyelographically demonstrated contraction and relaxation of the renal calyx that the pericalyceal muscles had a peristaltic function. Studying the histologic arrangement of muscle bundles, he proposed a theory of calyceal peristalsis *and* calyceal milking. (I refer you to p. 202 and 227 of his Renal Pelvis and Ureter). Narath quoted Henle who suggested in 1872 that these muscles had a milking effect on the papilla instrumental in the transportation of urine from the canalicular system of the renal papilla into the calyx.

Ureteral and Renal Nerve Function Possibly Related to Integrative Urodynamics

Thirty years ago, the same gross renal nerve trunks coursing in the renal pedicle were known to innervate both the renal vessels and the upper ureter, but with different branches.

Now we know that the upper ureter has an innervation, of still undefined physiologic significance in many species, but relative to its size, the kidney has as rich an innervation as any other organ. Electron microscopic and histochemical fluorescence methods have been used to demonstrate a predominantly adrenergic innervation of the afferent and efferent arterioles, the juxtaglomerular apparatus, the proximal and distal convoluted tubules and the thick ascending limb of the loop of Henle (Kopp and DiBona 1982; DiBona 1977, 1981, 1982; Gottschalk 1979; Kim et al. 1979).

Findings in both experimental animals and man indicate that the efferent renal sympathetic nerves can influence the renal tubular transport of sodium and water independent of changes in renal blood flow, glomerular filtration rate or circulating humoral agents. Studies in conscious unanesthetized unoperated animals demonstrate a role for the renal innervation in the regulation of renal tubular sodium and water transport and increase in urinary water and sodium excretion. These would alter urine volume flow and secretion and hence, pelvic distension and ureteral peristalsis.

Reflex increases or decreases in efferent renal sympathetic nerve activity influence renin secretion, the result depending on the inputs from carotid and aortic high pressure baroreceptors and cardiopulmonary low pressure baroreceptors and the degree to which the non-neural vascular baroreceptor and tubular macula densa receptor mechanisms are engaged.

Renal mechanoreceptor stimulation by increasing ureteral pressure can result in ipsilateral renal vasodilation and contralateral renal vasoconstriction.

The kidney is involved in overall blood volume and cardiovascular regulation and the maintenance of arterial pressure. Neural regulation of renal function represents an important control mechanism governing the contributions of the kidney to the maintenance of normal homeostasis. It is not isolated at all from the nerves near any postulated ureteral pacemaker.

Renal Micropuncture Evidence Relating to Ureteral and Pelvic Function

Lastly, the field of renal micropuncture may become the one most closely allied to that of ureteral physiology. Some recent experiments by Bodil Schmidt Nielsen (1980–1982) and her colleagues on renal papillary responses to peristaltic responses and changing urine flows in the hamster kidney may forge another link in the chain.

First, we must recognize the possibility that something might exist; then we can discover it. We never discover what exists if we do not believe it exists.

What is called the renal pelvis in monopapillary and crest-type kidneys (small rodents have the first type; cats, dogs and sheep, the latter type) is the funnel-shaped space and its extension surrounding the inner and outer medulla. In some multipapillary kidneys, such as those of man and pig, the structure is more complex, and different terminology is used. In this discussion, what is referred to as the renal pelvis is thus analogous to what is called the calyx in the human kidney.

Using micropuncture techniques, fiberoptics and movies, retrograde movements of the urine into the renal pelvic space, "pelvic refluxes" were studied in anesthetized Munich Wistar rats and hamsters. During constant urine flow, full refluxes did not occur. Urine either moved straight down the ureter after it exited from the ducts of Bellini or it briefly bathed the papillary tip. In rats, full pelvic refluxes started approximately 0.8 min after a bolus injection of 0.5 ml isosmotic saline i.v. at a time corresponding to a steep rise in urine flow. Full refluxes were also seen in the hamsters following a bolus injection, increased infusion rate; or increasing intrapelvic pressure by 1 cm H_2O also caused full pelvic refluxes. When full refluxes occurred, urine came into contact with all areas of the renal pelvis. Because full pelvic refluxes occur only during rising urine flow, this mechanism would bring urine with decreasing osmolality into contact with the outer medullary areas facing the pelvic space in the report of this group.

The urine was made green by a continuous i.v. infusion of lissamine green in saline, and the experimental kidney was either placed on a shallow trough or left in situ. The renal pelvis was exposed and illuminated with a fiber optic light, and urine movements were observed through the transparent but intact pelvic wall. Urine was collected from both kidneys in the rats. In both rats and hamsters, the inner medulla of the kidney was analyzed for solutes at the end of the experiment to show that the experimental procedures did not interfere with the normal function of the experimental kidney. The results were the same in rats and hamsters.

In the next study, the movements of urine in the medullary collecting ducts were observed and filmed through a dissecting microscope. Urine flow was determined also, indirectly, by measuring changes in the urinary bladder diameter, as the rate of urine formation was manipulated by changing the rate of lissamine green-saline infusion. Urine propelled by pelvic peristaltic waves, moved as discreet boluses in a pulsatile fashion through the papilllary collecting ducts. The length of the urine boluses and the percent of time the papillary collecting ducts were in contact with urine increased in direct proportion to the urine flow.

Next, these workers studied morphometry and fluid reabsorption during peristaltic flow in hamster renal papillary collecting ducts. Total cross sectional areas and circumferences of collecting duct lumina were measured in fixed renal papillae from diuretic and antidiuretic hamsters. In addition, the diameters of collecting ducts were determined in vivo from movies of papillae during peristaltic flows. The average diameter of collecting duct lumina on fixed tissue at various distances from the tip were found to be similar to those measured in vivo.

The hydraulic coefficient of absorption was at least one order of magnitude too low to account for the absorption rate and it was not until the final study that an explanation was postulated.

In the final study, with and without a snare around the renal papilla, changes in the fluid compartments of the hamster renal papilla were found to correlate with changes in peristalsis in such a manner as to suggest a medullary effect in the papilla by the calyceal peristalsis.

Morphometric measurements showed that the intercollecting duct volume was larger in the papillae with relaxed pelvis, but that cell volume of papillary epithelium was larger in the papillae with contracted pelvis, relatively to the other.

So, in conclusion, these workers suggested that fluid moves into the cells during contraction when urine flows through the collecting duct and into the interstitium during relaxation. This is consistent with the milking theory.

Ureteral physiology has gone through three historical stages of evolution: 1) The conduit or pipe theory, 2) the peristaltic organ, and 3) the adaptive system. Ureteral concepts have progressed from conduit to control system. The ureter exists to serve the kidney as well as the bladder and its physiology must be integrated into the physiology of homeostasis and the regulation of the internal environment, which is the first job of the kidney.

With growing chemical interest in endo-urology, ureteral physiology may become more important clinically than in the past. Certainly, calyceal physiology has now become an important frontier and deserves the close attention devoted to the bladder neck in the past decade.

References

DiBona GF (1977) Neurogenic regulation of renal tubular sodium reabsorption. Am J Physiol 233: F 73–81
DiBona GF (1981) The role of the renal sympathetic nerves in the control of renal function. In: Worcel M, Bonvalet JP, Langer SZ, Menard J, Sessard J (eds) New trends in arterial hypertension. INSERM Symposium No. 17. Elsevier/North-Holland, Amsterdam pp 225–240
DiBona GF (1982) The functions of the renal nerves. Rev Physiol Biochem Pharmacol 94: 76–157
Gottschalk CW (1979) Renal nerves and sodium excretion. Ann Rev Physiol 41: 229–240
Kim JK, Linas SL, Schrier RW (1979) Catecholamines and sodium transport in the kidney. Pharmacol Rev 31: 169–178
Kopp UC, DiBona GF (1982) The functions of the renal nerves in the kidney. The kidney: National Kidney Foundation, 15, No. 4: 17, July
Labay P, Boyarsky S (1974) Ureteral peristaltic response to renal compression and other maneuvers: Renal ureteral coupling as a physiological concept. J Urol III: 334–339
Narath P (1951) Renal pelvis and ureter. Grune & Stratton, New York, pp 202, 227
Reinking LN, Schmiedt-Nielsen B (1981) Peristaltic flow of urine in the renal papillary collecting ducts of hamsters. Kidney Internat 20: 55–60
Schmidt-Nielsen B, Graves B (1982) Changes in fluid compartments in hamster renal papilla due to peristalsis in the pelvic wall. Kidney Internat 22: 613–625
Schmidt-Nielsen B, Reinking LN (1981) Morphometry and fluid reabsorption during peristaltic flow in hamster renal papillary collecting ducts. Kidney Internat 20: 789–798
Schmidt-Nielsen B, Churchill M, Reinking L (1980) Occurence of renal pelvic refluxes during rising urine flow rate in rats and hamsters. Kidney Internat 18: 419–431

Subject Index

acetylcholine 35
acetylcholinesterase 294
actin 31
action potential 20, 24, 27, 287
adrenergic nerve fibres, ureter 292
– receptors 293
β-adrenergics 45, 204
α-adrenoceptor-agonists 51
– blockers 46, 229
anisotropy, in ureteral tissue 67
anticholinergics 51, 187, 204
aperistalsis, ureteral 165
benign prostatic hypertrophy 267, 269
bladder 188
– diverticula 251
– neck dyssynergy 212, 225
– – function 224
– – hypertrophy 219
– –, loop resection 230
– – obstruction 216, 246
– – relaxation 230
–, neurogenic 214
– outflow obstruction 212, 214
–, overdistended 188
– pressure 117, 123, 254, 275
–, small volume 188
– surface defenses 243
– volume, relation to flow rate 276
– wall 11
bolus 120
– pressure 123
–, propagation velocity 130
calcium 30, 31, 35, 39
– antagonist 40, 51
calibration 218
calyx 15
–, minor 30
cell unit, reactive 21
cholinergic nerve fibers in ureter 292
cholinesterase 289
cineradiography 139, 148, 154
collagen, in obstructed ureters 290
compression, effect on peristalsis 336
conduction, electrical 19, 60
conduit 74
contraction, isometric 16, 17
–, longitudinal 86, 114, 120
–, phasic 30

–, potassium induced 53
– rates 19
– ring 60, 69, 82, 88, 104, 114, 120, 153
–, spontaneous 11, 13, 36
–, tonic 30, 53, 85
contracture 33, 37
contrast medium 112
– –, influence on diuresis 114
coupling, electromechanical 39
–, pharmacomechanical 39
cystodynamogram 221
cystourethrography 221
depolarization 21, 32, 135
detrusor activity 168, 174
– dysfunction 212, 224, 227
– –, neuropathic 216
– electrostimulation 174
– instability 188, 213
– pressure 173
– -sphincter dyssynergia 223
dilatation, chronic 19
diuresis 112
–, effect on peristalsis 151
diverticulum, vesical 251
double ureter 164
ejaculate 230
electromyography 21, 24, 106, 117
electron microscopy 292
electrostimulation 126, 204
endoscopy 218
excitability, in obstruction 19
external sphincter, anatomy 193
– –, histochemistry 197
– –, innervation 193
flow, extraperistaltic 74, 83
– measurement 148
– meter 267, 270
fluororadiography 264
fluoroscopy 69, 102
frusemide 151
heterotopic extrasystolic activity 13, 19
hydronephrosis 15
–, structural and histochemical changes 290
hypertension 252
incontinence 205
infection 227
– and ureteral peristalsis 99
–, recurrent 241, 329

innervation of ureter 290, 292, 300, 338
intercellular connections 305
isotropy 3
jodine hippurate 148
kidney, monopapillary 16
–, multicalyceal 16
–, multipapillary 18, 40
– tumor 18
lumbopelic junction 79, 83
manometry 154
megaureter, motility 164
membrane potential 32
micropuncture, renal 338
micturition 263
–, physiology 193
– urography 329
myosin 31
nervous control, ureter 293
neuropathic detrusor dysfunction 216
nexus 288, 302
nocturia 227
nor-epinephrine 30, 35
nuclear medical space time matrix 154
obstruction 135, 146, 272, 276
–, chronic 19
– in female urethra 258
–, infravesical 188
–, urethral 215, 331
occlusion of renal vein, effect on peristalsis 336
– – – artery, effect on peristalsis 336
pacemaker 13, 18
– activity 48, 72, 288
– cells 45
– potential 45
panurography 327
papaverine 51
paraurethral glands 233
pelvis, renal 15
perfusion pressure measurements 177
peristalsis 13, 104, 292, 305
–, orthograde 18
–, retrograde 19
peristaltic contraction 69
– transport 102, 106
– wave, propagation velocity 67
pressure 96
– flow-relation 125
– flow-test 95, 169, 220
–, intravesical 117, 181
– measurement 124, 148, 169, 173, 263
–, pelvic 48, 96, 120, 124
profilometry 281
Progressive Autonomic Failure 228
prostatic enlargement 232, 234, 268
prostatism 212
prostatitis 227

pursinergic nerve fibres 298
pyeloureteral junction 14, 83
reflux, intraureteral 160
–, pelvic 339
–, vesico-ureteral 160, 164, 329, 331
residual urine 218, 243, 252
scintigram 155
scrotal flap technique 203
sexual activity 250
Shy-Drager-Syndrome 228
smooth muscle 51, 52, 57
– –, activity 13, 21, 30, 31
– –, ureteral 58, 288
sphincter, dyssynergy 222
–, external 193
– stricture 222
stress incontinence 258
teflon injection 204
time-distance-diagram 104, 155
trabeculation 219
trigone hypertrophy 188
tropomyosin 31
troponin 31
turbulence, within urethra 260, 278
upper urinary tract 30
– – –, bifid 73
– – –, dilatations 95
– – – mechanics 120
ureteral contraction 131, 134
– depot 160
– dynamics 139
– function 148
– ganglion 311
– morphodynamics 69
– motility 154
– peristalsis 45, 70, 155, 286, 289, 305
– physiology 340
– potential 48
– pressure 105
– tissue 20, 24, 28, 60, 67
– transport, kinematics and dynamics 102, 148
– ultrastructure 286
– wall 3, 28
ureterovesical ganglia 292, 306
– junction 168, 171
urethral profilometry 222, 258
– resistance 274
– stricture 268
urine bolus 3, 105, 118, 120, 142
– exit velocity 261
– flow 120
– transport 148
– viscosity 118
urodynamics 238, 263, 317, 333
urodynamogram, intravenous 220
urodynamometer 261

Subject Index

uroflowmetry 219, 228, 238
urography, excretion 102
–, kinetic 69, 81
uro-rheography 154, 317
vesicourethral suspension and angulation 204

viscoelasticity, ureteral 3, 11, 122
voiding 217
– disorders 228
– dysfunction in femals 258
– inefficency 217
Whitaker-procedure 325